Psychoanalytic Therapy and Behavior Therapy

Is Integration Possible?

Psychoanalytic Therapy and Behavior Therapy

Is Integration Possible?

EDITED BY
HAL ARKOWITZ
University of Arizona
Tucson, Arizona

AND
STANLEY B. MESSER
Rutgers University
New Brunswick, New Jersey

PLENUM PRESS • NEW YORK AND LONDON

Library of Congress Cataloging in Publication Data

Main entry under title:

Psychoanalytic therapy and behavior therapy.

Includes bibliographical references and index.

1. Psychotherapy—Addresses, essays, lectures. 2. Psychoanalysis—Addresses, essays, lectures. 3. Behavior therapy—Addresses, essays, lectures. I. Arkowitz, Hal, 1941- . II. Messer, Stanley B. [DNLM: 1. Behavior Therapy. 2. Psychoanalytic Therapy. WM 460.6 P9743]

RC480.5.P73 1984 616.89'14 84-9898

ISBN-13: 978-1-4612-9694-2 e-ISBN-13: 978-1-4613-2733-2

DOI: 10.1007/978-1-4613-2733-2

A Division of Plenum Publishing Corporation
233 Spring Street, New York, N.Y. 10013

Softcover reprint of the hardcover 1st edition 1984

Lovingly dedicated to our parents:
Ruth Arkowitz
William Arkowitz (*in memoriam*)
Sylvia Messer
Nathan Messer

Contributors

Hal Arkowitz, Ph.D., *Department of Psychology, University of Arizona, Tucson, Arizona*

Cyril M. Franks, Ph.D., *Graduate School of Applied and Professional Psychology, Rutgers University, Busch Campus, Piscataway, New Jersey*

Merton M. Gill, M.D., *Department of Psychiatry, University of Illinois, Chicago, Illinois*

Alan E. Kazdin, Ph.D., *Western Psychiatric Institute and Clinic, University of Pittsburgh School of Medicine, Pittsburgh, Pennsylvania*

Michael J. Mahoney, Ph.D., *Department of Psychology, Pennsylvania State University, University Park, Pennsylvania*

Eric Mendelsohn, Ph.D., *The New York Hospital-Cornell Medical Center, Westchester Division, White Plains, New York*

Stanley B. Messer, Ph.D., *Graduate School of Applied and Professional Psychology, Rutgers University, Busch Campus, Piscataway, New Jersey*

John M. Rhoads, M.D., *Department of Psychiatry, Duke University Medical Center, Durham, North Carolina*

Leon Salzman, M.D., *School of Medicine, Georgetown University, Washington, D.C.*

Thomas E. Schacht, Psy.D., *Center for Psychotherapy Research and Department of Psychology, Vanderbilt University, Nashville, Tennessee*

Lloyd H. Silverman, Ph.D., *New York Veterans Administration Regional Office, New York, New York and Department of Psychology, New York University, New York, New York*

Paul L. Wachtel, Ph.D., *Department of Psychology, City College of the City University of New York, New York, New York*

Meir Winokur, Psy.D., *Student Counseling Service, Hebrew University, Jerusalem, Israel*

Preface

This book has a question mark in its title because it aims to invite inquiry. The possibility of integrating psychoanalytic and behavior therapies has been controversial since it was first proposed about 50 years ago, and this has elicited a wide range of reactions from both psychologists and psychiatrists. It was with the hope of fostering constructive interchange that this book was conceived. We wanted to spark further thinking about the question in the title in a way that could lead either to conceptual and clinical progress toward an integrated approach or to a clearer sense of the obstacles involved. In either case, we hoped that it would present a healthy challenge to current forms of psychoanalytic and behavior therapies.

The present volume was stimulated by the appearance in 1977 of Paul Wachtel's book *Psychoanalysis and Behavior Therapy: Toward an Integration.* Although many reviewers did not necessarily agree with Wachtel's proposals for integration, they (and we) were highly laudatory of his attempt. After reading the book, Hal Arkowitz organized a symposium on integration that took place in Chicago at the November 1978 meeting of the Association for the Advancement of Behavior Therapy. The symposium included Cyril Franks, Merton Gill, Hans Strupp, Paul Wachtel, and Michael Merbaum as moderator. Arkowitz subsequently proposed to edit a book on integration and invited Messer to be coeditor. In this way, there was a joining of forces between one behaviorally oriented editor leaning toward integration (Arkowitz) and one psychoanalytically oriented editor leaning away from it (Messer).

The effort and involvement by the two editors of this book have been truly equal, and the order of editorship was determined alphabetically. Together, we selected contributors from the fields of psychiatry and clinical psychology who held different points of view about the possibility of integrating psychoanalytic and behavior therapies. We asked each to address the main question of whether integrating these two approaches was possible or practical and to spell out his position in some detail. The result was a range of thoughtful contributions that emphasized either theoretical, philosophical, empirical, or clinical issues.

To encourage an interchange of ideas further, we sent each contributor one of the chapters on which to comment. Chapter authors were given the opportunity to write a rejoinder to the commentary if they wished to do so. Some chose to respond, whereas others felt that a rejoinder was not necessary. The book begins with a chapter that gives a historical perspective on integration, and this is followed by a series of separately authored chapters, commentaries, and rejoinders. Each chapter is accompanied by a brief autobiographical statement giving the background of the author's interest in the question of integration. We hope that this provides a more personal touch and a context for their contributions. The book concludes with an overview of the central emergent themes, including the models of integration that are proposed and the controversies they raise.

We would like to thank a number of people who helped facilitate the task of preparing this book for publication. We especially appreciate the devoted help of our secretaries who were asked to prepare material that needed to be completed "no later than yesterday." At the University of Arizona, we wish to thank Rufulyn Andrew, Susan Diffenderfer, Nancy Hobbs, Alice Traut-Cavell, and Cathy Wylie, and, at Rutgers University, Karen Peterson and Sylvia Sorg.

Finally, we want to make special mention of our families. Hal Arkowitz would like to thank his daughters, Laura and Jennifer, for their enjoyable company and games of Centipede during breaks from working on the book. Stanley Messer would like to thank his wife, Donna, for her loving support and insightful comments on his work, and his daughters, Elana, Leora, and Tova, for their willingness to "play ball" with their sometimes distracted father.

HAL ARKOWITZ
STANLEY B. MESSER

Contents

1

Historical Perspective on the Integration of Psychoanalytic Therapy and Behavioral Therapy

HAL ARKOWITZ

Until 10 years ago, the idea of an integration between psychoanalytic and behavioral therapies was viewed by most with either disinterest or disdain, although a number of publications had appeared on this topic over a 50-year period. From the early 1970s to the present, there has been a marked acceleration of interest that is reflected in a dramatic increase in the number of books, conference papers, and articles on this theme. However, the earlier writings did not form a truly cumulative progression of thought but usually consisted of relatively isolated attempts to deal with limited aspects of this complex issue. Some of these earlier papers have now been anthologized in a book edited by Marmor and Woods (1980).

Most of the papers that appeared before 1970 were either neglected or reacted to in a negative and critical fashion by other therapists. An example of this was a paper by Birk (1970) that favored an integration, which was followed by two rejoinders (Levis, 1970; Rachman, 1970), both of which were quite critical. The title of Levis's rejoinder reflects this attitude: "Integration of Behavior Therapy and Dynamic Psychiatric Techniques: A Marriage with a High Probability of Ending in Divorce." Despite

HAL ARKOWITZ • Department of Psychology, University of Arizona, Tucson, Arizona 85721.

such criticisms, the interest in integrating behavioral and psychoanalytic approaches to therapy has been quite persistent over many years during which each separate approach was undergoing considerable growth and development.

From the early 1970s to the present, there has been a much stronger interest in integration, although the subject continues to generate considerable controversy. The 1977 appearance of Paul Wachtel's book entitled *Psychoanalysis and Behavior Therapy: Toward an Integration* was a major factor in this growing interest. In this book, Wachtel identified many of the problems facing such an undertaking and proposed a comprehensive integration at both the theoretical and clinical levels. Several other books related to integration have also recently appeared (Goldfried, 1982a; Marmor & Woods, 1980; Wachtel, 1982a). A group of papers was published in the journal *Behavior Therapy* that presented different positions on integration (Garfield, 1982; Goldfried, 1982b; Kendall, 1982; Wachtel, 1982b). In addition, an article by Messer and Winokur (1980) in the *American Psychologist* was followed by commentaries by Apfelbaum (1981) and Ellis (1981). Similarly, in England an article by Yates (1983) in the *British Journal of Clinical Psychology* was also followed by several commentaries (Davis, 1983; Messer, 1983a; Murray, 1983; Wachtel, 1983). Finally, there have been a number of symposia (e.g., Arkowitz, 1978) and public dialogues (e.g., Mahoney & Wachtel, 1982) on the topic. It is apparent that the integration of behavioral and psychoanalytic approaches is an issue that is stimulating even more thought and debate than ever before.

Integration among therapeutic approaches can take place at many levels (see Schacht, Chapter 4, this volume) and among many different therapeutic approaches. Related trends in the psychotherapy literature have included attempts to integrate other pairs of therapeutic approaches, such as behavioral and humanistic (e.g., Martin, 1971; Thoresen, 1973; Wandersman, Poppen, & Ricks, 1976) or psychoanalytic and humanistic (e.g., Appelbaum, 1976), a search for common factors that may cut across different therapeutic schools (e.g., Frank, 1961; Goldfried, 1980, 1982b), and eclecticism in psychotherapy (e.g., Beutler, 1983; Garfield, 1980). The history of these and other trends in integration has been reviewed by Goldfried (1982b). However, the possibility of an integration of psychoanalytic and behavioral approaches is one that seems to have intrigued many writers and therapists. This chapter will attempt to trace some of the main historical trends in the integration of these two approaches. Apart from setting the stage for the remaining chapters in this book, this chapter will also attempt to analyze the reasons for the persistent interest in this type of integration.

EARLY HISTORY

TRANSLATIONS BETWEEN FREUD AND PAVLOV

The earliest attempts at some form of integration appeared in the 1930s. These were primarily attempts to translate psychoanalytic concepts of psychopathology and treatment into the language of Pavlovian conditioning to see how well the latter could be used to explain the former. There was some hope that the use of another language might yield some new ideas as well.

In what may be the earliest such attempt, Ischlondsky (1930), in a book published in Germany, drew parallels between psychoanalytic and Pavlovian conditioning. His preliminary work was extended by Thomas French (1933) who published the first paper in English on the topic. French considered repression in terms of the Pavlovian concept of "inhibition" and object choice in terms of Pavlovian "differentiation." French even thought that conditioning and differentiation might constitute a rough approximation to insight. French's paper met with mixed reactions from a number of other prominent analysts such as Gregory Zilboorg, Paul Schilder, and Adolf Meyer whose commentaries were published along with French's original paper. Kubie (1934) elaborated on French's ideas and also extended his analysis to aspects of psychoanalytic treatment. He proposed that the passive-observer stance of the analyst and the encouragement of free association in psychoanalysis might operate by reducing Pavlovian inhibition so that previously repressed material could emerge into consciousness.

The 1930s and 1940s witnessed many important developments within learning theory and psychoanalysis, but little interest was expressed in integration during this time. Several new theories of learning were proposed that went significantly beyond earlier Pavlovian models (e.g., Guthrie, 1935; Hull, 1943; Mowrer, 1947; Thorndike, 1932; Tolman, 1948). In 1938, Skinner published his book *The Behavior of Organisms*, laying the foundations for the operant approach that has had such an important influence on learning and other fields of psychology.

Psychoanalysis was also undergoing changes during this time. Anna Freud's (1936/1967) book *The Ego and the Mechanisms of Defense* helped to spark the interest in ego psychology. Subsequently, Hartmann (1939/1958) and his associates (Hartmann, Kris, & Loewenstein, 1946) moved psychoanalysis more toward evolutionary theory in their examination of the adaptive capacities of the ego in its relationship to the social and physical environments. More interpersonal psychoanalytic theories also appeared during this time (e.g., Horney, 1945). The greater emphasis of ego psychology and interpersonal psychoanalysis on the environment was compatible, at a general level, with a similar emphasis of the learning theories. However, despite these new developments and potential points of overlap, this period was relatively barren of any interest in integration, with only occasional exceptions (e.g., Sears, 1944; Shoben, 1949).

In 1950, an important book by John Dollard and Neal Miller appeared that was entitled *Personality and Psychotherapy*. In some respects, Dollard and Miller's book can be viewed in the tradition of earlier attempts to translate psychoanalytic concepts into learning theory terms, using the more highly developed learning theory concepts of that time. To cite but a few examples, they attempted to explain the pleasure principle in terms of reinforcement, repression in terms of the inhibition of the cue-producing responses that mediate thinking, and transference as a case of generalization. In their book, they presented a rather sophisticated formulation of the dynamics of conflict and anxiety in neurosis by using learning theory terms and concepts. They also suggested the use of modeling, self-control strategies, homework assignments, and other procedures that have become part of present-day behavior therapy. The comprehensiveness and originality of their work is truly noteworthy, and it remains thought provoking even in the light of over 30 years of subsequent developments in the field. Despite this, their book did not have any major impact on an integration of psychoanalytic and behavioral views during the 1950s and 1960s, although it did influence Wachtel's (1977) later thinking. Although the book stimulated much research in learning theory, particularly on anxiety and conflict, it had little impact on the theory or practice of psychotherapy of that period.

In the decade following the publication of Dollard and Miller's book (1950–1960), little was written about integration. For the most part, each of the approaches seemed to be going their own separate ways. Important developments were occurring within each, but there was little communication between them.

The 1960s and Integration

The 1960s were a particularly significant period for the field of behavior therapy. Behavioral techniques were developed for a number of different problems, including childhood disorders (e.g., Lovaas & Simmons, 1969), anxiety disorders (e.g., Paul, 1969), and the behaviors of hospitalized schizophrenics (e.g., Ayllon & Azrin, 1968). Many of the exciting developments of this decade were reviewed and evaluated in a seminal book edited by Cyril Franks (1969) that was entitled *Behavior Therapy: Appraisal and Status*. Wolpe's (1958) book *Psychotherapy by Reciprocal Inhibition* was followed by another that was coauthored with Arnold Lazarus. This book spelled out behavior therapy techniques for a wide variety of problems (Wolpe & Lazarus, 1966). Much research and many case reports on both process and outcome in behavior therapy appeared during this decade, and Bandura (1969) presented an integrated learning theory to account for psychopathology and behavior change. Bandura's book also began to address the role of cognition in behavior therapy.

This period was one in which behavior therapists sought a definition and identification of behavior therapy that emphasized its differences from psychoanalytic theory and therapy. Perhaps because of this, some behavioral writings during the early 1960s were characterized by strong criticisms of psychoanalytic concepts (e.g., Eysenck, 1960; Ullman & Krasner, 1965; Wolpe & Rachman, 1960). For example, Wolpe and Rachman (1960) criticized the reasoning and evidence in Freud's (1909/1950) paper on Little Hans. They attempted to show that Little Hans' phobia could more parsimoniously be explained in terms of classical conditioning. Others, such as Eysenck (1960) and Ullman and Krasner (1965), were also highly critical and defined behavior therapy in large part by its differences from psychoanalysis. In this vein, Eysenck wrote:

> Freudian theory regards neurotic symptoms as adaptive mechanisms which are evidence of repression; they are the visible upshot of unconscious causes. Learning theory does not postulate any such unconscious causes, but regards neurotic symptoms as simple learned habits; there is no neurosis underlying the symptom, but merely the symptom itself. *Get rid of the symptom and you have eliminated the neurosis.* (Eysenck, 1960, pp. 8–9)

Undoubtedly, articles such as these served to widen the gap between psychoanalytic and behavior therapists at that time. Nonetheless, in the middle and later 1960s, as behavior therapists became more confident of their own identity and a considerable number of reports on the effectiveness of certain behavioral techniques began to appear, several behavioral and analytic writers began to reconsider the possibility of integration in a more positive vein.

During the 1960s, several psychoanalytic writers turned their attention to new developments in learning theory and behavior therapy and sought out points of overlap with psychoanalysis. Franz Alexander (1963) wrote that much of what happens in psychoanalytic treatment "can best be understood in terms of learning theory, particularly the principle of reward and punishment and also the influence of repetitive experiences" (p. 446).

Marmor (1964) provided a more detailed discussion of recent theories of learning as they related to psychotherapy. He was also one of the first psychoanalysts to advocate the use of behavior therapy techniques, particularly for problems that had been induced by traumatic experiences. Wolf (1966) believed that an integration between behavioral and psychoanalytic approaches was inevitable and desirable "however passionately some or many of us may chose to resist it" (p. 9). For the first time, psychoanalytic writers went beyond the translation attempts of French (1933) and Kubie (1934) and considered the possibility of integration at the applied clinical level.

Several other writers also began to focus their attention on the possibility of clinical integration during this period. Weitzman (1967) took an important step in this direction when he argued for the importance of cognitive processes in behavior therapy, a point that was made earlier by Breger and McGaugh (1965). Weitzman presented a cognitive and psychoanalytic interpretation of systematic densensitization. Whereas previous writings had emphasized learning interpretations of psychoanalytic concepts, Weitzman was one of the first to propose a psychoanalytic interpretation of a behavioral procedure. In Weitzman's view, "dynamically rich material," which was typically ignored by behavior therapists, was produced and could be utilized during the course of systematic desensitization. Anticipating later cognitive developments in behavior therapy, his analysis enhanced the possibility of an integration between the two approaches. Weitzman also presented several cases illustrating the use of such dynamic material during systematic desensitization. Along with Weitzman's paper, this period also witnessed the appearance of several other attempts to integrate psychoanalytic and behavioral approaches at the level of *applied clinical practice* (e.g., Brady, 1968; Leventhal, 1968; Stampfl & Levis, 1966; Wilson & Smith, 1968).

Behaviorally oriented writers were also becoming interested in the possibility of integration during the 1960s. Marks and Gelder (1966) made a strong case for rapprochement. They provided an objective assessment of similarities and differences between behavioral and psychoanalytic approaches and suggested that, for some clinical problems, one approach might be superior to the other and that a combination of approaches might be best in other cases. Sloane (1969) also explored the "converging paths" of psychoanalytic and behavioral therapies, finding more similarities than differences among them. In a thoughtful analysis of "insight" and "action" therapies, London (1964) analyzed the theoretical and philosophical assumptions of these two approaches. In a chapter entitled "The Multiplicity of Man: Integrating the Therapies," London discussed the importance of both insight and action in psychotherapy. Although he believed that action therapies were more successful in the treatment of symptoms, he also wrote that they have "tended, apparently somewhat unwittingly, to disregard the efficacy of thinking as a means of controlling human behavior" (1964, p. 128). He argued that a system that attempts to integrate insight and action might be more effective for a wider variety of problems than one that emphasizes only one of these approaches.

Not all behavior therapists were positive about such an integration. In an influential book, Bandura (1969) presented a revised and extended learning theory, giving a far greater emphasis to cognitive mediating factors in learning and behavior change than had most behaviorally oriented writers in the past. Nonetheless, Bandura was highly critical of psychoanalytic concepts and therapy and was clearly quite negative about the possibility of an integration. Bandura also reanalyzed the concept of "symptom substitution." He relabeled it "response substitution" and delineated conditions under which learning theory actually predicted that such substitution might occur. For example, new problem behaviors might emerge when anxiety-reducing responses were simply suppressed without removing the underlying anxiety. Without intending to do so, Bandura may have partially contributed to narrowing the gap between behavioral and psychoanalytic approaches by his cognitive emphasis and his acknowledgment of the behavioral phenomena that had previously been described as "symptom substitution."

A sign of the growing interest in integration was reflected in a symposium sponsored by the Ciba Foundation in 1968 on the role of learning in psychotherapy. The symposium was chaired by Neal Miller and brought together a number of prominent analysts (e.g., Lawrence Kubie and David Malan) and behaviorists (e.g., Albert Bandura and Arnold Lazarus). These symposium papers were later published in a book (Porter, 1968), with each one followed by commentaries from other participants. Although no major advances in integration resulted from this symposium, it did represent an important attempt to bring together people from the two schools for an open dialogue.

The end of the 1960s was marked by the publication of a unique paper in which a number of psychoanalytically oriented clinicians and researchers reported on their conclusions that were based on a week of intensive observations of two leading behavior therapists—Joseph Wolpe and Arnold Lazarus (Klein, Dittmann, Parloff, & Gill, 1969). The authors believed that the actual practice of behavior therapy was considerably more complex than the published literature indicated. They emphasized the role of suggestion in behavior therapy and demonstrated that the therapist–client relationship played a more important role than had been believed previously. They also stressed that the previously acquired clinical skills of these behavior therapists were important factors in their therapy, apart from the use of specific techniques. Although their paper did not propose an integration, it did argue against the development of behavior therapy as "yet another closed system of treatment." Finally, they believed that behavior therapy did have a contribution to make to psychotherapy, particularly in the behavioral emphasis on the objective evaluation of therapy outcome.

The decade of the 1960s was a diverse and seminal period for developments in the area of integration. There were further attempts to translate concepts from one language to another (e.g., Alexander, 1963), several broad pleas for integration (e.g., London, 1964; Wolf, 1966) as well as often heated criticisms of one approach by proponents of the other (e.g., Ullman & Krasner, 1965; Wolpe & Rachman, 1960). Another important development during this time was the appearance of a few articles illustrating how behavioral and psychoanalytic approaches might be combined in clinical practice (e.g., Leventhal, 1968; Wilson & Smith, 1968). It was a crucial period for behavior therapy with many new developments in theory, research, and practice (e.g., Franks, 1969). There were even some behavioral writers who began to favor cognitive constructs (e.g., Bandura, 1969), a direction that was to gain even further momentum in behavior therapy in the 1970s (e.g., Beck, Rush, Shaw, & Emery, 1979) and one that would make the possibility of integration more feasible. By the end of the 1960s, there was clearly a more substantial body of theory and clinical techniques in behavior therapy than ever before that could be considered for possible integration with psychoanalytic approaches.

Within psychoanalysis, there was increasing interest in object relations theory (e.g., Guntrip, 1969; Kernberg, 1966), which was based on the earlier work of Fairbairn (1952, 1955) and Winnicott (1953, 1971), among others. However, in the 1960s, the focus for most writers on integration was classical Freudian psychoanalysis and not on more recent versions of psychoanalytic theory and practice. With the exception of Paul Wachtel's (1977) work, which is discussed later in this chapter, it is still true today that writers on integration have concerned themselves almost exclusively with Freudian psychoanalysis and have not considered other versions of psychoanalytic theory.

RECENT DEVELOPMENTS

Interest in integration gained considerable momentum during the 1970s and has continued into the present. Although earlier writings were primarily either translation attempts or rather general statements about integration, the research published in the 1970s and afterward usually examined the issues in more depth. During this period, there were a number of case reports illustrating the application of an integrated approach to a variety of clinical problems (e.g., Birk, 1970; Lambley, 1976; Wachtel, 1975), intensive examinations of such issues as transference and resistance in both therapies (e.g., Rhoads & Feather, 1972), and a somewhat greater awareness by writers of one school of recent developments in the other. Behavior therapy was moving toward an increasingly cognitive emphasis (e.g., Mahoney, 1974; Meichenbaum, 1977), and some analytic writers were becoming more cognizant of this (Strupp, 1978). In addition, the work of Wachtel (1977) went beyond classical Freudian versions of psychoanalysis and examined the integration of interpersonal psychoanalysis with behavior therapy. The possibility of an integration between a more cognitive behavior therapy on the one hand and a more interpersonal psychoanalysis on the other seemed potentially more promising. This period was also marked by further applications of behavior therapy to more complex problems such as agoraphobia (e.g., Emmelkamp & Ultee, 1974), schizophrenia (e.g., Paul & Lentz, 1977), sexual dysfunctions (e.g., Lobitz & LoPiccolo, 1972; Masters & Johnson, 1970), and depression (e.g., Lewinsohn, 1975). The days of the snake phobia and public-speaking anxiety as hallmarks of behavior therapy were over.

Further Attempts at Integration

Broad Proposals for Convergence

Since 1970 there have been several behavioral and psychoanalytic writers who have made broad proposals for greater interchange and possible integration between the two approaches. For example, the growing interest in behavior therapy among psychodynamically oriented psychiatrists resulted in the formation of an American Psychiatric Association Task Force on Behavior Therapy (Birk, Stolz, Brady, Lazarus, Lynch, Rosenthal, Skelton, Stevens, & Thomas, 1974). The purpose of this task force was "to study the historical development of behavior therapy, its efficacy for the treatment of psychiatric problems , its current forms and uses as well as potential abuses, and its relationship to dynamic psychiatry" (p. xiii). Although the group was generally positive about behavior therapy, its recommendations fell short of any major attempt to integrate it with psychodynamic approaches. The members of the group did conclude that "there is general agreement that psychiatry has benefited and will benefit further from incorporating concepts and techniques derived from the behavioral tradition" (p. 83). They stated also that "there are many genuine points of contact between dynamic psychiatry and behavior therapy that we hope will continue to be explored productively by psychotherapists and behavior therapists" (pp. 83–84). However, the report also acknowledged that there were considerable differences in emphases, concepts, and procedures between the two approaches.

During the 1970s, a number of writers continued the plea to go beyond narrow school boundaries and toward a possible integration. For example, Birk (1970) advocated combining the "breadth and depth" of a psychodynamic approach with the "power and efficiency" of certain behavioral techniques. Ferster (1974) emphasized the complementarity of behavioral and psychodynamic approaches. Marmor (1971) was more forceful about an integrated approach and questioned the inevitability of symptom substitution when behavioral techniques were employed. Even further, he argued that removal of an "ego-dystonic symptom may, on the contrary, produce satisfying feedback from the environment that may result in constructive shifts within the personality system, thus leading to a modification of the original conflictual pattern" (p. 22). This potential interplay between behavior change and personality change was a theme that received further elaboration by Wachtel (1977). In addition, Woody (1971) published a book in which he advocated the selection and integration of techniques from both approaches on purely pragmatic grounds.

Unlike most earlier writers, Shectman (1975) specifically addressed the possibility of the integration of Freudian psychoanalytic concepts with operant conditioning. Shectman stressed some general similarities in the two approaches. He said that they were highly idiographic and looked to the past (although in different ways) to explain present behavior (e.g., early childhood conflicts in one approach and reinforcement history in the other). His article also pointed to some general similarities in techniques derived from the two approaches as well as similarities and differences in their views of man.

Several behavioral writers also began to move away from a narrow definition of behavior therapy and toward a more pragmatic eclecticism, drawing from many different therapeutic approaches. In advocating such eclecticism, London (1972) called for an "end of ideology" in behavior modification and argued that we should focus on finding effective treatments, regardless of their sources. Similarly, Arnold Lazarus, in a series of articles and books (1971, 1976, 1977, 1981), moved away from behavior therapy as a school and raised the question of whether "behavior therapy has outlived its usefulness" (Lazarus, 1977). In his own work, Lazarus moved toward a much more eclectic "multimodal" therapy. Although neither London nor Lazarus advocated a specific integration of behavioral and psychoanalytic approaches, their writings did seem to stimulate many behavior therapists to examine other points of view that were not specifically linked to a narrowly defined behavioral approach.

Specific Proposals for Integration

In recent years, a number of writers have addressed various clinical and theoretical issues more specifically in attempts to develop an integrated approach. In 1972, Feather and Rhoads published a series of papers that discussed their rationale for a "psychodynamic behavior therapy," along with several illustrative cases (Feather & Rhoads, 1972a,b; Rhoads & Feather, 1972), particularly for anxiety-based disorders. They argued that some phobias may be acquired in a relatively straightforward manner through classical conditioning (e.g., a driving phobia following an automobile accident). However, they believed that in many other cases, underlying repressed conflicts led to the behavioral symptoms. In particular, they focused on phobic and obsessive-compulsive disorders. They advocated an assessment that sought to discover the unconscious conflict, using directed fantasies in which patients were asked to imagine the most catastrophic outcomes they could that related to the situations that they feared. When their assessment suggested the presence of underlying conflicts related to the behavioral problems, Feather and Rhoads recommended a modified form of systematic desensitization, using a hierarchy in which the patient was asked to imagine progressively anxiety-arousing scenes involving enactment of the relevant fantasies (e.g., losing control). They suggested that systematic desensitization could be used to reduce anxiety to the drive-related images and thoughts underlying the behavioral symptoms. In the Feather and Rhoads approach, patients were also encouraged to expose themselves gradually to the feared situations in real life. However, patients were not encouraged to enact the impulses. Instead, the goal of therapy was to reduce anxiety to the thoughts and fantasies relating to the conflicts, rather than to act out the repressed impulses. Rhoads and Feather (1972) also discussed resistance and transference in behavioral and psychodynamic therapies as well as in their integrated approach. (For further developments of this work, see Chapter 7 in this volume.)

Birk and Brinkley-Birk (1974) also proposed an integrated model. They pointed out that, for the most part, the integration of behavioral and psychoanalytic techniques still lacked a solid conceptual foundation, and they tried to develop such a foundation in their essay. In their view, behavioral techniques may not be effective when the patient has "neurotic distortions" of the therapist or of the behavioral techniques. They saw insight as helping patients to discriminate current situations from past ones so that they could see that earlier maladaptive ways of responding were no longer necessary. In this way, insight could enhance behavior change by correcting distortions that might arise in the course of treatment. In turn, Birk and Brinkley-Birk suggested that behavior change effected through behavior therapy could lead to cognitive change. Like the later work of Wachtel (1975, 1977), Birk and Brinkley-Birk emphasized the therapeutically useful interplay between behavior change and insight, advocating a combination of behavioral and insight-oriented methods. They also suggested that transference can be analyzed even in the context of behavior therapy—a point that Wachtel (1977) subsequently developed in more depth.

Silverman (1974) presented a thoughtful analysis of the conditions under which it might be valuable to introduce behavioral techniques into analytic therapy and vice versa. Like Birk and Brinkley-Birk (1974), he argued that introducing some interpretation of the patient's possible misconceptions of behavioral techniques could facilitate therapy. As one example, he used the illustration of a patient's misperceiving desensitization as a sexual assault. In addition, Silverman (1974) more cautiously suggested the use of behavioral techniques in analytic treatment, at the same time focusing on interpretation of the patients' perceptions and an awareness of the impact of such techniques on the transference relationship. In the same year, Silverman, Frank, and Dachinger (1974) argued that the effectiveness of systematic desensitization could partially be accounted for by the activation of merging fantasies (e.g., symbiotic fantasies of merging with mother). In their experiment, women with insect phobias were subjected to a variant of systematic desensitization in which tachistoscopically presented cues relating to such merging fantasies were substituted for muscle relaxation in a modified desensitization procedure. They presented evidence for the effectiveness of this procedure. Silverman's work stimulated considerable interest, and he and others have pursued this line of thought (see Mendelsohn & Silverman, Chapter 5, this volume).

Murray (1976) argued for the use of behavior therapy for symptom removal when the symptoms developed in relatively healthy personalities through faulty learning, trauma, or cultural aberrations. He also argued that psychoanalytic therapy was indicated when symptomatic behaviors represented only one aspect of an underlying personality disturbance. However, even in such cases, Murray saw a possible role for behavior therapy because such symptomatic behaviors might persist due to external reinforcement, even when the initial conflict was resolved. He suggested a combined behavioral and psychoanalytic therapy in select cases.

In a highly influential book, *Psychoanalysis and Behavior Therapy: Toward an Integration,* Wachtel (1977) attempted to integrate behavioral and psychoanalytic approaches at both the theoretical and clinical levels. His discussion covered integration in a variety of areas, including assessment, therapy techniques, and images of man, to name just a few. He pointed out that there are many real obstacles involved in an integration, particularly if the attempt is to integrate a noncognitive behavior therapy with classical Freudian psychoanalytic theory. By bringing in more recent interpersonal psychoanalytic views such as those of Horney (1945) and Sullivan (1953), Wachtel believed that an integration with more cognitive versions of behavior therapy was much more possible.

Wachtel acknowledged the ability of behavior therapy to facilitate changes in behavior and of analytic approaches to provide an understanding of the often unconscious meanings in which these behaviors were embedded. He argued that psychoanalytic inferences about unconscious sources of anxiety could be useful for assessment of the problem. However, like Feather and Rhoads (1972b), Wachtel concluded that treatment interventions based on these inferences need not be limited to traditional psychoanalytic approaches but could include behavioral ones as well. At many points in the book, he demonstrated how behavioral interventions might facilitate insight and how, in turn, insight might facilitate behavior change further. However, Wachtel emphasized insight into *current* feelings and behaviors, rather than the early historical insight that was characteristic of Freudian psychoanalysis.

The role of transference and the therapeutic relationship received considerable attention in Wachtel's integration. He developed the thesis that the transference reactions could be clarified and the patient could be helped to understand dysfunctional feelings and behaviors, even in the context of a therapy involving greater directiveness and behavioral interventions on the part of the therapist. According to Wachtel, a "blank screen" posture was not necessary for helpful analyses of transference reactions. In his view, such analyses of the patient's behavior in therapy could facilitate behavior change outside of therapy and overcome resistances that might occur in a behavioral treatment that did not adequately attend to the therapeutic relationship.

A more complete summary of Wachtel's book is beyond the scope of this chapter. Wachtel's interweaving of behavioral and psychoanalytic approaches was both scholarly and clinically sophisticated. In addition, the comprehensiveness of his attempt at integration is truly noteworthy. Wachtel's book was probably the single most important work in the 1970s on the issue of integration, and it stimulated further interest, debate, and dialogue on the topic. The book received praise from several behavioral and psychoanalytic writers, although many did not agree with the main thrust of his attempt at integration.

Clinical Applications of Integrated Therapy Approaches

There was considerable progress during the 1970s in the development and application of an integrated clinical approach with a number of different clinical problems. One of the areas that received much attention was the treatment of sexual dysfunctions. During this period, Masters and Johnson (1970) published their important book on the treatment of sexual inadequacy, emphasizing behaviorally oriented interventions. Several clinicians began to question the utility of an exclusively behavioral therapy and raised the possibility that greater treatment effectiveness could be obtained with an integrated approach. For example, Levay and Kagle (1977) reported on patients who had been treated for sexual dysfunction by a Masters and Johnson's sex therapy but who returned for treatment because their sexual functioning had either deteriorated or was still not adequate. They illustrated their point that some couples need a combined psychodynamic and behavioral therapy in order to achieve lasting results. Levay, Weissberg, and Blaustein (1976) published a case report on the combined use of behavioral and psychoanalytic methods for treating sexual inadequacy, using different therapists for each.

Along similar lines, Helen Singer Kaplan (1974) presented a comprehensive treatment strategy for sexual inadequacy, using a combination of behavioral and psychodynamic methods. In Kaplan's approach, behavioral interventions are employed, but they constitute one, albeit major, treatment component. The goal of the treatment is the direct alleviation of the sexual inadequacy. However, underlying conflicts are examined in therapy, particularly when resistance, or any form of difficulty, arises in the course of the behavioral treatment. Kaplan also pointed to a synergistic effect that she had observed in using an integrated therapy. Kaplan's work has had an important influence on the practice of sex therapy, and it has served as a further impetus to clinical integration.

A number of case reports and illustrations appeared using an integrated approach with a variety of other clinical problems. These included Birk's (1970) case of homosexuality; Feather and Rhoads' (1972a) cases of anxiety attacks, compulsions, and public-speaking anxiety; Gullick and Blanchard's (1973) case of obsessional disorder; and Birk and Brinkley-Birk's (1974) cases of compulsive disorder and interpersonal anxiety. In addition, Wachtel (1975) discussed a case of social anxiety and isolation in which behavioral interventions facilitated psychodynamic exploration. Lambley (1976) used a combination of assertive training and insight-oriented therapy to treat a woman suffering from migraine headaches.

All of the clinical applications discussed thus far have dealt exclusively with individual therapy. During the 1970s, there were also a few attempts to extend clinical integration to other forms of therapy as well. Birk (1974) proposed an integrated form of group psychotherapy, arguing that patients who had shown little or no improvement with previous traditional psychoanalytic treatment showed marked improvement with his integrated approach. Gurman (1978) examined possible convergences among behavioral, psychoanalytic, and systems theory approaches to marital therapy. He concluded that they all shared some important similarities. According to Gurman, they all involved the therapist's structuring the flow of the therapy sessions, guiding the sequencing of goals, challenging assumptions and beliefs, clarifying communications, and assigning homework of different types outside of the therapy sessions. However, he did point to some important differences, paralleling those that have already been discussed regarding the role of the relationship in behavioral and psychoanalytic therapies. A more comprehensive attempt to integrate behavioral and psychoanalytic approaches to marital therapy appeared several years later in a book by Segraves (1982).

Integration and the Therapeutic Relationship

One issue that has persistently appeared in discussions of integration concerns the role of the relationship in psychoanalytic versus behavior therapy. In psychoanalytic therapies—and particularly in formal psychoanalysis—the relationship (through the emergence and analysis of the transference) is viewed as the major vehicle for therapeutic change, whereas in behavior therapy the relationship is relatively neglected, at least in the published writings of behavior therapists. When it is discussed, it is usually conceived of simply as a vehicle in which to implement the behavioral techniques. Rapport and cooperation are all that are seen as necessary in this regard. Marmor (1971) criticized behavior therapists for their neglect and oversimplification of the therapist–patient relationship. However, a few writers on integration have begun to address the relationship (e.g., Rhoads & Feather, 1972; Wachtel, 1977). Some earlier writers had observed phenomena like transference and resistance in behavior therapy (e.g., Crisp, 1966; Weinberg & Zaslove, 1963). Rhoads and Feather (1972) observed that failure to deal with relationship issues led to treatment failures in some cases but to more successful treatment when they were addressed.

A slight shift in emphasis in behavior therapy began during the 1970s, one in which behavior therapists began to pay somewhat greater attention to the relationship in therapy. As mentioned earlier, observers of behavior therapists (Klein *et al.*, 1969) believed that the behavior therapy relationship was more complex than the publications of behavior therapists suggested. In an influential clinical behavior therapy text, Goldfried and Davison

(1976) devoted a chapter to relationship issues in behavior therapy. Although still not advocating an approach based on analysis of transference, they did discuss some important relationship issues, such as resistance and the therapist's role as a "significant other" in behavior therapy. During this same period, behavior therapists also began to examine relationships in behavior therapy empirically (e.g., Morris & Suckerman, 1974a,b).

Wilson and Evans (1977) wrote a chapter on the relationship in behavior therapy. In it they questioned the validity of perceptions of behavior therapists as impersonal and mechanistic, a perception that had also been called into question by some data of Sloane, Staples, Cristol, Yorkston, and Whipple (1975). Wilson and Evans discussed several relationship issues relevant to behavior therapy, including attitudes toward the therapist as a role model, and patients' expectancies about therapy. Their discussion covered a range of behavioral techniques. Strupp (1979), in a discussion of the therapeutic relationship, stated that "the terminology of behavior therapists and psychodynamicists is different, but I submit that we are referring to identical or very similar psychological processes" (p. 128). The somewhat greater focus on the relationship in behavior therapy may provide yet another potential point of contact between behavioral and psychoanalytic approaches.

Developments in the 1980s

Even though we are but only a few years into the 1980s, there has already been much dialogue, debate, and intensive analyses of a number of theoretical and clinical issues pertaining to integration. It is clear from the number of books, chapters, articles, and presentations discussed later that the issue of integration is attracting even greater interest than ever before. One sign of this was the appearance of two books that reprinted earlier articles on integration (Goldfried, 1982a; Marmor & Woods, 1980). Apparently, many who had not read these papers when they were originally published are now examining them in the context of an emerging body of thought on the topic. Two books on clinical applications of an integrated behavioral and psychoanalytic approach also appeared during this time (Papajohn, 1982; Segraves, 1982). In addition, the issue of resistance, which had been a recurrent one in the literature on integration, has been examined in depth by a number of psychoanalytic and behavior therapists in a book edited by Wachtel (1982a). Although only three books relating to integration appeared prior to 1980 (Dollard & Miller, 1950; Wachtel, 1977; Woody, 1971), there have already been five that have appeared since that time. There have also been a number of articles (e.g., Goldfried, 1982b; Kendall, 1982; Messer & Winokur, 1980; Wachtel, 1982b; Yates, 1983), case reports (e.g., Cohen & Pope, 1980), and public presentations (e.g., Goldfried & Strupp, 1980; Mahoney & Wachtel, 1982; Meichenbaum, 1980). The atmosphere of spirited controversy and interchange surrounding the issue can be seen in the numerous commentaries that several articles have stimulated. For example, Apfelbaum (1981) and Ellis (1981) published responses to the article by Messer and Winokur (1980), and Davis (1983), Messer (1983a), Murray (1983), and Wachtel (1983) responded to the paper by Yates (1983). Although interest in common factors and eclecticism has continued, the question of integration of behavioral and psychoanalytic approaches has remained one that has generated strong interest.

A series of papers was published in *Behavior Therapy* that examined the pros and cons of an integration of behavior therapy with other approaches. After reviewing some of the issues surrounding such an integration, Kendall (1982) expressed some cautious interest:

> Behavior therapy has gained a sense of self-acceptance and can now be self-critical and self-evaluative. Behavior therapy has taken the perspective of others, has examined its worth, and is prepared for a useful sharing. The time is ripe for integration. But simply because the timing is right does not justify all forms of integration. (p. 560)

In this special section, Goldfried (1982b) and Garfield (1982) favored a broader examination of commonalities and mutual compatibilities across a variety of therapy approaches, but they did not specifically favor an integration of psychoanalytic and behavior therapies. Wachtel (1982b and Chapter 2 in this volume) has continued to advocate his integrative approach and has discussed issues relating to conflict, resistance, and normative and nonnormative assumptions in behavioral and psychoanalytic approaches.

In a book edited by Wachtel (1982a), a number of behavior therapists (e.g., Marvin Goldfried, Arnold Lazarus, and Donald Meichenbaum) and psychoanalytic therapists (e.g., Michael Basch, Paul DeWald, and Sidney Blatt) examined the role of "resistance" in psychotherapy. In the introduction, Wachtel (1982a) suggested that a consideration of the concept of resistance by behavior therapists used to be unthinkable. He believed that behavior therapists misunderstood the construct as implying that lack of progress in therapy was the client's fault or that the client was being intentionally uncooperative. Wachtel had hoped that the book would be a step toward rapprochement. Although several of the contributors examined possible points of overlap between the two approaches, most concluded that the differences were quite marked. Even Wachtel (1982a) acknowledged that his hope that the book would contribute to détente or mutual facilitation was largely unrealized. He wrote that "although the chapters are excellent and valuable clinical contributions, they are primarily inward looking rather than reaching to incorporate from outside the pale" and that they were often "defenses of the virtue of the writer's own point of view rather than efforts to see what could be learned from the other side of the boundary" (1982a, p. xvi). The book was reviewed by Messer who wrote that "therapist resistance to integration has its reasons which are no easier to dispel or analyze than resistance in therapy" (1983b, p. 112). Nonetheless, Wachtel (1982a) expressed continued commitment to an integration and believed that resistance could still serve as a point of contact between the two approaches, although that goal now seemed more distant.

During the 1980s, some writers on integration turned their attention to the philosophical assumption of psychoanalytic and behavior therapies. In a thoughtful paper, Messer and Winokur (1980) argued that behavioral and psychoanalytic approaches have many important differences in their perspectives on reality, with the analytic therapist focusing more on the inner world of "experience" and the behavior therapist focusing more on the outer world of "consensual reality." They also argued that they behavioral approach is characterized by a primarily "comic" vision of reality (in the sense of dramatic comedy). According to Messer and Winokur, this view sees conflict as resulting from situations that can be eliminated through some form of action, with the possibility of "gratification and happy endings" when the obstacles are gone. By contrast, they see the psychoanalytic approach as incorporating tragic, ironic, and romantic visions of reality along with some aspects of the comic vision as well. These three former visions relate to a recognition of the "inevitability and ubiquity of internal conflict, by the limits that an individual's early history places on the extent of possible change, and by an emphasis on contradiction and ambiguity in the process of therapy" (1980, p. 818). They also discussed how these differing perspectives and visions lead to differences in the practice of therapy. Nonetheless, they did not entirely rule out the possibility of some form of integration involving the "opportune" introduction of behavior therapy techniques into psychoanalytic therapy in order to help the patient translate insight into action. These views are developed further in their chapter in the present book (see Chapter 3). Their paper met with rather heated objections by Apfelbaum (1981) and Ellis (1981) who criticized them for either a narrow or misrepresented view of behavior therapy. By contrast, many of their views on obstacles to integration were heartily endorsed by Yates (1983).

Several prominent behavior therapists continued to express strong objections to integration during this period. Wilson (1982a) wrote that fundamental differences on basic conceptual and practical issues still divice the approaches of behavior therapy and psychoanalysis (p. 344). In another paper, Wilson (1982b) lauded the cognitive emphasis in behavior therapy. However, rather than seeing this as a useful point of contact with psychoanalytic therapy as others had, Wilson argued strongly that behavior therapy should retain its distinctive identity while testing its limits in the search for effective treatment methods. He urged that behavior therapists look toward experimental cognitive psychology for expansion rather than toward psychoanalytic concepts and methods. Wolpe (1981) also argued strongly for retaining a distinct definition of behavior therapy, at the same time answering several criticisms of behavior therapy.

Yates (1983) was also highly critical of integration on several grounds. He argued that claims for a combined or integrated therapy approach were not supported by any solid research evidence. He also endorsed Messer and Winokur's (1980) discussion of obstacles to integration based on differing views and perspectives on reality. Finally, Yates observed that most discussions of integration have centered around anxiety disorders. He stated his belief that the crucial test for integration lay elsewhere, in areas that more clearly highlighted differences in theory and therapy. He illustrated this with a discussion of the behavioral and psychoanalytic approaches to stuttering and enuresis, concluding that the differences between behavioral and psychoanalytic approaches" are not cracks that can be papered over, they are chasms that cannot be bridged" (p. 122). Several of the commentaries on his paper (e.g., Messer, 1983a; Wachtel, 1983) criticized Yates's exclusive use of Freudian conceptualizations of psychoanalysis and relatively noncognitive versions of behavior therapy. Others (Davis, 1983; Murray, 1983) argued that the fact that there is as yet no evidence to support the effectiveness of an integrated approach to therapy is no reason to reject it prematurely.

It is clear that we have seen a tremendous acceleration of interest in integration in recent years. Many earlier ideas are being reexamined, and a number of new ones proposed. Some of the reasons for the current interest have already been alluded to earlier in this chapter. They seem to have more to do with changes in learning theory and behavior therapy than with changes in psychoanalytic theory and practice. Learning theories have evolved from animal models based primarily on classical and operant conditions to more cognitive formulations of human learning and psychopathology (e.g., Bandura, 1977). Similarly, behavior therapy techniques have evolved from a few isolated demonstrations (e.g., Mary Cover Jones, 1924; Mowrer & Mowrer, 1938) to a considerable armamentarium of techniques applicable to a wide range of clinical problems. Demonstrations of the effectiveness of many behavior therapy techniques have made them more difficult to ignore by therapists of other orientations. There is now a much broader foundation of behavior theory and therapy from which the question of integration with psychoanalytic approaches can be considered. The recent cognitive behavior therapy emphasis also provides a point of possible convergence with psychoanalytic therapy. In addition, as Kendall (1982) has pointed out, behavior therapists are now more sure of their own identity so that they can more comfortably consider the possibility of integration with other approaches.

Changes in psychoanalytic theory and practice have also made the prospect of integration more feasible. The greater social and environmental emphases of ego psychology, interpersonal psychoanalysis, and object relations theory are potentially more compatible with behavior theory, and brief psychoanalytic therapy (e.g., Malan, 1976) may be more compatible with behavior therapy than is formal psychoanalysis. However, it appears that recent developments in behavior therapy have had more of an impact on the possibility of integration than have those in psychoanalytic theory and practice.

London (1983) has pointed out that many of the developments important for therapeutic integration and eclecticism were occurring "a generation before the trend was visible." He raised the interesting possibility that social and economic pressures may be the most important ones stimulating the current wave of interest. London wrote:

> The main "stuff" that legitimized eclecticism in therapeutic practice and ecumenism in theory, I believe, was the economic and social pressure of events created almost simultaneously by the behaviorist rebellion, the boom in professional practice via legal accreditation of psychologists and the mushrooming of their trade schools, the destigmatization of soul-searching for pay by growth centers and the encounter movement, and the outpouring of third party funding on both sides of the therapeutic counter—government paying for the doctors' training, and insurance companies financing the patients' treatment. These events, all set in place in the 1960's, [led to] a hyperinflation of brand-name treatments . . . on the one hand, and a tendency toward reconciliation among therapies belonging to the Mental Health Establishment, on the other. (London, 1983, p. 508)

Obviously, discussions and controversies about integration are continuing. The tone of the 1980s thus far seems to be one of more intense scrutiny of the issues but with more caution and pessimism about the possibility of integration.

THE FUTURE OF INTEGRATION

Although it has been a slow and uneven progression, the development of thought on integration has come a long way from Ischlondsky's (1930) and French's (1933) attempts to translate psychoanalytic concepts into

Pavlovian terms. In the past 50 years, we have moved well beyond this. Many obstacles confronting integration have been more clearly defined. There has been a greater focus on more specific issues such as the role of transference and the therapeutic relationship, resistance, and the theoretical and philosophical assumptions about the nature of man in the two approaches. There have also been several concrete illustrations of an integrated approach at the clinical level in such areas as anxiety disorders, sex and marital therapies, and group therapy. The nature and content of a clinical integration is beginning to take some shape.

Nonetheless, we still do not have any clear answers about the merits of such an integration. As we move away from broad polemics about integration to a more intensive exploration of substantive areas, we should be more clearly able to evaluate the strengths and weaknesses of an integrated approach. A number of issues need to be examined further, including transference, resistance, and models of man. Several others remain relatively unexplored. For example, Wachtel (1982b) has pointed to the need to examine the role of conflict and the "therapeutic contract" in discussions of integration. A consideration of the role of unconscious factors or the role of awareness in behavior change has been relatively neglected. A related concept that has received little attention is *insight.* Behavior therapists have examined the role of "covert self-statements" (e.g., Meichenbaum, 1977) and "self-monitoring" (e.g., Nelson, 1977) in behavior change. It may be useful to examine an integration of concepts such as these as well as other cognitive concepts (e.g., Bower, 1978) in behavior therapy with psychoanalytic conceptualizations of insight. The nature and role of *assessment* in an integrated approach is also one that deserves attention. These and other issues need a much closer scrutiny in the future to help us determine whether integration is either desirable or feasible.

It is also clear that relatively few therapists and writers from one orientation are very aware of recent developments in the other. The point was made earlier in the chapter that, with the exception of the work of Wachtel (e.g., 1977), discussions of integration have focused almost exclusively on Freudian psychoanalytic theory rather than on other psychoanalytic theories that more strongly emphasize ego functions and social and environmental influences. The possibilities of integration of behavior therapy with ego psychology, interpersonal psychoanalysis, and object relations theory remain to be fully explored. As one illustration of this point, Heinz Hartmann's (1939/1958) discussion of "autoplasticity" and "alloplasticity" has some important similarities to Bandura's (1977) concept of "reciprocal determinism." Both emphasize the reciprocal relationship between the individual and the environment in which a person both changes and is changed by the environment.

Discussions of therapeutic integration must also acknowledge that there are many forms of psychoanalytic treatment. For example, brief psychoanalytic psychotherapy (e.g., Alexander & French, 1946; Malan, 1976; Sifneos, 1979) places less emphasis on free association, dream interpretation, and complete resolution of the transference, and a greater emphasis on dealing with focal problems than does psychoanalysis. These trends in psychoanalytic treatment clearly provide a stronger potential possible link to behavior therapy than formal psychoanalysis.

Although discussions of integration need to acknowledge that psychoanalytic theory and therapy consist of more than what Freud proposed, they also need to take into account that behavior therapy is now something far more than the views of Pavlov and Skinner or even of Eysenck and Wolpe. Social learning theory (Bandura, 1977) is now an important base of behavior therapy, and cognitive constructs are far more prevalent now than ever before. In addition, cognitive behavior therapy approaches have been developed for a number of disorders (e.g., Foreyt & Rathjen, 1978). These recent emphases in behavior therapy need to be addressed if we are to have a fully informed discussion of the possibility of integration. The recent formation of a network of therapists of different orientations may help to overcome some of this mutual lack of awareness. In a recent paper, Goldfried has proposed a network of professionals

> who are interested in taking steps toward the ultimate achievement of some kind of rapprochement and consensus—to determine not only the common elements that may cut across different therapeutic orientations, but also to identify the unique contributions that any particular approach may have to offer. (1982b, p. 588)

Goldfried and Wachtel are currently coordinating this network, and they hope that it will help in breaking down some of the information barriers that have hampered many discussions of integration.

Another issue is that the clinical procedures that may grow out of an integrated approach have not yet been very clearly described. Some preliminary steps have been taken in some areas. Nonetheless, we need to spell out these clinical techniques and apply and evaluate them. We also need to consider the development of integrated therapy approaches for a wider variety of problems, as Messer has pointed out (Chapter 12, this volume). Many areas of psychopathology have been neglected, including childhood and personality disorders, schizophrenia, depression, and eating disorders, to name just a few. As Yates (1983) has indicated, most writers on integration have focused almost exclusively on anxiety disorders.

The current lack of quantitative research on questions relating to integration needs to be addressed. Most publications have consisted of theoretical or philosophical discussions or case illustrations. As Kazdin (Chapter 5, this volume) has pointed out, we need to generate and test hypotheses derived from an integrated approach. With the exception of the work of Silverman and his associates (see Chapter 9, this volume), such research has been seriously lacking. Similarly, we need outcome research on the effectiveness of an integrated approach to therapy. I agree with Yates (1983) that evidence for the superiority of an integrated approach over others is lacking. However, although Yates uses this lack to dismiss integration, I see it as a potentially rich research area for the future. For example, one area that seems ripe for such research is a test of the effectiveness of systematic desensitization using overt situational cues compared to desensitization directed at cues derived from inferred underlying psychodynamic conflicts. Although Silverman, Frank, and Dachinger (1974) have made a start in this direction, further studies would be useful.

A final question relates to the merits of a specific integration between psychoanalytic and behavioral approaches in contrast to attempts at convergence and eclecticism among many other forms of therapy as well. Whether a therapeutic marriage should be a monogamous one between behavioral and psychoanalytic partners or a polygamous one needs further thought.

Judging from the growing amount of interest and activity in the issue in recent years, it is clear that the question of integration of behavioral and psychoanalytic approaches will continue to occupy our attention in the future. Whether the outcome will be the development of new integrated approaches or the refinement of separate approaches based on challenges presented by the other, it seems clear that the controversy will continue to exert a healthy influence on theory, research, and practice in psychotherapy.

Acknowledgments

The author would like to thank Larry Beutler, George Domino, Stanley Messer, and Stephen Shanfield for their constructive comments.

AUTOBIOGRAPHICAL STATEMENT

My interest in integration can partially be traced to my course work as an undergraduate at New York University. I took a course in abnormal psychology that was taught by a dedicated Skinnerian who used B. F. Skinner's *Science and Human Behavior* as the sole text! Although I gained a respect for this approach, I was also left feeling that it was limited in capturing some of the depth and complexity of psychopathology and psychotherapy. Because of this, I decided to take abnormal psychology once again, but this time from an instructor who was completing her training as a psychoanalyst. Although I did indeed find the depth and complexity I had sought, I was once again not completely satisfied. These two courses contributed to the development of what I have sometimes experienced as a professional "split personality" in my subsequent career.

In graduate school at the University of Pennsylvania, I was exposed to an exciting group of faculty members who provided me with excellent training in empirical research and a healthy appreciation for rigor in thinking. At Pennsylvania, my interest in behavior therapy was further stimulated by a seminar on systematic desensitization taught by James Geer. To demonstrate the procedure, Geer asked for a "volunteer phobic" from the class. In what might be described as "counterphobic behavior," my hand shot up, reflecting as much my long-standing and intense fear of snakes as it did my interest in volunteering as a subject. The desensitization, conducted in front of the class by my good friend and fellow student Robert Leff, was so successful that I later bought my own snake for a research project.

Nevertheless, I was still drawn to what a psychoanalytic approach had to offer, and I pursued this interest in an internship at Langley Porter Neuropsychiatric Institute. There, I was exposed to a number of instructors and therapy supervisors from whom I learned much about psychoanalytic theory and therapy. But, once again, it seemed to me that there were some important limitations to a purely psychoanalytic therapy, particularly in helping patients translate "insight" into "action." The following year, I took a postdoctoral fellowship at the State University of New York at Stony Brook where I received excellent training in behavior therapy from Gerald Davison and Marvin Goldfried, among others. At Stony Brook, I observed that what many of my supervisors said and did in therapy reflected a grasp of psychodynamic and relationship factors that went well beyond what was described in the published reports of behavior therapists. My experiences and observations thus far strengthened my conviction that both behavioral and psychoanalytic perspectives had much to offer.

In my subsequent faculty positions at the University of Oregon and the University of Arizona, I pursued a more behavioral focus in my research and practice. During this time, I also felt that I was developing an approach to therapy based on an integration between psychoanalytic and behavioral models. However, it seemed easier to me to practice such an integration than to articulate it in my teaching. Then I read *Psychoanalysis and Behavior Therapy: Toward an Integration* by Paul Wachtel, a book that has had a strong influence on my thinking and practice. Wachtel articulated many of the issues I had been struggling with over the years. Reading this book helped me to resolve many conflicts that had contributed to the "split" in my professional personality. Although I clearly support integration, I also believe that there are many serious obstacles confronting it. Some may believe that an integration may incorporate the worst of both possible worlds; I believe that it is equally likely that it can lead to the best of both.

HAL ARKOWITZ, PH.D.

REFERENCES

Alexander, F. The dynamics of psychotherapy in light of learning theory. *American Journal of Psychiatry*, 1963, *120*, 440–448.

Alexander, F., & French, T. M. *Psychoanalytic therapy*. New York: Ronald, 1946.

Apfelbaum, B. Integrating psychoanalytic and behavior therapy. *American Psychologist*, 1981, *36*, 796–797.

Appelbaum, S. A. A psychoanalyst looks at gestalt therapy. In C. Hatcher & P. Himmelstein (Eds.), *The handbook of gestalt therapy*. New York: Aronson, 1976.

Arkowitz, H. (Chair). *Behavior therapy and psychoanalysis: Compatible or incompatible?* Symposium presented at the convention of the Association for Advancement of Behavior Therapy, Chicago, November 1978.

Ayllon, T., & Azrin, N. *The token economy: A motivational system for therapy and rehabilitation*. New York: Appleton-Century-Crofts, 1968.

Bandura, A. *Principles of behavior modification*. New York: Holt, Rinehart & Winston, 1969.

Bandura, A. *Social learning theory*. Englewood Cliffs, N.J.: Prentice-Hall, 1977.

Beck, A. T., Rush, A. J., Shaw, B. F., & Emery, G. *Cognitive therapy of depression*. New York: Guilford, 1979.

Beutler, L. E. *Eclectic psychotherapy: A systematic approach*. New York: Pergamon, 1983.

Birk, L. Behavior therapy: Integration with dynamic psychiatry. *Behavior Therapy*, 1970, *1*, 522–526.

Birk, L. Intensive group therapy: An effective behavioral-psychoanalytic method. *American Journal of Psychiatry*, 1974, *131*, 11–16.

Birk, L., & Brinkley-Birk, A. Psychoanalysis and behavior therapy. *American Journal of Psychiatry*, 1974, *131*, 499–510.

Birk, L., Stolz, S. B., Brady, J. P., Brady, J. V, Lazarus, A. A., Lynch, J. J., Rosenthal, A. J., Skelton, W. D., Stevens, J. B., & Thomas, E. J. *Behavior therapy in psychiatry: A report of the American Psychiatric Task Force on behavior therapy*. New York: Aronson, 1974.

Bower, G. H. Contacts of cognitive psychology with social learning theory. *Cognitive Therapy and Research*, 1978, *2*, 123–146.

Brady, J. P. Psychotherapy by combined behavioral and dynamic approaches. *Comprehensive Psychiatry*, 1968, *9*, 536–543.

Breger, L., & McGaugh, J. L. A critique and reformulation of "learning theory" approaches to psychotherapy and neurosis. *Psychological Bulletin*, 1965, *63*, 338–358.

Cohen, J. H., & Pope, B. Concurrent use of insight and desensitization therapy. *Psychiatry*, 1980, *43*, 146–154.

Crisp, A. H. Transference, symptom emergence, and social repercussions in behavior therapy: A study of 54 treated patients. *British Journal of Medical Psychology*, 1966, *39*, 179–196.

Davis, J. D. Slaying the psychoanalytic dragon: An integrationist's commentary on Yates. *British Journal of Clinical Psychology*, 1983, *22*, 133–144.

Dollard, J., & Miller, N. E. *Personality and psychotherapy*. New York: McGraw-Hill, 1950.

Ellis, A. Misrepresentation of behavior therapy by psychoanalysis. *American Psychologist*, 1981, *36*, 798–799.

Emmelkamp, P. M. G., & Ultee, K. A. A comparison of "successive approximation" and "self-observation" in the treatment of agoraphobia. *Behavior Therapy*, 1974, *5*, 606–613.

Eysenck, H. J. Learning theory and behaviour therapy. In H. J. Eysenck (Ed.), *Behaviour therapy and the neuroses*. London: Pergamon, 1960.

Fairbairn, W. *Psychoanalytic studies of the personality*. London: Tavistock, 1952.

Fairbairn, W. Observations in defense of the object-relations theory of personality. *British Journal of Medical Psychology*, 1955, *28*, 144–156.

Feather, G. A., & Rhoads, J. M. Psychodynamic behavior therapy: I. Theory and rationale. *Archives of General Psychiatry,* 1972(a), *26,* 496–502.

Feather, B. W., & Rhoads, J. M. Psychodynamic behavior therapy: II. Clinical aspects. *Archives of General Psychiatry,* 1972(b), *26,* 503–511.

Ferster, C. B. The difference between behavioral and conventional psychology. *The Journal of Nervous and Mental Disease,* 1974, *159,* 153–157.

Foreyt, J. P., & Rathjen, D. P. *Cognitive behavior therapy: Research and applications.* New York: Plenum Press, 1978.

Frank, J. D. *Persuasion and healing.* Baltimore: Johns Hopkins, 1961.

Franks, C. M. (Ed.). *Behavior therapy: Appraisal and status.* New York: McGraw-Hill, 1969.

French, T. M. Interrelations between psychoanalysis and the experimental work of Pavlov. *American Journal of Psychiatry,* 1933, *89,* 1165–1203.

Freud, S. [The analysis of a phobia in a five-year old boy.] *Collected papers* (Vol. 3). London: Hogarth Press, 1950. (Originally published, 1909.)

Freud, A. *The ego and the mechanisms of defense* (Rev. ed.). New York: International Universities Press, 1967.

Garfield, S. L. *Psychotherapy: An eclectic approach.* New York: Wiley, 1980.

Garfield, S. L. Eclecticism and integration in psychotherapy. *Behavior Therapy,* 1982, *13,* 610–623.

Goldfried, M. R. Toward the delineation of therapeutic change principles. *American Psychologist,* 1980, *35,* 991–999.

Goldfried, M. R. *Converging themes in psychotherapy: Trends in psychodynamic, humanistic, and behavioral practice.* New York: Springer, 1982(a).

Goldfried, M. R. On the history of therapeutic integration. *Behavior Therapy,* 1982(b), *13,* 572–593.

Goldfried, M. R., & Davison, G. C. *Clinical behavior therapy.* New York: Holt, Rinehart & Winston, 1976.

Goldfried, M. R., & Strupp, H. H. *Empirical clinical practice: A dialogue on rapproachement.* Paper presented at the meeting of the Association for the Advancement of Behavior Therapy, New York, November 1980.

Gullick, E. L., & Blanchard, E. B. The use of psychotherapy and behavior therapy in the treatment of an obsessional disorder—an experimental case study. *Journal of Nervous and Mental Disease,* 1973, *156,* 427–431.

Guntrip, H. *Schizoid phenomena, object relations, and the self.* New York: International Universities Press, 1969.

Gurman, A. S. Contemporary marital therapies: A critique and comparative analysis of psychoanalytic, behavioral, and systems theory approaches. In T. J. Paolino & B. S. McCrady (Eds.), *Marriage and marital therapy: Psychoanalytic, behavioral, and systems theory perspectives.* New York: Brunner/Mazel, 1978.

Guthrie, E. R. *The psychology of learning.* New York: Harper, 1935.

Hartmann, H. [Ego psychology and the problem of adaptation] (David Rapaport, trans.). New York: International Universities Press, 1958. (Originally published, 1939.)

Hartmann, H., Kris, E., & Loewenstein, R. Comments on the formation of psychic structure. *Psychoanalytic Study of the Child,* 1946, *2,* 11–38.

Horney, K. *Our inner conflicts.* New York: Norton, 1945.

Hull, C. L. *Principles of behavior.* New York: Appleton-Century-Crofts, 1943.

Ischlondsky, N. E. *Neuropsyche und Hirnride: Bank II. Physiologische Grundlagen der Tiefenpsychologie unter besonderer Berücksichtigung der Psychoanalyse.* Berlin: Urban und Schwarzenberg, 1930.

Jones, M. C. A laboratory study of fear: The case of Peter. *Pedagogical Seminary,* 1924, *31,* 308–315.

Kaplan, H. S. *The new sex therapy.* New York: Brunner/Mazel, 1974.

Kendall, P. C. Integration: Behavior therapy and other schools of thought. *Behavior Therapy,* 1982, *13,* 59–571.

Kernberg, O. Structural derivatives of object relations. *International Journal of Psychoanalysis,* 1966, *47,* 236–253.

Klein, M., Dittmann, A. T., Parloff, M. B., & Gill, M. M. Behavior therapy: observations and reflections. *Journal of Consulting and Clinical Psychology,* 1969, *33,* 259–266.

Kubie, L. S. Relation of the conditioned reflex to psychoanalytic technique. *Archives of Neurology and Psychiatry,* 1934, *32,* 1137–1142.

Lambley, P. The use of assertive training and psychodynamic insight in the treatment of migraine headaches: A case study. *Journal of Nervous and Mental Disease,* 1976, *163,* 61–64.

Lazarus, A. A. *Behavior therapy and beyond.* New York: McGraw-Hill, 1971.

Lazarus, A. A. *Multimodal behavior therapy.* New York: Springer, 1976.

Lazarus, A. A. Has behavior therapy outlived its usefulness? *American Psychologist,* 1977, *32,* 550–554.

Lazarus, A. A. *The practice of multimodal therapy.* New York: McGraw-Hill, 1981.

Levay, A. N., & Kagle, A. A study of treatment needs following sex therapy. *American Journal of Psychiatry,* 1977, *134,* 970–973.

Levay, A. N., Weissberg, J. H., & Blaustein, A. B. Concurrent sex therapy and psychoanalytic psychotherapy by separate therapists: Effectiveness and implications. *Psychiatry,* 1976, *39,* 355–363.

Leventhal, A. M. Use of a behavioral approach within a traditional psychotherapeutic context: A case study. *Journal of Abnormal Psychology,* 1968, *73,* 178–182.

Levis, D. Integration of behavior therapy and dynamic psychiatry: A marriage with a high probability of ending in divorce. *Behavior Therapy,* 1970, *1,* 531–537.

Lewinsohn, P. M. The behavioral study and treatment of depression. In M. Hersen, R. Eisler, & R. Miller (Eds.), *Progress in behavior modification* (Vol. 1). New York: Academic Press, 1975.

Lobitz, W. C. & LoPiccolo, J. New methods in the behavioral treatment of sexual dysfunction. *Journal of Behavior Therapy and Experimental Psychiatry,* 1972, *3,* 265–271.

London, P. *The modes and morals of psychotherapy.* New York: Holt, Rinehart & Winston, 1964.

London, P. The end of ideology in behavior modification. *American Psychologist,* 1972, *27,* 913–920.

London, P. Ecumenism in psychotherapy. *Contemporary Psychology,* 1983, *28,* 507–508.

Lovaas, O. I., & Simmons, J. Q. Manipulation of self-destruction in three retarded children. *Journal of Applied Behavior Analysis,* 1969, *2,* 143–157.

Mahoney, M. J. *Cognition and behavior modification.* Cambridge: Ballinger, 1974.

Mahoney, M. J., & Wachtel, P. L. *Convergence of psychoanalytic and behavioral therapy.* Paper presented at the Institute for Psychosocial Study, New York, May 1982.

Malan, D. H. *The frontier of brief psychotherapy.* New York: Plenum Press, 1976.

Marks, I. M., & Gelder, M. G. Common ground between behavior therapy and psychodynamic methods. *British Journal of Medical Psychology,* 1966, *39,* 11–23.

Marmor, J. Psychoanalytic therapy and theories of learning. In J. Masserman (Ed.), *Science and psychoanalysis* (Vol. 7). New York: Grune & Stratton, 1964.

Marmor, J. Dynamic psychotherapy and behavior therapy: Are they irreconcilable? *Archives of General Psychiatry,* 1971, *24,* 22–28.

Marmor, J., & Woods, S. M. (Eds.). *The interface between the psychodynamic and behavioral therapies.* New York: Plenum Press, 1980.

Martin, D. G. *Learning-based client-centered therapy.* Monterey, Calif. Brooks/Cole, 1971.

Masters, W., & Johnson, V. *Human sexual inadequacy.* Boston: Little, Brown, 1970.

Meichenbaum, D. H. *Cognitive behavior modification.* Morristown, N.J.: General Learning Press, 1977.

Meichenbaum, D. *Nature of conscious and unconscious processes: Issues in cognitive assessment.* Paper presented at the meeting of the Eastern Psychological Association, Hartford, Conn. April 1980.

Messer, S. B. Integrating psychoanalytic and behavior therapy: Limitations, possibilities, and trade-offs. *British Journal of Clinical Psychology,* 1983(a), *22,* 131–132.

Messer, S. B. The resistance to integration. *Contemporary Psychology,* 1983(b), *28,* 111–112.

Messer, S. B., & Winokur, M. Some limits to the integration of psychoanalytic and behavior therapy. *American Psychologist,* 1980, *35,* 818–827.

Morris, R. J., & Suckerman, K. R. The importance of the therapeutic relationship in systematic desensitization. *Journal of Consulting and Clinical Psychology,* 1974(a), *42,* 148.

Morris, R. J., & Suckerman, K. R. Therapist warmth as a factor in automated systematic desensitization. *Journal of Consulting and Clinical Psychology,* 1974(b), *42,* 244–250.

Mowrer, O. H. On the dual nature of learning—A reinterpretation of "conditioning" and "problem solving." *Harvard Educational Review,* 1947, *17,* 102–148.

Mowrer, O. H., & Mowrer, W. M. Enuresis: A method for its study and treatment. *American Journal of Orthopsychiatry,* 1938, *8,* 436–459.

Murray, E. J. Beyond behavioral and dynamic therapy. *British Journal of Clinical Psychology,* 1983, *22,* 127–128.

Murray, N. E. A dynamic synthesis of analytic and behavioral approaches to symptoms. *American Journal of Psychotherapy,* 1976, *30,* 561–569.

Nelson, R. D. Assessment and therapeutic functions of self-monitoring. In M. Hersen, R. M. Eisler, & P. M. Miller (Eds.), *Progress in behavior modification* (Vol. 5). New York: Academic Press, 1977.

Papajohn, J. C. *Intensive behavior therapy: The behavioral treatment of complex emotional disorders.* New York: Pergamon, 1982.

Paul, G. H. Outcome of systematic desensitization II: Controlled investigations of individual treatment, technique variations, and current status. In C. M. Franks (Ed.), *Behavior therapy: Appraisal and status.* New York: McGraw-Hill, 1969.

Paul, G. H., & Lentz, R. J. *Psychosocial treatment of chronic mental patients: Milieu versus social-learning programs.* Cambridge: Harvard University Press, 1977.

Porter, R. *The role of learning in psychotherapy: A Ciba symposium.* Boston: Little, Brown, 1968.

Rachman, S. Behavior therapy and psychodynamics. *Behavior Therapy,* 1970, *1,* 527–530.

Rhoads, J. M., & Feather, B. W. Transference and resistance observed in behavior therapy. *British Journal of Medical Psychology,* 1972, *45,* 99–103.

Sears, R. R. Experimental analysis of psychoanalytic phenomena. In J. McV. Hunt (Ed.), *Personality and the behavior disorders.* New York: Ronald Press, 1944.

Segraves, R. T. *Marital therapy: A combined psychodynamic-behavioral approach.* New York: Plenum Press, 1982.

Shectman, F. A. Operant conditioning and psychoanalysis: Contrasts, similarities, and some thoughts about integration. *American Journal of Psychotherapy,* 1975, *29,* 72–78.

Shoben, E. J. Psychotherapy as a problem in learning theory. *Psychological Bulletin,* 1949, *46,* 366–392.

Sifneos, P. *Short-term dynamic psychotherapy: Evaluation and technique.* New York: Plenum Press, 1979.

Silverman, L. H. Some psychoanalytic considerations of non-psychoanalytic therapies: On the possibility of integrating treatment approaches and related issues. *Psychotherapy: Theory, Research, and Practice,* 1974, *11,* 298–305.

Silverman, L. H., Frank, S. G., & Dachinger, P. A psychoanalytic reinterpretation of the effectiveness of systematic desensitization: Experimental data bearing on the role of merging fantasies. *Journal of Abnormal Psychology*, 1974, *83*, 313–318.

Skinner, B. F. *The behavior of organisms*. New York: Appleton-Century-Crofts, 1938.

Sloane, R. B. The converging paths of behavior therapy and psychotherapy. *American Journal of Psychiatry*, 1969, *125*, 877–885.

Sloane, R. B., Staples, F. R., Cristol, A. H., Yorkston, N. J., & Whipple, K. *Psychotherapy vs. behavior therapy*. Cambridge: Harvard University Press, 1975.

Stampfl, T. G., & Levis, D. J. Essentials of implosive therapy: A learning-theory-based psychodynamic behavioral therapy. *Journal of Abnormal Psychology*, 1967, *6*, 496–503.

Strupp, H. A psychodynamicist looks at behavior therapy. *Psychotherapy: Theory, Research, and Practice*, 1979, *16*, 124–131.

Strupp, H. H. *Are psychoanalytic therapists beginning to practice cognitive behavior therapy or is behavior therapy turning psychoanalytic?* Paper presented at the meeting of the American Psychological Association, Toronto, August 1978.

Sullivan, H. S. *The interpersonal theory of psychiatry*. New York: Norton, 1953.

Thoresen, C. E. Behavioral humanism. In C. E. Thoresen (Ed.). *Behavior modification in education*. Chicago: University of Chicago Press, 1973.

Thorndike, E. L. *The fundamentals of learning*. New York: Teachers College Press, 1932.

Tolman, E. C. Cognitive maps in rats and men. *Psychological Review*, 1948, *55*, 189–208.

Ullman, L. P., & Krasner, L. (Eds.). *Case studies in behavior modification*. New York: Holt, Rinehart & Winston, 1965.

Wachtel, P. L. Behavior therapy and the facilitation of psychoanalytic exploration. *Psychotherapy: Theory, Research, and Practice*, 1975, *12*, 68–72.

Wachtel, P. L. *Psychoanalysis and behavior therapy: Toward an integration*. New York: Basic Books, 1977.

Wachtel, P. L. (Ed.). *Resistance: Psychodynamic and behavioral approaches*. New York: Plenum Press, 1982. (a)

Wachtel, P. L. What can dynamic therapies contribute to behavior therapy? *Behavior Therapy*, 1982, *13*, 594–609. (b)

Wachtel, P. L. Integration misunderstood. *British Journal of Clinical Psychology*, 1983, *22*, 129–130.

Wandersman, A., Poppen, P. J., & Ricks, D. F. (Eds.), *Humanism and behaviorism: Dialogue and growth*. Elmsford, N.Y.: Pergamon, 1976.

Weinberg, N. H., & Zaslove, M. "Resistance" to systematic desensitization of phobias. *Journal of Clinical Psychology*, 1963, *19*, 179–181.

Weitzman, R. Behavior therapy and psychotherapy. *Psychological Review*, 1967, *74*, 300–317.

Wilson, A., & Smith, F. J. Counterconditioning therapy using free association: A pilot study. *Journal of Abnormal Psychology*, 1968, *73*(5), 474–478.

Wilson, G. T. Clinical issues and strategies in the practice of behavior therapy. In C. M. Franks, G. T. Wilson, P. C. Kendall, & K. Brownell (Eds.), *Annual review of behavior therapy* (Vol. 8). New York: Guilford, 1982. (a)

Wilson, G. T. Psychotherapy process and procedure: The behavioral mandate. *Behavior Therapy*, 1982, *13*, 291–312. (b)

Wilson, G. T., & Evans, I. The therapist–client relationship in behavior therapy. In A. S. Gurman & A. M. Razin (Eds.), *Effective psychotherapy: A handbook of research*. New York: Pergamon, 1977.

Winnicott, D. W. *Playing and reality*. New York: Basic Books, 1971. (Originally published in 1953.)

Wolf, E. Learning theory and psychoanalysis. *British Journal of Medical Psychology,* 1966, *39,* 1–10.

Wolpe, J. *Psychotherapy by reciprocal inhibition.* Stanford: Stanford University Press, 1958.

Wolpe, J. Behavior therapy vs. psychoanalysis: Therapeutic and social implications. *American Psychologist,* 1981, *36,* 159–164.

Wolpe, J., & Lazarus, A. *Behavior therapy techniques: A guide to the treatment of neuroses.* New York: Pergamon, 1966.

Wolpe, J., & Rachman, S. Psychoanalytic evidence: A critique based on Freud's case of Little Hans. *Journal of Nervous and Mental Disease,* 1960, *131,* 135–148.

Woody, R. H. Toward a rationale for psychobehavioral therapy. *Archives of General Psychiatry,* 1968, *19,* 197–204.

Woody, R. H. *Psychobehavioral counseling and therapy: Integrating behavioral and insight techniques.* New York: Appleton-Century-Crofts, 1971.

Yates, A. J. Behavior therapy and psychodynamic psychotherapy: Basic conflict or reconciliation or integration? *British Journal of Clinical Psychology,* 1983, *22,* 107–125.

2

On Theory, Practice, and the Nature of Integration

PAUL L. WACHTEL

It is really not very difficult to argue against an integration of psychodynamic and behavioral approaches. All one has to do is to define psychodynamic and behavioral in the right way, and they will indeed be incompatible. This the critics of integration have done, sometimes with flair and considerable sophistication. It will be the burden of this chapter to argue, however, that such criticisms do not really address the kind of integration I have proposed. They are, I suggest, articulate defenses of a less than satisfactory status quo and they impede the creative fusion that I believe is necessary for a major advance in psychotherapeutic efficacy and in the theoretical understanding on which such enhanced efficacy must be based.

To some degree I myself have abetted the definitional confusion. For a variety of reasons, partly syntactic and aesthetic, partly having to do with the term *psychoanalysis* being more familiar and widely recognized and partly, I confess, to arrest potential readers with a starker, more provocative challenge, I referred in the title of my book to psycho*analysis* and behavior therapy. It would have been less confusing to indicate (as I did do in the body of my book) that I was concerned with an integration of psycho*dynamic* and behavioral approaches. The term *psychodynamic* is a broader—and less jealously guarded—one that includes not only Freudian theory

PAUL L. WACHTEL • Department of Psychology, City College of the City University of New York, New York, New York 10031.

and those variations of it that have been included in what might be called the official psychoanalytic movement but also points of view that, although originally rooted in Freudian thought, have presented direct challenges to certain assumptions still widely held by Freudians.

It could reasonably be argued that psychoanalysis *is* the correct term for the points of view on which I rely. Horney and her followers did describe what they did as psychoanalysis, and many Sullivanians describe themselves as analysts. (Indeed, the journal of the William Alanson White Institute, the major Sullivanian training center, is called *Contemporary Psychoanalysis.*) Nonetheless, I do believe that it is more accurate—or at least less confusing—for someone like myself, who relies as much on Horney and Sullivan as on Freud, to describe my point of view as *psychodynamic* rather than specifically as psychoanalytic.

Freud himself varied on what he considered the essential defining features of psychoanalysis. In 1914 he said:

> Any line of investigation, *no matter what its direction,* which recognizes [the facts of transference and resistance] and takes them as the starting point of its work may call itself psychoanalysis, though it arrives at results other than my own. (Freud, 1914/1959, p. 298, italics mine)

A few years later a harder-line, more restrictive statement was offered—one that both upped the ante as to what a psychoanalyst must pay obeisance to and that was cast in a syntax of prohibition rather than of permission:

> The assumption that there are unconscious mental processes, the recognition of the theory of resistance and repression, the appreciation of the importance of sexuality and of the Oedipus complex—these constitute the principal subject-matter of psycho-analysis and the foundations of its theory. *No one who cannot accept them all* should count himself a psycho-analyst. (Freud, 1923/1959, p. 247, italics mine)

Freud's efforts to define the "sine qua nons" of the tradition he had launched were related to sectarian battles within the psychoanalytic movement. Fairly early, Freud was confronting the consequences of the extraordinarily stimulating effect his discoveries and theories produced; he spawned intellectual progeny he was eager to disown. He had, of course, every right to distinguish between his own theories and those of others whose ideas might be confused with his. I would largely agree with him that he is

> justified in maintaining that even to-day no one can know better than I what psycho-analysis is, how it differs from other ways of investigating the life of the mind, and precisely what should be called psycho-analysis and what would better be described by some other name. (Freud, 1914/1959, p. 287)

But if Freud could attempt with some justification to control what was to be called psychoanalysis, he had neither the right nor the power to control more generally how others were to reinterpret or selectively make use of his work. The more broadly psycho*dynamic* tradition consists of all those efforts to build a psychology starting from at least some of the central premises of Freudian thought, even if they diverged from Freud in substantial ways. After more than four decades of post-Freudian development, psychoanalysis itself—that is, modern Freudian orthodoxy—is hard to delineate precisely, and controversy (e.g., over whether Kohut's [1977] theorizing is properly Freudian psychoanalysis) abounds. The broader psycho*dynamic* umbrella is, of course, even harder to define. It is the essence of much of it that different proponents see different aspects of Freud's thought as the most crucial or most valuable. What is to one an unfortunate anachronism in Freud's otherwise brilliant work is to another the heart and soul of what makes psychoanalysis of continuing value.

Nonetheless, it is useful to delineate a broader psychodynamic point of view, many of whose proponents are steeped in Freud but are also critical of aspects of the Freudian mainstream. Despite the diversity of theoretical perspectives and of evaluations of Freud's own contribution, the notion of a psychodynamic tradition, encompassing Freudian psychoanalysis but including considerably more, is not really that vague. Agreement as to who would belong within such a category would be rather high. (And clearly, present-day behavior therapists would not fit within it.)

MISLEADING CHARACTERIZATIONS OF PSYCHODYNAMIC THOUGHT

There are certainly features of some versions of psychodynamic thought that would make an integration with behavior therapy rather difficult. Critics have seized upon these as if they were the essential defining features of a psychodynamic point of view. Some of these are almost totally red herrings. The contention, for example, that, unlike behavior therapy, psychoanalysis is a medical or disease model is thoroughly without merit. The close association of the official psychoanalytic organization in the United States with the medical profession was a matter of economics and guild protectionism and was counter both to the general policy of the International Psychoanalytic Association and to Freud's (1926a/1959) own arguments. The psychoanalytic situation, in fact, was largely set up to *avoid* the kinds of interactions and expectations that are encountered in medicine. The psychoanalytic model is a psychological, not a medical model (Wachtel, 1977a).

More respectable, but still off the mark, is the contention that integration is impossible because psychoanalysis attributes causation to the past and because behavior therapy focuses on the present. It is certainly true that many analysts do contend that an exploration of the patient's past is essential for lasting and meaningful change. Such a view, however, though it was held by Freud, is not an essential characteristic of a psychodynamic point of view (Horney, 1939; Wachtel, 1977a).* Concern with unconscious motivation, with conflict—and even with the enormous shaping influence of early experience—can as readily be pursued via a model of cumulative skewing of development that gives great weight to present environmental input (Wachtel, 1973, 1977b, 1981) as it can with a model that makes the influence of the past impervious to present realities. That is, one can trace how early experiences skew the kinds of later experiences one encounters, with the effect of maintaining the psychic structures previously existing. One can also trace how those psychic structures in turn lead to still further skewing of experience and to still further confirmation of existing structures in a continuing circle that at each point takes place in what is then the present. The mediational events in this continuing process can include unconscious conflicts and wishes, but they are always present wishes and conflicts, no matter however much they resemble those of the past.

A third objection is more interesting because it is based on a characterization that is indeed true for a very large majority of psychodynamic thinkers, whatever their specific persuasion. Franks (1978; Franks & Wilson, 1979) has described a methodological or epistemological difference between psychodynamic and behavioral thinkers. For the former, he suggests that "subjective data derived entirely from the clinical situation are typically regarded as valid." The latter, he says, play by different rules.

The general picture this characterization presents of two groups of thinkers is largely accurate. Psychodynamic thinkers often do take as evidence for a particular formulation or general concept data that most behavior therapists do not find persuasive. As some analysts are beginning to articulate (e.g., Schafer, 1976), psychoanalysis is based on a methodology and epistemology that is more akin to that of history or literary studies than it is to that of the natural sciences. It seeks to explain by offering formulations that account for coherences in a diverse range of phenomena. It seeks also to show how the pictures offered by dreams, by slips of the tongue, by omissions and failures of memory, and by various otherwise

* Indeed, one can argue that even where a strong concern with the past does characterize a particular psychodynamic thinker's approach, that does not preclude the use of behavioral measures. It is only where a strong stance of nonintervention is taken in order to permit the transference to emerge or unfold that a concern with the past is problematic for the purposes of integration (Wachtel, 1977a, 1982a).

puzzling behavioral patterns all converge—that is, to articulate unities behind the manifest diversity. The explanation is, to a large degree, one that *makes sense* out of the flux of events and that gives order and coherence. It is a latticework of evidence in which each strand supports the others and in which each piece of evidence *becomes* evidence only in the context of the other pieces.

The dream, for example, that gives weight to an interpretation that an overly solicitous son in fact harbors warded-off hostile feelings toward his mother might *not* be evidence for such a view if the other data (slips, "inadvertent" behavior patterns, particular trends in the sequence of associations, etc.) did not also point that way. Indeed, in another context, the same dream might be usable as evidence for a *different* line of interpretation. And the same holds, by and large, for *each* piece of evidence. To a very great degree, pieces of evidence gain meaning and evidential gravity *from each other.*

This does not mean that evidence is used arbitrarily, that you can use anything to prove anything. Unfortunately, there are more dynamically oriented clinicians than one would wish who do make of their formulations a procrustrean bed in which any potentially disturbing observations are put to rest; and it is probably also true that the mode of evaluating evidence in psychodynamic work makes it easier to "cheat" or to fool oneself that one has proven what one has not than is the case for behavior therapists.* But there is a discipline available that helps to minimize such occurrences if it is properly used. There *are* pieces that do not fit, that serve a cautionary or discomfirming function. When the paradigm is properly applied, such new observations can—in the fashion suggested before—lend a different cast to all the data previously seen as supportive of one's first formulation and force a new formulation that provides a coherent picture of this newer, larger body of data.

Thus the "good" psychoanalyst discards prior hypotheses just as the experimenter does when new results require it. And among the followers of both methodological paradigms, there are those whose ideas show a remarkable immunity to new observations, and there are those who actually learn from what they do. But if one can make a case that the methodologies and epistemologies are equally defensible, they are nonetheless different. Indeed, I have at times been astounded at how refractory some behavior therapists can be to what I regard as solidly convincing configurational evidence.

There is thus something useful in Franks and Wilson's distinction

* It really does not take all that much ingenuity—or wrongheadedness—to cheat within the behavioral paradigm either. Behavior therapy, too, has begun to develop divergent schools with mutual bitterness and accusations of highly selective renderings and interpretations of data.

between the methodological or epistemological orientation of psychoanalysts and behavior therapists. If you define the essence of the psychodynamic and behavioral approaches as they do, the case for integration does look shaky.

Even here, it should be noted, their distinction refers to something statistical rather than essential. That is, although it is true that *most* psychoanalytic thinkers have a different orientation to evidence than do *most* behavior therapists, there is at least a small minority in each group whose canons of evidence overlap considerably. There are, for example, a number of psychoanalysts who have felt a need to establish psychoanalytic concepts by experimental evidence as well as by the more common configurational kind of evidence (see, for example, Shevrin, 1980; Silverman, 1976; Wolitzky & Wachtel, 1973). And, I suggest, in clinical practice many behavior therapists show at least some inclination to think configurationally rather than requiring anything like experimental confirmation before they regard a hypothesis as confirmed. (They are much more likely to require such confirmation with regard to general *principles,* but as I have noted elsewhere [Wachtel, 1982b], the relation between those general principles and their actual clinical functioning is far looser than is usually suggested.)

Now, of course, one could say that to the degree that they deviate from experimental canons of evidence they are not really behavior therapists. But this is winning the anti-integration argument by tautology. Or perhaps it would be fairer to say that Franks and Wilson argue against a different kind of integration than what I have advocated. Methodological or epistemological integration—that is, integration of ideas about evidence—may or may not be possible, but it is at the least very difficult. Certainly it is far more difficult than the kind of integration I have advocated.

Franks and Wilson suggest that at times it may be useful to attempt an integration at the level of clinical practice but not at a "conceptual" level. Even here they are rather skeptical and refer to this possibility as "technical opportunism," a term that could conceivably be defended as merely descriptive but whose connotation is hard to ignore. It is certainly true that there is yet scant evidence that an integration at the level of clinical practice will yield superior results. Though my own guess is obviously different, I regard as perfectly reasonable Franks and Wilson's hunch that in the long run advancement in clinical practice is more likely to follow from pursuing one of the presently established systems than from attempting an integration of techniques. But when they contrast their preferred scenario with "an indiscriminate deployment of what seems to work," I hope it is clear to the reader—and to them—that they are no longer referring to the kind of effort I have advocated.

My aim is not simply the practical application of a combination of clinical procedures but rather to work toward a thorough conceptual integration. The particular way of proceeding clinically that I have developed out of my integrative efforts seems to me useful for now, but I am sure it will change. What seems more likely to be of enduring value is the construction of a frame of reference in which the ideas and the observations emanating from both* broad approaches can find a coherent place and in which the discoveries of each can push the other to expand. That frame of reference too is not a final or finished product; it continues and *must* continue to change and evolve in order to accomodate further observations and ideas. But, in my view, it is the development of a coherent way of thinking about clinical problems, a way open to input from a variety of sources, that will enable really effective clinical work at the practical level to proceed most expeditiously.

The development of a conceptual integration is, I think, usefully distinguished from a methodological or epistemological integration. Franks and Wilson conflate these two levels in arguing that a "conceptual" integration is impossible. They are quite right that "one's belief system" is hard to integrate with another that feels alien. Psychoanalysts and behavior therapists—to the degree that separate schools persist in coming years—will continue to hold different ideas about what constitutes "proof," as they will continue (at least as distinguishable statistical aggregates) to evidence different "visions" of life (see Messer & Winokur, 1980, and their commentary at the end of this chapter). But an integration at the conceptual—rather than the ideological or epistemological—level remains a useful and achievable goal. I will have more to say shortly about what such an integration is like, but first I would like to return to its constituents. I have said something about what I think are *not* the essential defining features of a psychodynamic or behavioral view and about what I think are misleading or irrelevant differences for present purposes. Let me now indicate, at least briefly, what I do take to be the most significant characteristics of each approach.

THE PSYCHODYNAMIC POINT OF VIEW

I have argued that a number of characteristics commonly claimed to be essential to the psychodynamic point of view are not really essential after all. The "medical model," the emphasis on the past, and (to a lesser

* Although the integration of psychodynamic and behavioral approaches in particular is both the focus of this chapter and the starting point of my integrative efforts, other perspectives, such as that of family therapists, of Piaget, or of gestalt therapists have also begun to be included in the integrative effort under discussion here and will probably continue to be to an increasing degree. (See, for example, Wachtel, 1981b.)

degree) a particular epistemological orientation are, I suggest, misleading or unnecessarily constraining as defining properties of psychodynamic thought. To this negative list I would add such other candidates as the libido theory, Freud's mental geography, the requirement of neutrality or nonintervention by the therapist, and the insistence on insight as the primary source of psychological change (cf. Wachtel, 1977a, 1982b, in press-b). Have I then succeeded in draining the term *psychodynamic* of all meaning and left just a hollow shell with no substance? I believe not. There remain a number of crucially important characteristics shared by all psychodynamic thinkers that clearly distinguish them from those in the behavioral tradition and represent, in my view, the most significant legacy of Freud's pioneering efforts.

Clearly, the single most essential defining property is a concern with unconscious processes. If anything is a sine qua non of the psychodynamic point of view, this is it. What Freud illuminated, more than anything else, was the degree to which we do not really know ourselves. Further, he points us to inquire into the *motives* for our self-deceptions and into their consequences: Our lack of awareness is not merely a failure to notice or to register. We *try* not to notice, and we *dare* not notice.* And, unfortunately, the immediate comfort this turning away brings us quite frequently has as its heir a disruption of our lives that is far out of proportion to the initial gain. The price of comfort is very high.

A second critical feature of the psychodynamic point of view is a focus upon *conflict*. What we want, it turns out, is not as simple as we would wish. In the prism of psychoanalysis our unitary actions or expressions of desire are resolved into components that, alone, would lead us in rather differing directions. Conceptions of conflict pervade the psychodynamic approach to motivation and, implicitly, suggest a quite different way of understanding what happens when a behavior therapist attempts to use reinforcements (Wachtel, 1977a, Chapter 11; 1982b). The psychodynamic conception of conflict is closely related to the concern with what is dynamically unconscious as well as to an increasing emphasis on the role of anxiety (Freud, 1926b/1959; Dollard & Miller, 1950). It need not, however, imply a strictly intrapsychic view of how conflict is generated or maintained (Wachtel, 1977a, 1982a).

A related feature of most psychodynamically oriented clinical work (though not as crucially defining a feature) is a concern with the *compromises* that conflict, anxiety, and self-deception lead to. From a psychodynamic perspective, even patterns of behavior or aspirations and guiding assump-

* Sometimes, of course, simple failures to notice do occur. Freud distinguished between the dynamic and the descriptive unconscious. It is the former that plays such a key role in psychological difficulties and which Freud dedicated himself to illuminating.

tions with which the person seems comfortable are likely to be called into question. This can at times be overdone, as behavior therapists have appropriately pointed out; the patient has a right to keep his goals and focus narrow, and some version of informed consent seems called for if the person's comfortable assumptions are to be systematically challenged. But if the analyst is attentive to the ethical complexities, this broader and deeper inquiry is one of the most valuable characteristics of the psychodynamic approach. Ignoring what the person is explicitly telling you is deplorable. But refusing to hear what cannot yet be put into words is unfortunate as well.

The psychodynamic perspective points not only to unconscious motives and to motivational conflict but to *unusual* and *nonnormative* motives as well. Freud's researches have alerted us to the importance and the prevalence of wishes that differ substantially from what would conventionally be expected. Viewed psychodynamically, what people actually seek—as opposed to what they *say* they are seeking—can be rather surprising. Behavior therapists, in contrast, tend to assume that what people want is what they say they want and/or what is normatively expectable (Wachtel, 1977a, Chapter 7).

Finally, a crucial feature of the psychodynamic approach is the rules of inference whereby such nonobvious, nonnormative motives can be identified. It is these rules that make claims regarding such motives not simply arbitrary assertions. Unfortunately, many of these rules have been passed along primarily by an oral tradition, and there is little good, explicit written material on the rules themselves. This has made it easy for opponents of psychoanalysis to view psychoanalytic claims about unconscious motives and thoughts as being essentially arbitrary. I have already indicated briefly some of the reasons why I think these inferences are *not* arbitrary. I hope before too long to complete a paper which examines this matter in more detail. For now, I simply wish to indicate that I regard such rules as essential contributions from the psychodynamic end to the synthesis under discussion in this chapter.

The reader will notice that such bellweather concepts as "transference" and "resistance"—the ideas Freud first designated as the essential defining characteristics of psychoanalysis—do not appear in the preceding list. Unlike "libido" or "neutrality," this is not because I think them faulty or inessential. In the case of resistance, it is merely that it is already subsumed under what has been outlined sketchily. Resistance is simply the manifestation in the therapy session of the conflict and motivated self-deception referred to previously (Wachtel, 1982c). The concept of transference—or at least the phenomena and concerns to which it refers—is certainly essential to address if one hopes to depict the psychodynamic point of view accurately. The term has, however, accumulated so much excess freight over the years and is so closely related to notions I do want to question, such as neutrality and nonintervention, that it cannot simply be listed without elaborate discussion. I have spelled out elsewhere alternative ways of understanding transference phenomena and how transference can be conceived so as to lend itself to the kind of integrative effort being discussed here (Wachtel, 1981b, 1982a).

THE BEHAVIORAL APPROACH

Indicating what I take to be the essential features of a behavioral approach is in some ways a more difficult task. As Franks and Wilson indicate, "there is much less of an abiding core to which all behavior therapists would subscribe." For present purposes, though, what is most important is to indicate those features of the behavioral approach that are central in the effort to achieve a psychodynamic and behavioral integration.

Perhaps most important in this regard is the emphasis on *active intervention*. Behavior therapists employ a wide variety of techniques to intervene in and alter maladaptive patterns of behavior. In their own way, so do analysts—both more and less than they think. They do more, in the sense that neutrality is a myth and influence is exerted in every choice to interpret, to remain silent, or to say, "Why do you ask?". They do less, in the sense that the clinical procedures of psychoanalysis are not nearly as powerful as one might hope and that they could be notably enhanced by the use of the intervention techniques developed by behavior therapists.

In psychoanalysis and in most psychodynamic therapy, the inquiry into the patient's difficulties and the intervention techniques are essentially the same. Understanding *is* the therapy. In behavior therapy, the understanding that is attained—by both patient and therapist—is *applied*. Explicit methods are utilized to assure that the patient garners the experiences that will enable him or her to change. These methods can also be used, I have argued, to make it more likely that the insights attained from a psychodynamic point of view in fact lead to the changes the patient is seeking (Wachtel, 1975, 1977a).*

* One can, of course, define psychodynamic therapy so as to include as an essential feature the presently common one of the therapist's striving for neutrality and/or an exclusively interpretive approach. To do so would, of course, make the use of active interventions incompatible with anything psychodynamic. Clearly, that is not the notion of psychodynamic therapy under discussion here. I regard the prevalent emphasis on neutrality as unfortunate and in no way required by the logic of the psychodynamic point of view *per se* (Wachtel, 1977a, 1982a).

A second feature of behavior therapy that is important in the present context is its concern with the environmental context of behavior, with relating the patient's behavior and experience to what is going on around him or her. Again, this is not something unique to behavior therapy. Even some versions of psychodynamic thought do this to a substantial degree (Wachtel, 1973), though usually not as thoroughly as behavior therapy. Family therapists, of course, are particularly concerned with relating behavior to context and have made valuable contributions in this regard that the present approach is still working to assimilate.

A third relevant feature is the emphasis by behavior therapists on an explicit contract between patient and therapist and a corresponding concern with specific target complaints. This leads, in conjunction with the emphasis on relating patients' difficulties to environmental events, to a kind of inquiry that has considerable merit both on ethical grounds and on practical ones. As discussed before, the articulation of a more explicit contract between patient and therapist need not exclude a concern with conflict or with examining the compromises and self-deceptions in the patient's life. But it does permit the patient to be a partner more fully in the therapeutic effort.

It is a common psychodynamic stereotype of behavior therapy that behavior therapists are authoritarian and manipulative and that they *work upon* the patient. Actually, in many respects the behavior therapist is *less* guilty of such an orientation. The emphasis by many dynamic therapists on therapeutic anonymity, the frequency with which questions are not explicitly answered, and other related features of most psychodynamic approaches contribute to an atmosphere in which the patient is in a child-like, one-down position. Behavior therapists, by and large, rather than dynamic therapists, are the ones who share explicitly with the patient what the rationale is for each thing that is being done and who concern themselves most explicitly with whether the work is moving in a direction that is consonant with the patient's own aims. Once anonymity and the idea that the transference should "emerge" or "unfold" without interference from the therapist are excluded as defining features of a psychodynamic approach (Wachtel, 1982a), it becomes possible to be similarly collaborative with the patient while maintaining a recognition of the important role of unconscious processes and motivational conflict.

As I noted earlier, I think it is misleading to identify a greater concern for evidence as an essential defining feature of behavior therapy, though I would agree that, as a group, behavior therapists are probably more alert to the need for, and pitfalls in gathering, such evidence. The characteristics of behavior therapy just noted, however—the effort to specify very clearly and precisely what changes the patient wants to achieve and the effort to relate particular patterns of behavior to particular environmental contexts—do facilitate the evaluation of therapeutic efficacy. The effort to discuss patients' difficulties and the goals of the work in terms at least potentially amenable to evaluation—although sometimes leading to excessive narrowness or unwillingness to address what cannot be immediately measured—is a valuable feature of the behavioral approach that is capable of being incorporated into an integrated model. The goals of psychodynamic therapy are often discussed in such terms as *autonomy, structural change,* or *resolution* of conflicts or of the transference—notions that are notoriously hard to evaluate (Wachtel, in press-b).

MESSER AND WINOKUR'S OBJECTIONS

The most interesting and sophisticated objection that has yet been made to the integration of psychodynamic and behavioral approaches has been offered by Messer and Winokur (1980). I believe that their objection can be effectively answered and that it really reflects a *comparative* orientation to psychodynamic and behavioral therapies rather than one that fully takes into account the selective and emergent properties of a true integration. That is, they look at similarities and (especially) differences between psychodynamic and behavioral approaches but do not as explicitly address how an integration—as a new, third orientation—might yield conceptions that reconcile those differences that presently exist. Nonetheless, their argument is an important one that must be addressed by any proponent of integration.

Messer and Winokur attempt to show that the values and the grounding vision that characterize psychoanalysts and behavior therapists are basically different. Even between the most ego- and reality-oriented analysts and the most cognitive or broad-spectrum behavior therapists there is, they suggest, a "nagging breach" that is based on different conceptions of what is important in human life and what is possible. They pursue their comparative analysis by considering how an analytically and a behaviorally oriented therapist would pursue the same case as well as by a more general consideration of the basic orientation of each approach. Their descriptions seem to me, for the most part, to be fair minded and accurate, and they do reveal ~~some very~~ significant differences. In some respects I have sensed similar differences myself in my own interactions with proponents of these two broad schools of thought. There are, however, a few points at which I would question their characterization, and I would like to address these before going on to consider my main objection to their line of argument—that differences *between* approaches do not necessarily preclude an integration *of* them.

In depicting the difference between the psychoanalytic and the behavioral vision, Messer and Winokur rely on a paper by Schafer (1976) that uses Northrup Frye's categories of mythic forms (Frye, 1957). Schafer argues that psychoanalysis can be seen as being characterized by four complementary visions of reality—the romantic, the ironic, the tragic, and the comic—and he elaborates the nature of each. This mode of characterization is useful in conveying various aspects of the psychoanalytic world view *per se.* But when it is employed by Messer and Winokur in an effort to compare the psychoanalytic vision with that of the behavior therapist, it is far less satisfactory. For *this* purpose, this set of categories has some insurmountable problems.

To begin with, the choices offered by this particular fourfold scheme lead to the vision of the behavior therapist being characterized as "comic." Messer and Winokur state explicitly that in this context the term is not meant to connote "funny," "in a light vein," or "not serious." But surely, as analysts they must recognize that connotations are not so easily dispelled. Whatever verbal disavowal may be offered, to characterize an entire approach to human problems simply as comic cannot fail to detract from any sense that that approach has something profound or serious to offer. Yes, Shakespeare's comedies can indeed be viewed as both profound *and* serious, but what Shakespearean scholar, writing commentaries on those plays, would be pleased at having his or her *own* work described simply as comic?

Moreover, even Messer and Winokur's explicit definition of comic, meant to dispel the aforementioned connotation, is really a loaded one. In the comic vision, they say, conflict "can be eliminated by effective manipulative action or via the power of positive thinking." Why do they speak of effective *manipulative* action? Why do they not say effective action only? This is a small point perhaps but is not the word *manipulative* here both unnecessary and possessed of a possibly negative connotation? Similarly, "the power of positive thinking" is, after all, the title of a book that is not a scholarly work but a bit of pop preachiness for the *Reader's Digest* set—and, moreover, it is a book written by one of the favorite preachers of our most disgraced president, the man who presided over the wedding of Julie Nixon. In a paragraph devoted to dispelling the idea that comic implies a lack of seriousness or profundity, was there not a phrase with more scholarly associations that could have conveyed the same idea?

Further, Messer and Winokur go on to say about the comic vision that "endings are happy ones free from guilt and anxiety." This may be a more or less accurate picture of the structure of dramatic comedy. But does not the term "happy endings" nonetheless evoke the superficiality of Hollywood at its worst, where even films not intended as comedies have foolish, hard-to-take-seriously happy endings? And does this really—

as it seems to by the associative link they develop—characterize not just the comic vision but the world view of behavior therapists as well? By and large, behavior therapists do seem to be more optimistic in their outlook. They are less certain that tragedy and the involution of desire must haunt our days. But do they really expect simply happy endings, and do they really claim that after therapy patients are completely free from guilt and anxiety?

Finally, we come to a more subtle bias that is introduced as a consequence of the scheme Messer and Winokur use to analyze the competing visions. As an artifact of how they choose to slice the pie, it appears that psychoanalysis has *four* separate visions, whereas behavior therapy has but one. That alone, it seems, would make psychoanalysis far more comprehensive. Behavior therapy, with its single vision, seems superficial just by virtue of that. Of course, a vision of reality is not a "thing." It makes no sense to count visions or add them up. Yet, there is something initially compelling about seeing that the vision that guides behavior therapy is but one of the four visions guiding psychoanalysis.*

The problem, of course, lies in the terms in which the comparison is framed. The psychoanalytic world view is neatly dissected by this scheme, and the multiplicity of its perspectives is revealed. But the various facets of the behavioral vision are not similarly captured by this particular way of slicing things, so it is left with just "one" vision. In fact, the comic view of behavior therapists is a quite different one from the comic view of the analyst. Whereas for analysts this concept of Frye's intersects with but a small portion of their total world view, it is forced, within the constraints of this scheme, to cover the totality of the behavior therapist's vision. The behavior therapist's comic vision, however—being coterminous with the behavior therapist's vision *per se*—is (not suprisingly therefore) more complex. There is a sense, in fact, in which it can be said to be the container for the behavior therapist's sense of tragedy, of irony, and of romance. His or her vision is not totally devoid of these elements. Rather, they are organized differently; they are subsumed under a general orientation toward meliorating suffering rather than enduring it and under a basically optimistic (but not necessarily Pollyannaish) view of human possibilities.

Consider, for example, Messer and Winokur's discussion in their paper of the psychodynamic approach to a hypothetical patient, Mrs. J.

* I do not mean to imply here that Messer and Winokur themselves count visions and argue on that basis. They do not. Rather, the point is that the scheme they use is likely to lead the *reader* to be struck by the seeming fact that the behavior therapist's vision is but one of the four visions of the analyst and to be led, perhaps without even recognizing it, to perceive behavior therapy in a way that introduces a negative bias.

> When the dynamic therapist allows Mrs. J. to experience grief, mourn her losses, see the death of her father and loss of her husband in their tragic grimness, the thrust is to help her change by facing the loss, reexperiencing it and working it through, with all the pain involved. Only rarely, the dynamic therapist would say, does growth in therapy, as in childhood, take place without some suffering. In all this, the tragic element in life is recognized. (p. 824)

This certainly is a different picture than one would expect from a behavior therapist. Yet the gulf is not as thoroughly unbridgeable as it first might seem. After all, it is the essence of many behavioral measures to enable the patient to expose himself or herself to the experiences and situations he or she has previously avoided. Often, as in systematic desensitization, the attempt is made to minimize the pain, but some pain is almost inevitable and in certain techniques, such as flooding, things are arranged so that the pain is considerable. Behavior therapy is not predicated on avoidance of the painful but on confrontation and mastery.

WHAT IS AN INTEGRATION?

My point is not to deny the differences between the psychoanalytic and behavioral visions; the differences are real and in some ways substantial. My preceding objections notwithstanding, I regard Messer and Winokur's characterizations as largely accurate and in essence to be fair minded. I do not think that the instances of bias I have pointed out were conscious efforts to mislead. They reflect, rather, an almost inevitable influence on our language of the passionate convictions that sustain any good work. I discussed them both to attempt a corrective and to indicate that the gap is not thoroughly beyond the reach of any conceivable effort at bridge building. At this point, however, I wish to approach the issue from a different angle. Let me alert the reader to the fact that it is in the following paragraphs that the most important part of my argument can be found.

Arguments showing that psychoanalysis and behavior therapy are *different* do not really bear on the question of whether they can be integrated. Indeed, were they not rather different there would be little point in an integration. It is the very fact that each stresses certain things that the other does not that makes an integration more useful than either separately. And, of course, it is their differences that make an effort at integration interesting and challenging. It is no feat to put together what seems compatible and alike to everyone.

As I conceive it, an integration is not just a hodgepodge of eclecticism, a salad with a little of this and a little of that tossed in. The goal, rather, is the development of a new coherent structure, an internally consistent approach both to technical intervention and to the construction of theory. An integrative or synthetic effort is built on both an admiring and a critical attitude toward each separate approach. It is admiring in the sense that each has something useful and important to contribute, and it is critical in the sense that each is seen as *omitting* something useful and important (for the most part something that is part of what is valuable about the other approach).

Messer and Winokur (1980), for example, capture well some of what I find valuable in psychoanalysis and somewhat missing in behavior therapy. They indicate, for example, that they could not approve of any approach that "denies complexity, ambiguity, and the ubiquity of conflict in human affairs" (p. 825). Neither could I.*

But I have come to feel that an approach that fails to appreciate the enormous significance of present contextual cues and contingencies, that fails to consider the therapist's responsibility to help the patient systematically to apply the lessons learned in the sessions to his or her daily life, that underestimates the factors that make it difficult for the patient to make that application spontaneously, or that has a deep-rooted bias against active intervention by the therapist is also unacceptable. As things stand now, we have the choice of embracing one set of follies (and of course strengths) or the other. The aim of an integration is to build upon the strengths of each without the limiting blinders. This can seem a grandiose aim (and in Messer and Winokur's terms it is comic—an effort to transcend the limitations, to take only the good). But one need not feel that the millennium is around the corner to strive for something better than we have or to expect some tangible gain from an integrative effort.

It is important to be clear that one can value the unique contributions of each approach without endorsing each and every feature of either. As a proponent of integration, I am frequently in the position of trying to persuade my behavioral colleagues of the virtues of a psychodynamic point of view and vice versa. In this task I am at times embarrassed by things that are written by representatives of one or the other school. But that embarrassment stems from tactical rather than logical considerations. That is, it stems from a recognition that foolish excesses from either side make it harder to get people from the other side to see or hear what really is

* I wish to make it clear that I do not endorse the implicit message that behavior therapists deny all complexity and ambiguity. Messer and Winokur's specific way of stating their point here seems to me a bit unfair. But I do agree that there are complexities to which behavior therapists give *insufficient* attention, and my own inclinations are closer to those of Messer and Winokur. With regard to conflict in particular, a more categorical criticism of most behavior therapists does seem in order (cf. Wachtel, 1977a).

useful, and thus they play into an attitude of "See, I told you that stuff is worthless." But these embarrassing impediments to the *practical* task of persuading people on either side of the great divide are not necessarily impediments to the *theoretical* task of devising a new synthesis that incorporates the best of both. I agree with my psychoanalytic colleagues about many of the things they find objectionable in behavior therapy and vice versa with regard to my behavioral colleagues. My charge as an integrationist is not to defend everything that analysts or behavior therapists say or do but rather to show that each side contributes *something* useful that the other omits or plays down and to show how these *selected* features can be put together in a logically coherent fashion.

The total package that presently constitutes behavior therapy is indeed incompatible with the total package that is called psychoanalysis. One cannot be a psychoanalyst *and* a behavior therapist—at least not simultaneously. Messer and Winokur have helped to clarify further the nature of the differences. But one can take *elements* of each and combine them into a new synthesis that is still a *third* package, as it were.

The fallacy in most arguments against integration is a failure to appreciate that a synthesis is a different entity than either of its constituents. It is a clinical and theoretical approach with its own structure. It can be selective in what aspects of each approach it incorporates, drawing upon what seems potentially useful in constructing a new synergistic strategy, rather than upon what proponents of each as *separate* therapies regard as most important. The major constraint is that the elements must not be incompatible in the context of the new structure.*

Messer and Winokur state that behavior therapists are primarily interested in the external reality of their patients' lives and that psychoanalytic therapists are primarily interested in (conscious and unconscious) subjectivity. Representatives of each school might object to this, pointing to ways in which they do manifest the opposite perspective. But, as a broad characterization of emphasis, it is probably accurate. In the integrative approach discussed here, *both* perspectives are given substantial weight. This occurs not by striving for a balance by doing a little of this, a little of that—a kind of one-perspective–one-vote rule—but through the utilization of a conceptual structure that unites the two perspectives and reconciles their differences. That conceptual structure, for me, has centered

* What makes the approach described in this chapter an integration rather than a third approach is, first of all, the fact that its elements come primarily from the approaches being integrated rather than being original to it; what is unique is how they are put together. Secondly, this approach, rather than being a new "school," is founded on the conviction that schools have become more limiting than facilitating at this point. Finally, this approach is based upon respect for the earlier approaches rather than opposition to them.

on an effort to describe people's difficulties in terms of vicious circles, in which neither impulse nor defense and neither internal state nor external situation is primary; they are continually determining each other in a series of repeated transactions. I have described that conceptual structure as one of *cyclical psychodynamics* (Wachtel, 1982a, in press-a) and have tried to show how it makes possible the reconciliation of what seem like opposing viewpoints (see also Wachtel, 1973, 1977a, 1977b).

When the sharp dichotomy between "inner" and "outer" is challenged, one can see how even the deepest levels of subjectivity reflect, frequently in a symbolic way, the person's life situation. Thus, one patient began to dream of melting into his girl friend and of being swallowed by her. Such fears and experiences of merger and boundary dissolution are frequently described by analysts as "deep" or "early" and are attributed to the intrapsychic residue of early experiences with mothering. The experiences the patient reported, however, could also be understood as symbolizing his present way of life: He was very inhibited and unassertive and felt unable to say no to his girl friend or to spend any evenings alone or with friends if she wanted to see him. As he became more able to do so, he felt less swallowed up by her, and his sense of ego boundaries became firmer. Regardless of the origins of the experience he reported, it was not a purely intrapsychic event but a function as well of manifest events in his daily life.

At the same time, the situations one finds oneself in can often be understood not as thoroughly external events but as products of one's subjective particularities. That is, the events do not simply "happen" to us but are a predictable consequence of our internal state and the behavior it leads to. The stark impassiveness of a dominating husband, for example, both contributes to the wife's fear of assertiveness and stems from it. One woman I worked with was stunned to discover how much of a "pushover" her husband was once she started asserting herself. As she spontaneously put it, "I thought he was the situation I faced, but he was the situation I *made*."

Recently, the social learning formulations that have provided the theoretical background for much of the work in behavior therapy have stressed similar circular causal chains under the rubric of "reciprocal determinism" (Bandura, 1978). This seems to reflect an incorporation of earlier criticisms of social learning theory (Wachtel, 1973) and of earlier formulations of "social behaviorism," which Staats has argued—in a paper with extraordinary claims and an even more extraordinary history—have systematically preceded similar, more frequently cited formulations by Bandura (Staats, 1983).

Messer and Winokur note that "where the behavioral approach, consonant with the comic view, leads to action, the psychoanalytic approach, following the tragic view, leads to reflection and inquiry." For an integrative approach, *both* action and reflection are central. Messer and Winokur suggest this combination may be difficult to effect because of "the radical shift in perspective and vision involved" (1980). I would agree: It *is* difficult. My own efforts thus far, though encouraging, still remain far from the fully integrated ideal toward which I strive. But the difficulty is not so much the seemingly intractible one of irreconcilable visions as it is a practical one of finding just what is the best way to proceed (a difficult, painstaking task but one that it is reasonable to expect might yield to continued effort). After all, by Messer and Winokur's own account, psychoanalysis has managed to contain and integrate four rather different visions of reality. As a synthesis of several visions, psychoanalysis is itself evidence that a powerful overarching vision can reconcile polarities among its constituent elements.

The challenge is to achieve a new sustaining vision of sufficient breadth and power. That task has only begun. I am optimistic about the possibilities of a synthesis rooted in the study of vicious circles, of how defensive efforts contribute to the very wishes and feelings they defend against, of how significant people in the present serve as "accomplices" in maintaining neurotic patterns, of how recognition of this can enable a conception of skewing of development to replace earlier notions of fixation and developmental arrest, of how such a perspective permits a transcendence of the dichotomy between an inner world and outer reality, of how conceptions of transference are altered by the application of Piagetian notions of "schema," "assimilation," and "accommodation," and finally, of how all of these conceptual modifications point to a greater variety of ways to intervene in the processes that produce neurotic misery.

The references cited in this chapter point to some of my own efforts in this direction. These efforts have been preceded and paralleled (and greatly aided) by important work on the part of a relative handful of innovative theorists and clinicians (see Goldfried & Padawer [1982] for a good review of this body of work). There are indications now of interest in the possibilities of integration on the part of a larger number of people. This greatly increases the likelihood of significant advances. The challenge will soon have to be faced of how to coordinate and bring together these various efforts. Working between rather than within established traditions is difficult, personally as well as intellectually. A support group that provided workers on the interface with a shared identity would be very useful. Both a journal and an organization could help to give this work a home, to attract young researchers and clinicians to this effort, and to enable a wider audience to become aware of the work and of new developments in it. But there are dangers as well. It would be unfortunate if integrative psychotherapy were to become a new "school," with gradually encrusting borders. Its strength lies precisely in its continued openness to the work of others. Devising the proper organizational framework to represent such a multifaceted and open-ended effort may be as important a challenge as is the development of the ideas and techniques themselves.*

AUTOBIOGRAPHICAL STATEMENT

The origins of my interest in integration are complex and manifold. In the spirit of integration itself, I should surely trace them both to early parental influences and to later reinforcement contingencies. Among more conscious influences, I would include among the earliest my experience as an undergraduate at Columbia. I became a psychology major only in my senior year, which is probably fortunate, for the general richness and diversity of a Columbia education did not tend to be matched by the specific offerings of the Columbia Department of Psychology in those days. As an undergraduate institution, Columbia was a wonderful intellectual cornucopia, but the psychology department was monolithically Skinnerian, and it was a shock to discover how different was the psychology I was being taught from what I had imagined and sought. (Indeed, so overweening was the Skinnerian influence that for some part of that year I seriously wondered whether the Great Man's initials accounted for the fact that psychology books were listed in the library under the call numbers "BF.")

Among the effects of that experience were an abhorrence for closed systems of thought and (nonetheless) a grudging respect for the utility and potential applicability of the principles being explored in the learning laboratory. Both have remained with me (though the respect for learning principles is no longer grudging). When, later in my career, I encountered psychoanalytic communities that matched my Skinnerian Columbia professors in their ability to generate intellectual claustrophobia, I was prepared.

Clearly, being a graduate student at Yale at a time when John Dollard and Neal Miller were both active in the department also contributed to my readiness to seek an integrative path. Their influence in my later work is plain to see, but for a time it was submerged in the effort to master the intricacies of psychoanalytic theory and technique. I immersed myself in a postdoctoral psychoanalytic training institute that billed itself as being open to a wide range of views, but it proved, instead, to harbor a less-than-friendly coexistence between Freudians and neo-Freudians. That experience was a disillusioning one with regard to the possibilities of intellectual openness in a psychoanalytic institute, but it provided me with intensive clinical training and the opportunity for contact with a number of individuals whom I continue to respect greatly despite my disagreements with them on many matters.

*Shortly after the completion of this chapter, the Society for the Exploration of Psychotherapy Integration (SEPI) was founded, whose membership includes many of the contributors to this volume.

My explorations of the interpersonal tradition in psychoanalytic thought increasingly impressed me both with the possibilities they presented for applying Freud's insights in new ways and with the failure of most interpersonal therapists to carry through on these possibilities.* When, for reasons that were largely fortuitous, I began to read the literature in behavior therapy more closely, I was intrigued to discover that—when the parochial rhetoric of each was put in the background—the outlines of a convergence between certain strands in the behavioral approach and important themes in the interpersonal approach began to become apparent. I began to see how the active intervention methods of behavior therapists and their emphasis on observing the connections between our actions and the events that preceeded and followed them could help to activate the potential I saw in the interpersonal point of view.

Over the years, my approach to integration has changed. Initially, I used the basic behavioral techniques in their original form more than I do today. Now, although I still use them at times, I am more likely to recast them in ways that better fit in a therapy that is guided by a psychodynamic point of view; they are more subtle, less visible, but nonetheless important (Wachtel, in press-a). I have also paid greater attention to integrating still other points of view into the evolving approach, such as those of gestalt therapy and family therapy. Finally, I have become increasingly interested in how the point of view I have been developing can be applied to larger social issues, such as the claim that we are a narcissistic society (Wachtel, 1981) or the overemphasis on economic considerations in our national life (Wachtel, 1983).

There is a price to be paid for leaving the safe shores of an established point of view. One can feel like a man without a country. But if one finds one's roots in the commitment to learn, to change, and to help, the journey can be a rewarding one.

PAUL L. WACHTEL, PH.D.

REFERENCES

Bandura, A. The self-system in reciprocal determinism. *American Psychologist*, 1978, *33*, 344–358.

Dollard, J., & Miller, N. E. *Personality and psychotherapy*. New York: McGraw-Hill, 1950.

Franks, C. M. On the importance of conceptual integrity and its mutual advantages to two fundamentally incompatible systems. Paper read at the annual meeting of the A.A.B.T., Chicago, November 17, 1978.

Franks, C. M., & Wilson, G. T. Behavior therapy: An overview. In C. M. Franks & G. T. Wilson (Eds.), *Annual review of behavior therapy*. New York: Brunner/Mazel, 1979.

Freud, S. On the history of the psycho-analytic movement. In *Collected papers* (Vol. 1). New York: Basic Books, 1959.(Originally published, 1914.)

Freud, S. Two encyclopaedia articles. *Standard edition* (Vol. 18). London: Hogarth, 1959. (Originally published, 1923.)

* This latter theme is one in which I have become particularly interested in the past few years (e.g., Wachtel, 1979, 1982a).

Freud, S. Inhibitions, symptoms, and anxiety. *Standard* edition (Vol. 21). London: Hogarth, 1959.(Originally published, 1926b.)

Frye, N. *Anatomy of criticism.* New York: Athaneum, 1957.

Goldfried, M. R. & Padawer, W. Current status and future directions in psychotherapy. In M. R. Goldfried (Ed.), *Converging themes in psychotherapy.* New York: Springer, 1982.

Horney, K. *New ways in psychoanalaysis.* New York: Norton, 1939.

Kohut, H. *The restoration of the self.* New York: International Universities Press, 1977.

Messer, S. B., & Winokur, M. Some limits to the integration of psychoanalytic and behavior therapy. *American Psychologist,* 1980, *35,* 818–827.

Schafer, R. *A New Language for Psychoanalysis.* New Haven: Yale University Press, 1976.

Shevrin, H., & Dickman, S. The psychological unconscious: A necessary assumption for all psychological theory? *American Psychologist,* 1980, *35,* 421–435.

Silverman, L. H. Psychoanalytic theory: "The reports of my death are greatly exaggerated." *American Psychologist,* 1976, *31,* 621–637.

Staats, A. W. *Science standards or separatism? Questions on the conduct of psychology.* Unpublished manuscript, University of Hawaii, 1983.

Wachtel, P. L. Psychodynamics, behavior therapy, and the implacable experimenter: An inquiry into the consistency of personality. *Journal of Abnormal Psychology,* 1973, *82,* 324–334.

Wachtel, P. L. Behavior therapy and the facilitation of psychoanalytic exploration. *Psychotherapy: Theory, Research and Practice,* 1975, *12,* 68–72.

Wachtel, P. L. *Psychoanalysis and behavior therapy.* New York: Basic Books, 1977. (a)

Wachtel, P. L. Interaction cycles, unconscious processes, and the person-situation issue. In D. Magnusson & N. Endler (Eds.), *Personality at the crossroads: Issues in interactional psychology.* Hillsdale, N.J.: Lawrence Erlbaum Associates, 1977. (b)

Wachtel, P. L. Internal and external determinants of behavior in psychodynamic theories. In L. A. Pervin & M. Lewis (Eds.), *Perspectives in interactional psychology.* New York: Plenum Press, 1978.

Wachtel, P. L. Karen Horney's ironic vision. *The New Republic,* 1979, *106*(1), 22–25.

Wachtel, P. L. The politics of narcissism. *The Nation,* January 3–10, 1981, pp. 13–15. (a)

Wachtel, P. L. Transference, schema, and assimilation: The relevance of Piaget to the psychoanalytic theory of transference. *The annual of psychoanalysis* (Vol. 8). New York: International Universities Press, 1981. (b)

Wachtel, P. L. Vicious circles: The self and the rhetoric of emerging and unfolding. *Contemporary Psychoanalysis,* 1982, *18,* 259–273. (a)

Wachtel, P. L. What can dynamic therapies contribute to behavior therapy? *Behavior Therapy,* 1982, *13,* 594–609. (b)

Wachtel, P. L. Resistance and the process of therapeutic change. In P. L. Wachtel (Ed.), *Resistance: Psychodynamic and behavioral approaches.* New York: Plenum Press, 1982. (c)

Wachtel, P. L. *The poverty of affluence: A psychological portrait of the American way of life.* New York: Free Press, 1983.

Wachtel, P. L. Integrative psychodynamic therapy. In S. Lynn & J. Garske (Eds.), *Contemporary psychotherapies: Models and methods.* Columbus, Ohio: Chas. E. Merril, in press. (a)

Wachtel, P. L. The philosophic and the therapeutic: On the goals of psychoanalysis and psychotherapy. In R. Stern (Ed.), *Science and psychotherapy* (Vol. 4). New York: Haven Press, in press. (b)

Wolitzky, D. L., & Wachtel, P. L. Perception and personality. In B. Wolman (Ed.), *Handbook of general psychology.* Englewood Cliffs: Prentice-Hall, 1973.

2

Psychoanalytic Therapy versus Psychodynamic Therapy

Commentary on Paul L. Wachtel

STANLEY B. MESSER and MEIR WINOKUR

There is much we agree with and appreciate in Paul Wachtel's presentation, as readers of our chapter will readily discern. In that chapter we asserted that some psychoanalytic and behavior therapists may be prepared to effect an integration of the kind Wachtel proposes because of their willingness to compromise on the perspectives, visions, and values that are inherent in their preferred approaches. Others, we said, will not be so inclined. Wachtel points the way to integration by emphasizing certain aspects of psychoanalytic (or psychodynamic) theory and practice while deemphasizing others. Although we agree with his choice of elements for *inclusion* in a definition of the psychodynamic approach, we feel that he has *excluded* elements quite as central that we cannot readily forego. By focusing on our objections, we hope to clarify what makes integration difficult for many psychoanalytic therapists.

THE DEFINITIONAL PROBLEM

Referring to psychodynamic and behavioral therapies, Wachtel writes that "all one has to do is to define psychodynamic and behavioral in the

STANLEY B. MESSER • Graduate School of Applied and Professional Psychology, Rutgers University, Busch Campus, Piscataway, New Jersey 08854. MEIR WINOKUR • Student Counseling Service, Hebrew University, Jerusalem, Israel.

right way and they will indeed be incompatible." But the reverse is true as well: Define these approaches in the right way, and they will indeed be compatible. Wachtel, wisely and correctly we believe, now labels his approach "psychodynamic" rather than "psychoanalytic." This is quite consistent with the elimination of certain Freudian and ego psychological assumptions from his model. Most psychoanalytic therapists would agree with him about the centrality in psychoanalysis of unconscious phenomena, the ubiquity of conflict, its nonnormative assumptions, certain rules of inference, and its exemplifying a psychological rather than a medical or disease model. There are, however, other elements excluded that we, and probably many psychoanalytic therapists, regard as very important and would be loath to drop. These include Freud's mental geography or structural viewpoint that we find directly helpful in clinical and theoretical formulation, drive theory, the central role and force of the past, and the relative neutrality or noninterventionist stance of the therapist. By deemphasizing these elements, Wachtel makes integration easier for some, but he simultaneously loses another part of his psychoanalytic audience. Two of these elements we regard as particularly important: The role of the past and the therapist's noninterventionist stance.

The Role of the Past

Past traumas, repressed feelings and thoughts, and the unconscious fantasies to which they give rise do continue to lumber about the psyche like "woolly mammoths" (to use Wachtel's beguiling metaphor), notwithstanding present external situations. Clearly, we are talking about a relative emphasis because we do not wish to deny the importance of present contextual clues, just as Wachtel does not ignore the influence of the past. But the role of the past is conceptualized differently in psychoanalysis and in Wachtel's psychodynamic schema. By employing a model of cyclical psychodynamics or a cumulative skewing of development, Wachtel diminishes the role of unconscious fantasy, developmental arrest, fixation, and repetition compulsion. In his view, the past is carried along by the person's behavior and the response that it in turn elicits in others, rather than by a sticky intrapsychic engram of experience. His theory paves the way for integration, whereas the latter classical constructs make integration a rougher, even impassable, road to travel. However, these latter concepts continue to have central theoretical and practical importance in our clinical work.

To take Wachtel's example of a patient's dream of melting into his girl friend and of his being swallowed by her. Does it primarily symbolize his present way of life in which he is unable to resist any or all of his girl friend's wishes? If so, then change in his willingness to say no as a result of assertiveness training may indeed rectify his sense of ego boundaries, as Wachtel claims. Or, is his fear of merger and being swallowed a reflection of an early arrest of development, a fixation, or a regression in which the present situation with his girl friend is primarily a reminder or cue? Within this view of psychoanalytic theory, we find it hard to imagine how a course of assertiveness training could bring about a fundamental change in this man's sense of ego boundaries and fear of merger. It is precisely in patients with these kinds of boundary and merger problems that the developmental concepts of *arrest, fixation,* and *regression* seem so essential to a correct and useful interpretive formulation. Furthermore, our experience tells us that patients with chronic merger and boundary problems are not likely to be helped substantially by any kind of brief intervention, be it behavioral, psychodynamic, or psychoanalytic.

Elimination or deemphasis of concepts like *developmental arrest* and *repetition compulsion* downplays the tragic elements in psychoanalytic theory and practice. It seems to us a tragic fact that people with boundary and merger problems are in a very real sense stuck in the past and that behavioral exercise does not result in any easy transformation. Wachtel's cyclical psychodynamic view of development is certainly more optimistic but in many cases does not seem to fit the facts as we perceive them.

Therapist Neutrality versus Activity

The influence of the therapist's behavior on the process of therapy raises the important question of the place of therapist neutrality versus active intervention. Although we, like Wachtel, view the therapeutic process as interactional and believe that the real and not only fantasied or distorted view of the therapist influences process, we do not arrive at Wachtel's conclusion—namely, that active intervention can be readily accomplished without endangering the therapeutic process as viewed from a psychoanalytic perspective. By instituting assertiveness training or systematic desensitization, one loses one's basically neutral, nonevaluative stance, and this raises problems for the development and interpretation of the transference, as Gill has stated so well (see Chapter 6). And, to reiterate a point we have made previously, to intervene actively is to lessen the exploration of inner conflict and its resolution through interpretation in favor of more immediate behavioral change. Active intervention also curtails ironic and romantic aspects of the therapy and thereby compromises visions and values held by many analytic therapists, including ourselves. (See Chapter 3 for an expansion of this point.)

Parenthetically, a more neutral therapeutic stance need not place the patient in a childlike, one-down position (in the sense of keeping the patient in the dark as to what is going on), as Wachtel claims. If the latter comes about, it is due to a therapeutic misalliance rather than a necessary result of the analytic ambience. In a different sense of the word *childlike,* analytic therapy aims to reach the child in the adult that need not be demeaning but, on the contrary, should constitute regression in the service of ego growth and development. This is consonant with the romantic vision that aims at temporary regressive detachment from reality with the ultimate aim of restoration at a more mature level.

WACHTEL'S COMMENTS ON MESSER AND WINOKUR

In essence, Wachtel, although finding our previous analysis of the visions of reality meritorious, questions our description of behavior therapy as solely comic and objects to the implications of the term. In our current chapter we have broadened our own view of behavior therapy and have tried to show that it too contains elements of some of the other visions. It is in a relative rather than absolute sense that the four visions apply. Nevertheless, we continue to feel that there is a remarkably good fit between the structure of dramatic comedy as analyzed by the literary critic Northrop Frye and the theory, process, and view of outcome of behavior therapy. Both dramatic comedy and behavior therapists, in what they write and do, stress manipulation of people and events, the power of positive thinking, and the possibility of happy endings. We see no reason to put a gloss on it because this is an emphasis to which many behavior therapists themselves proudly ascribe. To describe the behavioral approach with terms such as "effective action" or "optimism" in the place of "manipulation" and "happy endings" does not change the basic outlook it embodies. We did not introduce these terms—which, admittedly, have a somewhat pejorative connotation—with any sinister intention but rather drew them from another field in which they were employed. Similarly, we do tend to regard the psychoanalytic view as more complex, and this is reflected in the fact that it draws more heavily on several visions of reality than does the behavioral approach.

Finally, we agree with Wachtel that we have pursued a comparative approach to the two therapies, but we do not agree that the considerable differences that we unearth "do not really bear on the question of whether they can be integrated." If analytic therapists share romantic and tragic visions and behavior therapists do not, if analytic therapists are more dialectical and poetic and behavior therapists more demonstrative and scientific in their way of knowing and reasoning, if analytic therapists prefer the hermeneutic—and behavior therapists the natural science—method of knowing, and if analytic therapists emphasize transference interpretation, therapist neutrality, and the past, and if behavior therapists emphasize transference manipulation, therapist activism, and the present, the prospects for integration are diminished. To the extent that analytic therapists will adopt more of the demonstrative and analytic styles of knowing, embrace experimental and correlational versus configurational methods, put less emphasis on neutrality, transference, and developmental arrest and on the tragic vision of man's makeup and adopt a more comic view of the prospects for change, to this extent psychoanalytic therapists will be amenable to an integration of psychoanalytic and behavior therapies.

2

A Rejoinder to Stanley B. Messer and Meir Winokur

PAUL L. WACHTEL

No doubt, from the perspective of many psychoanalytic therapists an integration with behavior therapy implies a "compromise" as Messer and Winokur suggest. And their description, in the last paragraph of their commentary, of the modal views and preferences of psychoanalytic and behavioral therapists is largely an accurate one. But the issue I have been addressing is not whether one can reconcile the beliefs, attitudes, or visions of the particular *individuals* who are presently psychoanalytic or behavioral therapists. Such a reconciliation is necessarily limited by the habits, group identifications, personalities, and vested interests of the people involved. As the physicist Max Planck put it,

> a new scientific truth does not triumph by convincing its opponents and making them see the light, but rather because its opponents eventually die, and a new generation grows up that is familiar with it.

Whether integration deserves to be regarded as "a new scientific truth" is certainly far from proven. But it should be clear that the criteria for evaluating it should not be whether those presently immersed in a particular view are likely to be converted. If it is hard to do in physics, what are the odds in a field like ours, where new observations can so readily be interpreted as consistent with old paradigms?

PAUL L. WACHTEL • Department of Psychology, City College of the City University of New York, New York, New York 10031.

My concern, rather, is with whether it is possible to construct a logically consistent integration that—in its own way—builds on selected aspects of the theories and practices that these individuals employ. That some are poetic and some scientific, some inclined toward believing they are neutral and others toward a frank activism, is not in itself an impediment to integrating key elements in each's approach. Indeed, the tendency toward a dichotomous split in their characteristics as individuals is one of the reasons why an integration is likely to be fruitful. Each tend to activate only a part of the potential in their approach, not seeing possibilities incompatible with their private philosophical visions.

Messer and Winokur are correct: I point the way to integration by emphasizing certain aspects of psychoanalytic (or psychodynamic) theory and practice while deemphasizing others. Rhetorically, their reversal of my comment that if you define the two approaches in the right way you can make them incompatible has a nice ring; they are good writers. But it is not as telling as the well-turned phrasing might suggest. *Of course* I view these approaches in ways that permit compatibility. The reason I think that an integration is feasible and desirable is because I have a particular vision of what are the really significant contributions of the psychodynamic (or behavioral) point of view.

The additional elements Messer and Winokur (along with most psychoanalysts, to be sure) would like to include as essentials would indeed make integration difficult. It is precisely because I regard Freud's mental geography, drive theory, the emphasis on the past, and (especially) the notion of neutrality as to a greater or lesser degree missteps in the building of a psychodynamic point of view that I see integration in the positive light I do. Certainly, I "lose part of my psychoanalytic audience" as a result. Those analysts who regard the aforementioned as just as crucial and valuable as Freud's insights into unconscious motivation and fantasy, conflict, and defense, and so forth are not likely to agree with me. I would not expect to persuade them. They hold a different image of what the contribution of psychoanalysis is (or should be).

One correction is in order regarding Messer and Winokur's otherwise accurate depiction of my view. I do, indeed, in my own theorizing diminish the roles of developmental arrest, fixation, and repetition compulsion. But I do not downplay unconscious fantasy. I view such fantasies differently—as symbolizations of continuing interpersonal experiences rather than as frozen remnants of the past—but I regard them as crucially important. Actually, even developmental arrests and fixations find a place in my view, or at least the *observations* on which these concepts rest. Where I differ is in how to explain those observations, preferring a transactional account rather than the static account embodied in notions of fixation and developmental arrest.

Messer and Winokur dichotomize too sharply, I believe, in saying that in my view "the past is carried along by the person's behavior and the response that it in turn elicits in others, *rather than* [italics added] by a sticky intrapsychic engram of experience." As I see it, what makes the intrapsychic engram "sticky" *is* that it is confirmed over and over by interpersonal experiences in the evolving present. I have elaborated this view elsewhere by depicting what Messer and Winokur call an "engram" in terms of Piaget's notion of "schema" and by spelling out the differing implications of this theoretical strategy (Wachtel, 1981).

Messer and Winokur assert that "to intervene actively is to lessen the exploration of inner conflict and its resolution through interpretation in favor of more immediate behavioral change." I would disagree. Frequently, by encouraging the patient to take new steps in his or her daily life, one finds that he or she is first in a position to explore the previously warded-off feelings that are thereby evoked. It is true that the approach I advocate does place less emphasis on the resolution of conflict via *interpretation* (as it does on insight). That is not due to less of a concern with conflict or its resolution but to a different view of *how* conflicts are resolved, indeed of what "resolution" consists of. I believe that Dollard & Miller (1950) introduced a major clarification in their emphasis on approach–avoidance conflicts as being at the heart of what psychoanalysis is about. Such conflicts are resolved most of all by *becoming less afraid* of what is no longer dangerous, so that previously warded-off feelings and inclinations can find fuller expression. Elsewhere (Wachtel, 1982), I have discussed this in more detail as part of an effort to indicate how contemporary psychoanalytic theorists have failed to capitalize on the important new emphasis introduced by Freud in *Inhibitions, Symptoms, and Anxiety* (Freud, 1926/1959).

I am appreciative of Messer and Winokur's challenging and articulate discussion. Most at issue is not logical error or oversight on either of our parts but rather different visions of what were the really valuable features of Freud's contribution. The test of time will determine which (if either) of our visions is the most fruitful.

REFERENCES

Dollard, J., & Miller, N. E. *Personality and psychotherapy.* New York: McGraw-Hill, 1950.

Freud, S. Inhibitions, symptoms, and anxiety. *Standard edition* (Vol. 21). London: Hogarth Press, 1959. (Originally published, 1926.)

Wachtel, P. L. Transference, schema, and assimilation: The relevance of Piaget to the psychoanalytic theory of transference. *The annual review of psychoanalysis* (Vol. 8). New York: International Universities Press, 1981.

Wachtel, P. L. Vicious circles: The self and the rhetoric of emerging and unfolding. *Contemporary Psychoanalysis,* 1982, *18,* 259–273.

3

Ways of Knowing and Visions of Reality in Psychoanalytic Therapy and Behavior Therapy

STANLEY B. MESSER and MEIR WINOKUR

In an article exploring limits to the integration of psychoanalytic and behavior therapies (Messer & Winokur, 1980), we suggested that the barrier between them resides primarily in the contrasting perspectives on reality and the different visions of life they embody. Psychoanalytic therapists, we argued, focus on the inner world of experience, emphasizing clients' introspection and subjectivity. By contrast, behavior therapists were seen as more preoccupied with the outer world of consensual reality, approaching clients within a more objective and external framework. We tried to show how these perspectives influence, in turn, the nature of the techniques employed and the treatment goals emphasized in each form of therapy.

In the first section of this chapter we pursue and extend the implications of these perspectives. We see not only the techniques and goals of psychoanalytic and behavior therapy as affected by these different vantage points but also the very ways of knowing and reasoning that are typically employed in each. The psychoanalytic way of knowing is based

STANLEY B. MESSER • Graduate School of Applied and Professional Psychology, Rutgers University, Busch Campus, Piscataway, New Jersey 08854. MEIR WINOKUR • Student Counseling Service, Hebrew University, Jerusalem, Israel.

on an internal perspective utilizing empathy and union with the client (an approach that is sometimes called *intuitive* or *poetic*) and a dialectical mode of reasoning. Behavior therapists, by contrast, more typically embrace an external perspective based on observing the client at a distance along with a demonstrative way of reasoning (an approach often called *scientific* or *analytic*). Following this distinction, we spell out how each group of therapists leans more heavily toward a particular model of understanding and organizing data—natural science or hermeneutics—that affects what they accept as data, where they look for it, and ultimately, how they treat their clients.

Despite our emphasis on the differences between psychoanalytic and behavior therapies in the vantage points from which their proponents view reality and the limits these set for complete integration, we have also stressed the merit of psychoanalytic therapists' maintaining a dual perspective on psychological events; that is, shifting their attention back and forth between clients' fantasies, memories and feelings, and the external events of their lives; making psychoanalytic data public; and at times specifying the goals of treatment and measuring outcomes objectively. Similarly, we believe that behavior therapy stands to gain by adopting, to some extent at least, a style of knowing and an attitude toward data employed by psychoanalytic therapists. By recognizing and delineating some fundamental differences between the approaches, we do not mean to close the door to integration. Rather, we hope that further exploration will lead to a more realistic appraisal of the possibilities and limits involved in such an effort.

The second section of this chapter focuses on the different visions of reality embodied in behavior therapy and psychoanalysis. Whereas *perspectives* imply an angle or position from which reality is viewed, *visions* comprise assumptions about the very nature and content of human reality. We previously used four visions of reality—*romantic, ironic, tragic,* and *comic*—as a basis for contrasting the behavioral and psychoanalytic world views (Messer & Winokur, 1980). These visions were originally proposed by Northrop Frye (1957) as mythic forms in the context of literary criticism and were applied by Roy Schafer (1976) to psychoanalysis. The four visions are explored in detail later, but some brief definitions are in order at this juncture.

Within the *romantic* vision, life is a series of quests—"a perilous, heroic, individualistic journey . . . which ends after crucial struggles with exaltation" (Schafer, 1976, p. 31). The *ironic* vision is characterized by a readiness to seek out contradictions, ambiguities, and paradoxes and involves "spotting the antithesis to any thesis" (p. 51). Whereas the *tragic* vision emphasizes the dangers, conflicts, and absurdities of human existence, the *comic* vision stresses the familiar, controllable, and predictable aspects of situations and people. Conflict within the comic vision is viewed as centered in situations, and it can be eliminated by effective manipulative action; whereas, within the tragic viewpoint, conflict is due to implacable and sinister forces that cannot be eliminated but only confronted with the muted hope of partial mastery. (Note that use of the term *comic* in this chapter is not meant to imply *funny* or *nonserious*.)

Our position was that behavior therapy operates primarily within a comic vision of reality in that it emphasizes the possibility of nonambiguous happy endings leading to security and gratification through direct action and removal of situational obstacles. In psychoanalytic therapy, the comic and ameliorative thrust is tempered by a tragic recognition of the inevitability and ubiquity of human conflict and the limits placed by the individual's early history on the extent of possible change, by an ironic emphasis on contradiction and ambiguity in the process of therapy, and by a romantic openness by the therapist to new and unexpected developments in the therapeutic adventure and quest. A more exclusively comic view of reality that denied the ubiquity of conflict and misfortune in human affairs was, we felt, inconsistent with our therapeutic and life experiences. Although it may be that behavior therapists do not really believe in uncomplicated happy endings, in what they write they either imply it or say nothing to dispel such a conclusion. Furthermore, we viewed the behavioral interventions recommended by Wachtel (1977a) following the partial working through of conflict as possibly representing a trade-off between immediate relief and deeper resolution of problems, giving pause to the prospects for integration.

In reacting to our viewpoint, some therapists felt that we had succeeded in capturing the essence of the difference between the two approaches and had put our finger on issues that they had sensed all along (e.g., Fay & Lazarus, 1982; Geller, 1981; Yates, 1981, 1983). Other correspondents, such as Ellis (1981), retorted that cognitive behavior therapy was quite as subjective, introspective, and idealistic (vs. realistic) as psychoanalytic therapy, and that it embodied ironic elements and an attitude of curiosity and adventure dictated by the romantic vision. In responding to Ellis (Messer & Winokur, 1981), we continued to insist on the validity of the distinctions drawn, but his comments and those of others have stimulated us to consider further the ways in which visions of reality affect how therapy is conceived of and conducted. In the second part of this chapter, we offer a more thorough consideration of how psychoanalytic and behavior therapies intersect with the four visions. We then take up the question of the integratability of the therapies in light of our explorations and discoveries.

STYLES OF KNOWLEDGE IN PSYCHOANALYTIC THERAPY AND BEHAVIOR THERAPY

We begin by examining styles of knowledge in the psychoanalytic and behavioral approaches in a way that highlights the differences between them. We will then demonstrate that within the broad reach of each of these two therapies are alternative modes of knowing that somewhat narrow the gap between them.

Knowledge from "Without" and Knowledge from "Within"

The different perspectives on reality embodied in the behavioral and the psychoanalytic approaches can be characterized as explanation "from the outside," or understanding "from the inside," respectively (Dilthey, quoted in Radnitzky, 1973, p. 213). In the mode typically employed by the behavior therapist, we experience what we know as an object, which is something outside of ourselves and which stands in opposition to us. In the mode more characteristic of the psychoanalyst, our knowledge comes through a feeling or sympathy with something, a knowing something through a form of union with it. "The first implies that we move round the object; the second that we enter into it" (Bergson, quoted in Stern, 1965, p. 43).

Karl Jaspers (Stern, 1965) also talked of a similar polarity that we can relate to ways of viewing and treating psychopathology.

> *Understandable* connections within the psychic have also been called causality from within; this indicates an unbridgeable abyss between this kind of causality on the one hand and *causal* connections on the other—i.e., causality from without. (p. 45)

Causality from within involves comprehending ("taking into"), whereas in causality from without, the observer explains ("lays outside"—which is opposite to comprehension).

Consider, in this connection, the etiology and treatment of stuttering by traditional behavioral and psychoanalytic therapists. From a certain behavioral perspective, stuttering is regarded, according to a prominent behavior therapist,

> as an acquired speech dysfluency which can be treated by operant conditioning techniques, or as resulting from a faulty servocontrol system for speech output to be treated by over-riding or correcting the faulty system by the use of various techniques. (Yates, 1983)

Thus, Goldiamond (1965) employs conditioned aversive stimuli to eliminate stuttering. Note how, in this instance, causal factors are determined from the outside—either acquired through externally prompted learning or consisting of a neuropsychological deficit that is directly correctable from the outside. Neither intuition nor empathy, or union, with the stutterer need be involved in either arriving at the etiological explanation or in carrying out the treatment procedures. (Here too, some behavior therapists might argue that if one is to gain a detailed picture of a client's learning history, then intuitive and empathic listening is necessary. This is rarely acknowledged or emphasized in the behavior therapy literature.)

The traditional psychoanalytic understanding of stuttering, on the other hand, is derived from an intimate knowledge of the stutterer in psychoanalysis. According to analytic findings, the speech function has become suffused with aggression; that is, words are potential weapons that the speaker, who is conflicted about the expression of anger, defends against by inhibiting his or her speech (Fenichel, 1945). Such a formulation can only be arrived at in the first place by eliciting the stutterer's fantasy life and conflicts and their developmental origins in the context of a therapeutic relationship. The knowledge acquired and the relationship established help the stutterer work through the conflict. Thus, the psychoanalytic and behavioral approaches differ in three interrelated ways: How the causal factors are identified, the nature of the causes, and the meliorative techniques to be employed. In the psychoanalytic view, the causal factors are seen as coming from within; they are derived from entering into an intimate transaction with the subject, whereas in the behavioral approach, the causal factors are identified through observation "from the outside." In the former, the cause is seen to reside in a dynamic conflict versus (in the latter) a faulty habit or neurological functioning gone awry. Different therapeutic techniques logically follow—interpretation of defenses against recognition of the conflict or a technique to correct the deficit directly. We should emphasize that we are not evaluating, for the moment, the validity or utility of either kind of explanation or therapy but are pointing to the perspective taken to arrive at each and the consequences for treatment that result.

Ways of Knowing

Closely allied to knowing which comes from "laying outside" the subject is a style of knowledge called *discursive, analytic,* or *scientific.* In it, one proceeds from premises to conclusions in a series of linear, logical steps. The hypothetico-deductive method is an example of such a style. It may be contrasted to that mode of knowledge called *intuitive, poetic,* or in Husserl's terms (quoted in Stern, 1965, p. 44) *wesensschau*—an immediate beholding of essences. Karl Stern (1965) reviews this basic polarity and demonstrates our current pejorative attitude toward "poetic insight" or intuition—our viewing it as archaic, prerational, and childlike. He posits that we tend to label this mode of thinking "feminine" because knowledge by connaturality (which comes from sharing a similar experience with fellow human beings) originates in the early mother–child relationship. All knowledge by union and incorporation has its primary bond with the mother. Thus, "the skeptic warns the believer not to 'swallow' things and not 'to be taken in' " (p. 54).

The pervasiveness of this antinomy runs through Oriental as well as Occidental thinking.* Chinese Taoism, for example, contains the principle of yin (the feminine-receptive mode, relying on intuition) and yang (the masculine-active mode, allied with analytic thinking). A contemporary example of this polarity that shares some of its attributes is the distinction between right and left cerebral hemisphere information-processing modes. The right hemisphere has been described as operating with instantaneous, spatial, and global strategies, whereas the left hemisphere uses sequential, verbal, and analytic modes of knowing (Zaidel, 1979). Cognitive styles also may be referable to the same duality, for example, field independence and reflectivity (the more analytic and active styles) versus field dependence and impulsivity (the more global and passive styles) (Messer & Schacht, in press; Witkin, Dyk, Faterson, Goodenough, & Karp, 1962).

The psychoanalytic technique employed to understand various problems such as stuttering relies both on poetic insight—on listening with the "third ear" (Reik, 1949) and on analytic thinking. Greenson (1977) captures very nicely the balance between the two toward which the analytic therapist strives:

> He listens consciously, intellectually and detachedly, at the same time from the inside as a participant. This kind of listening requires that the analyst have the capacity to shift from participant to observer, from introspection to empathy, from intuition to problem solving thinking, from a more involved to a more detached position. It is necessary for him to oscillate, make transitions and blendings of these different positions. (pp. 100–101)

The psychoanalytic way of knowing, then, is a disciplined subjectivism (Stein & Kayzakian-Rowe, 1978). Behavioral explanations, by contrast, are derived from the application of a series of experiments using the hypothetico-deductive method and highly controlled and structured observation and analysis—an attitude carried forward into behavior therapy. Nor is a passive-receptive stance much in evidence in the behavioral strategy employed to extinguish problems such as stuttering.

* These modes have been described in different ways with different emphases, and although not all contrasting pairs are quite the same, they bear enough resemblance for us to consider them together. We thank Etienne Perold for making us aware of some of the parallels we will describe.

Ways of Reasoning

Rychlak (1968) discusses two modes of reasoning—the dialectical and the demonstrative—that parallel to some extent the two modes of knowing that are embodied in psychoanalytic and behavior therapies. The dialectic involves discourse and dialogue, knowing things through transaction with them. It stresses an active role for the mind, in which meanings are generated and allowed to emerge. We can easily discern a link between knowing things from the inside—the dialogue of psychoanalytic therapy—and the dialectical mode of reasoning.

In demonstrative thinking,

> The theorist begins his reasoning with assumptions or items of information that he takes (or "knows") to be primary and true from the outset. . . . The attitude of the operationist who says that "for my purposes, we shall define x as so and so" is in line with demonstrative reasoning, for he has his meaning confidently in mind before he proceeds. (Rychlak, 1968, p. 305)

Truth is found in the immediately identifiable, the facts as defined operationally and demonstrably before one's eyes. The "demonstrator" is William James's tough-minded thinker and, in our view, the behavior therapist: The dialectician is tender-minded, and this term aptly describes the psychoanalytic therapist. Note the link of the words tough- and tender-minded to what is stereotypically considered masculine and feminine, much as described in the yin and yang of Taoism and in Stern's sex-linked characterization of ways of knowing.

Psychoanalytic Therapists' Style of Knowledge

What is the picture of psychoanalytic therapists that emerges from the ways of knowing and reasoning by which we have characterized them? Psychoanalytic therapists operating in these modes attempt to project themselves into patients' subjective and phenomenological worlds, acquiring knowledge of them through empathy and intuition.

> The essential mechanism in empathy is a partial and temporary identification with the patient. In order to accomplish this, it is necessary to regress from the position of the detached, intellectual observer, to a more primitive kind of relationship in which the analyst becomes one with the person he is listening to. . . . It requires the capacity for controlled reversible regressions. (Greenson, 1977, p. 101)

Consonant with the therapist's "prerational" attitude, the patient is not only allowed but is encouraged to regress to earlier modes of thinking. What is archaic and primitive, global, unstructured, and impressionistic is valued (Balint, 1968). In short, psychoanalytic therapists are at times immersed in the subjectness and subjectivity of their patients, but they alternate this mode with one that is more intellectual and distant.

> When we work with patients as psychoanalysts we do so from a position that is both objective and subjective. That is, to explore and expand the scope of a personal theory one must, to some degree, get outside it. . . . Yet, since the stuff of analysis is personal and emotional, there is a sense in which it can only be known subjectively. (Breger, 1981, p. 267)

Psychoanalysts are also involved in a dialogue, a dialectical transaction with the patient from which new meaning emerges from old problems that, it is hoped, will set the person free. In fact, patients tend to be viewed as producers of subjective meanings, and their pathology is seen to derive from certain patterns of ideas, wishes, and precepts involving their hidden inner life.

Although we have stressed the poetic and dialectical styles of knowledge in psychoanalytic therapy and the scientific and demonstrative styles in behavior therapy, the case, admittedly, is not quite so straightforward. Holt (1972), for example, has convincingly demonstrated that there are both humanistic and mechanistic images of man in Freudian psychology that, in the terms used here, predispose some psychoanalytic therapists to emphasize poetic and dialectic modes, whereas others prefer scientific and demonstrative styles of knowing. At the same time as penetrating from within, the latter may appear as neutral or even slightly detached—"blank screens" onto which patients can project their transference predispositions. Their focus is on analyzing the patient's verbal productions and offering interpretations based on a more demonstrative mode of reasoning. They may view their patients (a) as replete with cathexes and countercathexes, based on an energy model adapted from 19th-century physics; (b) as relating to objects of their drives (i.e., other people) in order to reduce internal tensions; (c) as being entirely determined by early events over which the patient had no control; and (d) as the object of unconscious forces. In all, patients seen in this way are proper objects of natural science and a demonstrative approach, much as are other objects in the universe. At least on the dimensions we have been describing regarding styles of knowing, there is somewhat less distance, then, between behavioral and psychoanalytic therapists when the classical instinct model is adhered to.

A recent article by Bettleheim (1982) is enlightening on the origins of the more mechanistic and medical stream within American psychoanalysis. Although admitting that Freud saw psychoanalysis at some moments in his life as a natural science, he argues that, especially later in his life, Freud wanted us to accept psychoanalysis as basically a humanistic enterprise. Freud's translators, for example, wishing to perceive psychoanalysis as a scientific and medical specialty, translated the German *ich* into the impersonal noun "ego," rather than the more personal and richly associative word "I". They also translated *die Seele* into "mind" or "psyche," rather than "soul," as Freud apparently intended. Thus, the famous psychoanalytic dictum describing the aim of psychoanalysis—"Where id was, there shall ego be"—becomes "Where it was there should become I." The point is that "if 'I' [rather than my ego] am driven by fear or ambition or greed, 'I' can do something about it" (p. 89). In this way, conscious recognition and deliberate alteration become more possible.

Psychoanalysis, in recent times, has shown signs of moving away from the more mechanistic model of man. Instinct theory has given ground to object relations theory, centering less on the control of drives and more on the development of the ego in the matrix of a good mother–infant relationship (Guntrip, 1971). Sublimating sexual and aggressive drives then becomes secondary to the need to maintain an optimal level of human relatedness. Similarly, Kohut (1977)—who has a large following among psychoanalytic therapists—has made the "self" the cornerstone of his psychoanalytic theorizing, viewing it as a cohesive unit of the personality, an independent center of initiative, competence, and power. Also, Stolorow and Atwood (1979) take the subjective, representational world of the individual as the focus of their approach, which they call "psychoanalytic phenomenology." For them, the proper units of analysis are the configurations of mental representations of the self and of others that include both cognitive and emotional aspects. In these recent trends, there is the unmistakeable stamp of the humanistic approach: a stress on the organic unity of the individual (vs. stress on individual parts), on the interpersonal aspects of his or her psychological functioning (vs. the intrapsychic only), on his or her subjectivity (vs. objective status), and on the role of empathy and relatedness in psychotherapy.

Holt describes the antitherapeutic effect of the physicalistic residue of Freudian metapsychological language.

> The mechanistic image encourages treating the patient in the way so many patients want to be treated: as a passive machine, to be manipulated back into chugging properly, rather than as a partner in a joint enterprise of trying to increase his ability to function for himself in a free, mature, responsible way. (p. 15)

The metapsychological concepts "give the illusion of deep and exact 'scientific' understanding when in fact they are blurs" (Schafer, 1970, p. 438). (For a very different view of the importance of metapsychology, see Ricoeur, 1977). As Bettleheim (1982) evaluates it, the translation of Freudian terms into Latin or Greek pronouns created emotional distance from the impact of personal English pronouns. (Interestingly, the French translate *das Ich* as the personal *le moi.*) Psychoanalysis is partially shedding its mechanistic cloth woven with the scientific mode of knowing and the demonstrative way of reasoning.

Paralleling this clash in the realm of psychoanalytic theory is an ongoing debate on the proper stance of the psychoanalytic therapist. On the one side are those who have emphasized the importance of the "real relationship" between patient and therapist in which the therapist's benignity and humanness are considered exemplary (e.g., Ferenczi, Rank, Reik, Alexander, and, in more recent times, Stone, 1961). On the other are psychoanalysts (including Fenichel, Hartmann, Rapaport, and, most recently, Brenner, 1979) who stress the importance of therapist neutrality. Brenner (1979), in refuting Stone's position, wrote:

> [If] a patient suffers a catastrophe, or a success in life, it is not the best for his analyst to express sympathy or congratulations before "going on to analyze" [as Stone says he would do]. . . . As an example, for his analyst to express sympathy for a patient who has just lost a close relative may make it more difficult than it would otherwise be for the patient to express pleasure or spite or exhibitionistic satisfaction over the loss. (p. 153)

According to Malcolm (1981), Stone's humanistic view of the analyst's role is now very much in the ascendancy in psychoanalytic circles. All in all, one suspects that personality as much as ideology determines the stance taken by an individual psychoanalytic therapist.

Behavior Therapists' Style of Knowledge

Turning our attention to behavior therapists, what has been their traditional attitude toward knowing and reasoning? Here, too, the picture is not unimodal. Many have prided themselves on emphazing that which is most readily knowable from the outside in their clients ("moving around the object")—their behavior, overt symptomatology, verbal self-reports, and physiological responses. They mistrust their clients' more fanciful productions—their dreams, fantasies, projections, and distorted views of the therapist. Rather than capitalize on what allies them—"conatures" them—with their clients, they prefer to stand outside the relationship to avoid introducing their subjective biases. Their model of man stems originally from the animal laboratory, particularly Pavlov's, Watson's and Skinner's, which inclines them less to what is unique to human beings. As part of this heritage, they look to environmental causes of their client's distress ("causality from without") and try to help them change these as much as to change themselves internally. The behaviorist, Watson (1914) wrote, "recognizes no dividing line between man and brute." It is possible to define psychology as

> the "science of behavior" . . . never to use the terms consciousness, mental states, mind, content, will, imagery, and the like. . . . In a system of psychology completely worked out, given the responses, stimuli can be predicted; given the stimuli, the responses can be predicted. (pp. 1, 9–10)

Just as there is some latitude of style possible within the domain of psychoanalytic therapy, allowing for individual differences in therapist predilection, there is variation in ways of knowing among behavior therapists. Some cognitive and multimodal behavior therapists are interested in knowing their clients from the inside—especially their beliefs, expectancies, plans, attributions, and attitudes. They acknowledge the importance of the relationship between them and their clients—trying to create a warm, friendly, helping atmosphere (Goldfried, 1982; Wilson & Evans, 1977). Less likely to zero in on a particular discrete behavior than the traditional behavior therapist, they will range over many aspects of the client's conduct in a multimodal fashion (Lazarus, 1981). The client may be encouraged to engage in a dialogue with the therapist, the two of them arriving, for example, at a mutually agreeable contract for therapy (Meichenbaum & Gilmore, 1982). In line with this mode, client's self-efficacy (Bandura, 1977a) is emphasized as well as their wishes for self-control. Connotative, and not just denotative, meaning of events is taken into consideration (Goldfried, 1979).

In contrast to the psychoanalytic therapist's emphasis on the intuitive way of knowing and the dialectical mode of reasoning, however, both kinds of behavior therapists that we have described continue to stress rational and demonstrative styles. Ellis (1970), for example, wrote:

> The rational-emotive therapist . . . can almost always put his finger on a few central irrational philosophies of [the client]. . . . He can often induce him . . .to replace them with scientifically testable hypotheses about himself and the world.

Similarly, Mahoney (1974), in his earlier writings, advocated that we train clients as personal scientists. He proposes that "we should model and teach an 'intimate empiricism' replete with skills training in problem analysis, hypothesis generation, evaluative experimentation and so on" (p. 274). Eschewing the dialectical mode of reasoning, the behavior therapist prefers the demonstrative—what can be pointed to, operationalized, and measured. A scientific, demonstrative, and analytic way of knowing is encouraged not only for the therapist but for the client as well. Reasoning along similar lines, Zeldow (1979) contrasts "psychodynamic sociotherapy" and "rational (behavioral) sociotherapy" as they are applied to the milieu of psychiatric hospital wards.

The adoption of this style by behavior therapists is neither casual nor accidental. In an elegant analysis of behavior therapy's world view, Woolfolk and Richardson (in press) demonstrated that behavior therapy is

> a system of thought that adopts a radically scientific and technological perspective on human conduct and on the enterprise of behavior change. . . . It prizes expertise over wisdom, utility over aesthetic appeal, fact over value. (pp. 21, 24, 30)

In these respects, the authors point out, it is the most faithful embodiment of modernity whose world view is dominated by science, technology, and *their modes of thought.*

Even in the realm of modes of thought, however, there is the beginning of a slight breach in the wall of the behavior therapist's rational-demonstrative style. In a recent article, Mahoney (1980, p. 159) has expressed his concerns about current cognitive therapies and in a substantial leap toward a humanistic image of man and the poetic way of knowing, he has advocated that more attention should be paid by behavior therapists to unconscious processes and to feelings that, he says, should not be viewed "as phenomenal artifacts that are to be controlled rather than experienced" (cf. Messer & Winokur, 1980). Concomitantly, he recommends decreased attention to the role of rationality in adaptation. Congruent with movement toward the mode of "knowing from within," he advocates that cognitive behavior therapists would do well to consider supplementing self-reported thoughts with such assessment techniques as (a) ongoing experiential diaries, (b) dream reports, (c) projective fantasies, and (d) memory recall of personally significant experiences. He stands with Polanyi in stating that "the core beliefs in a personal paradigm may be predominately tacit" and that "since the cognitive foundations of one's place in [and relationship to] the world are probably developed in childhood, it would not be surprising if they were nonverbal and unrealistic" (p. 175). Bowers (1980) agrees with Mahoney and recognizes that it is often "beneficial to circumvent the patient's willful active efforts to control the contents of thought and, instead, to engender a psychological state of passive receptiveness" (p. 184). Herein lie some potent possibilities for integration.

Similarly, Weimer (1980) has called therapists to task who adopt what he calls the "rationalist constructionist" ideal of scientific practice that includes, among other attributes, a demonstrative way of knowing. The kind of specificity and exactness called for in this approach, he argues, constitutes "scientistic methodolatry" because it does not apply to the subject matter of clinical psychology. He notes that we possess skills that our explicit awareness and rationality cannot explain or improve upon. In presenting a view of science and therapy as a rhetorical process involving "argumentative use of discourse and action" and one that "never seeks final form or ultimate proof," he is backing up those who advocate the dialectial mode of reasoning.

METHODS OF KNOWING: NATURAL SCIENCE AND HERMENEUTICS

Weimer (1980) then asks the question of how we should change the client and answers it by suggesting the idea of therapy as a rhetorical transaction. "The *rhetorical interchange,* taking place over time, *will create and change the meaning of events and actions for both client and therapist.* The result will be a client whose behavior and perspective has been changed as much by his or her own activity as by the intervention of the therapist" (italics ours, p. 389). His point of view is remarkably close to that of Steele (1979) who argues that the hermeneutic method typically applied to literary and historical texts is more appropriate than the natural science model for psychoanalytic therapy in particular.

Hermeneutics is the art and science of interpretation and, in Steele's opinion, offers a challenge to the hegemony of the methods of investigation in social science that are based on the natural sciences. It is the study of understanding, and its task is to aid communication so as to facilitate that understanding. As Palmer (1969) says, " The keys to understanding are not manipulation and control but participation and openness . . . not methodology but dialectic" (p. 215). (Any method of study in fact—be it hermeneutics or natural science—determines what we see, and in this sense Palmer is correct in saying that all method is interpretation). We transform an object into a subject when we allow it to speak and to have meaning to us. The goal of interpretation within hermeneutics is to bring meaning to light that has been hidden even to the author of a text or to a person whose life events are interpreted in therapy. The truth that is established through hermeneutic understanding is not the "correct" fact of the natural sciences, but rather, it is a *construction* of something that makes sense, something that emerges, for example, out of the psychoanalytic dialogue (Steele, 1979).

How does one evaluate the constructions that are arrived at by this route. "By their logical consistency, their coherency and by their configuration—the harmony of the parts with the whole. One moves towards a consensus between interpreter and partner that maximizes shared meaning" (Steele, p. 392). Wachtel (1977b) has made a similar defense of the psychoanalytic method in emphasizing inner consistency and a network of converging observations that determine the form of psychoanalytic interpretations. Interpretations can be further checked by investigating parallel productions by the same person (e.g., Rorschach and TAT responses, diaries, etc.) and knowing the personal, social, and historical contexts in which the person lives. In an article describing and encouraging the use of investigative reporting as a research method in clinical psychology, Levine (1980) emphasizes its focus on the meaning—feeling dimension of experience in contrast to the social sciences' emphasis on abstraction. He points to the social sciences' renewed interest in and acceptance of clinical and qualitative methods and the attempt to be as scientific as possible about subject matter that is made up of human meanings, not natural phenomena.

Just as hermeneutics stands to some extent in contrast to natural science so does a coherence theory of truth challenge a correspondence theory (Adler, 1927). The correspondence theory bases itself on empiricism and holds that truth is what fits the facts, whereas the coherence theory asks whether a piece of information coheres with a corpus of knowledge. Rychlak (1968) equates the latter position with the dialectical mode of knowing and the former with the demonstrative. Similarly, Waelder (1977) describes these differences in terms of the German philosophers' distinction between *nature* (the physical universe) and *Geist* (mind of culture). *Nature* can be described by a finite number of quantifiable variables, whereas *Geist* can only be comprehended as a totality. "From this point of view, experimental or statistical investigations in matters of *Geist* betray a fundamental misunderstanding of the subject; they are something like intellectual original sin" (p. 160).

Although an approach encompassing hermeneutics, *Geist,* and the coherence theory is quite acceptable to most psychoanalytic therapists and, most important for our present purposes, influences their daily therapeutic attitudes and behaviors, it may leave most behavior therapists cold. Where, they may ask, is the careful experiment with its specified procedures, discrete operationalized variables, and controls? Where is the order, lawfulness, and causality of normative science? Where are the goals of prediction and control, and where are the behavioral science rules of reliability, validity, and replicability? In the words of a prominent chronicler of behavior therapy, "For data to be acceptable, they must conform to the hypothetico-deductive or some related methodology of the behavioral scientist. . . . We are playing by certain rules about the nature of data and methodology" (Franks, Chapter 8, this volume). Although Franks grants that "there may be more to the study of human beings than slogans about objectivity, measurement, prediction and controlling variables," he points out that

> It might also be difficult in actual practice for behavior therapists *to abandon their customary objective approach to all patients* and proceed largely in terms of the more subjective, intuitive feeling, and interpretative style of the psychodynamic clinician. (Franks, Chapter 8)

How clear it is in this statement that the behaviorists' approach to methodology defines not only their work as researchers but influences their attitudes toward clients as well.

This controversy as to what constitutes proper methodology for the subject matter of psychotherapy has a considerable effect on what kinds of data we allow and on where we look for them, both within and outside the therapy hour. Congruent with his psychodynamic background and perspective, Wachtel (1977b), in his attempt to integrate psychoanalytic and behavior therapy, has stressed the importance and validity of naturalistic observation, clinical data, and other sources of nonexperimental evidence. It is on this very point, however, that Phillips (1978, p. 132), a behavior therapist, takes him to task. "One's view of the nature of acceptable scientific evidence and inference cannot be converted so readily . . . this is where he is least likely to influence the behavioral therapist."

ROUTES TO INTEGRATION

Phillips's skepticism notwithstanding, we believe that there are some grounds here for an innovative integration of psychoanalytic and behavior therapies, even though the differences will continue to set limits to such an endeavor. As therapists, the kinds of data we accept and which journals we read have a major impact on how we construe the therapy hour and on what we decide to do in it. Behavior therapists like Mahoney, Goldfried, and Bowers seem to appreciate the ways of knowing that are classically associated with psychoanalytic (and experiential) therapies. We believe that a shift by behavior therapists in the direction of a dialectical or rhetorical transaction and a willingness to learn more about their clients from the inside through intuition and passive receptivity will expose them to new sources of data that could lead to new therapeutic possibilities. Just as scientists and philosophers have begun to recognize the role of personal values, intuition, and precritical elements in science (Jones, 1981), so should behavior therapists recognize that rationality and objectivity as guiding principles have their limits. Polanyi (1964) wrote:

> Objectivism has totally falsified our conception of truth by exalting what we can know and prove, while covering up with ambiguous utterances all that we know and cannot prove, even though the latter knowledge underlies and must ultimately set its seal to, all that we can prove. (p. 286)

To use Bakan's (1956) apt phrase, such objectivism leads to "epistemological loneliness."

Behavior therapy need not adopt specific psychoanalytic concepts *per se* so much as the characteristic psychoanalytic mode of knowing and reasoning and the kind of evidence generated in this way. We wonder why, for example, behavior therapists rarely attend to clients' dreams, even though there are empirical data of the kind they most readily accept attesting to their meaning and importance (Fisher & Greenberg, 1977). If they were to be more accepting of the poetic-intuitive-receptive mode of knowing, we suspect their attitude toward dream research and toward their clients' dreams would be quite different. Similarly, a greater stress on the configurational approach to coping with clinical data in line with hermeneutic understanding would tend to lead to a more complex, integrated, and holistic image of man in behavioral theory.

Just as behavior theorists and therapists limit their access to a broad range of data from their clients by a too-exclusive reliance on the scientific way of knowing and doing research, psychoanalytic therapists and theoreticians have tended to rely too heavily on hermeneutics alone. What emerges from this mode is what Sherwood (1969) has called "narrative fit" and Spence (1982a; 1982b), "narrative truth."

> A good narrative explanation may be useful because it brings together disparate pieces of a patient's life in an appealing way, but what might be called its narrative truth may depend more on its aesthetic properties . . . than on its historical validity. (p. 49)

In emphasizing coherence and continuity, Spence argues, psychoanalysts may leave out data that disconfirm hypotheses, thus leading to a weaker and less valid theory. At least one kind of corrective (but not the only kind), we suggest, is corroborating evidence from more rigorously controlled naturalistic and experimental studies.

That is, we think that psychoanalysts' view that the scientific method exemplified in behavioral science research is déclassé (Malcolm, 1981) or worse is unwarranted. Controlled research does have potential relevance for clinical practice even if psychoanalytic theory does not require validation from extraclinical sources. Such research, for example, has shown that the superego develops more through identification with the loving attributes of parents (Aronfreed, 1968) than through fear of punishment and castration as Freud (1924/1961) proposed. That dreams may sometimes not be wish fulfillments but rather attempts at problem solving (Hawkins, 1969) and that manifest, and not just latent, content can convey important meaning (Fisher & Greenberg, 1977) are the sort of "tough-minded" research findings that can inform the analytic clinician. Systematic, naturalistic observation—leading, for example, to the delineation of early stages of development (Mahler, 1972)—that takes place outside of the analytic hour has obvious relevance for psychoanalytic therapy. Insofar as both types of therapists give more credence to *both* ways of knowing and reasoning and to *both* methods of generating data, there are bound to be bridges built between them. Several of the authors who have addressed themselves to such styles of knowledge (e.g., Chessick, 1977; Rychlak, 1968; Waelder, 1977) point out that, although these are contrasting modes, they are also complementary approaches that need not and should not preclude one another.

Many behavior therapists and analytic therapists, however, will be strongly inclined toward a preferred way of knowing their clients and a preferred (and related) methodology that will dominate their theoretical orientation, their clinical interaction, and their research. For example, we still find it hard to employ behavioral techniques such as systematic desensitization, assertiveness training, or biofeedback as Wachtel (1977a) would have dynamic therapists do. Yet, we recognize the usefulness of these approaches in the hands of others or when conducted alongside psychoanalytic therapy. Self-reflection leads us to speculate that our allegiance to the dialectical process of analytic therapy and the deepening of understanding it entails, the mixture of visions it incorporates, and the kind of autonomy of the client it advocates make it difficult for us to shift into the other mode. These considerations may hamper some but not others for whom integration may be easier to attain.

Thus, the limiting factors to integration for individual therapists may be the extent to which they are attracted to one mode, to the other, or to something in between as a function of their own personality dispositions and value structures. Aspiring therapists may "resonate" more to a way of knowing and to a vision of reality that is characteristic of a certain theory. Stolorow and Atwood (1979) have used the concept of "resonance" to illustrate how the kind of personality theory that psychologists (such as Freud, Jung, and Reich) formulated was inevitably linked to their particular life experiences and subjective concerns. In a similar vein, Mark (1980) has demonstrated the close link of therapist orientation and personal concerns in a study of already-committed behavioral and psychoanalytic therapists.

> Both groups of therapists incorporated the terms, language and perspective of their therapeutic orientation as an integral component of their identity. In most cases it was clear that the adoption of a therapeutic stance serves an important purpose in the person's life and characteristic coping styles. Once fully incorporated, the orientation acts as a template through which life experience can be understood. (p. 175)

Mark found, for example, that among behavior therapists a vision of the self as in control was central and that it had arisen as a manifestation of a power struggle with the parents. The psychoanalytic therapists had a pronounced concern for understanding origins and history of the self, especially aspects involving interpersonal closeness and how to achieve it. Mark claims that these attitudes typically preceded adoption of a theoretical and therapeutic orientation.

As a result, we can expect that some therapists will want to practice squarely within one mode, resonating strongly as they will to its perspective, vision, and value position (e.g., see Franks, Chapter 8 and Gill, Chapter 6, this volume). Others, by virtue of somewhat different values and personality dispositions, may be comfortable incorporating features of more than one therapy even while maintaining a basic attachment to a particular therapy (e.g., see Wachtel, Chapter 2 and Rhoads, Chapter 7, this volume).

Parenthetically, we wonder whether differences among therapists in what we have referred to as masculine and feminine ways of knowing may be due to their specific early experiences and identifications with the same- and opposite-sex parents (Mark, 1980; Perold, 1981). The psychological nature and developmental origin of such differences, including the form of therapy one practices, is, in itself, a topic worthy of study as a branch of the psychology of knowledge.

VISIONS OF REALITY IN PSYCHOANALYTIC THERAPY AND BEHAVIOR THERAPY

We turn now from perspectives and styles to a consideration of how the four visions of reality—tragic, comic, romantic, and ironic—are embodied in behavioral and psychoanalytic therapy. The visions may be reflected in three general aspects of therapy: (a) the postulates of the *theory* from which it derives, (b) the structure and themes of the *therapeutic process* and relationship, and (c) the *goals,* or outcome criteria, emphasized. Different therapies within the spectrum of a given orientation (psychoanalytic, behavioral, humanistic) seem to embody the different visions to different degrees in different aspects of the therapies, and these will be explored later.

In literature and drama, Frye's (1957) mythic forms (Schafer's visions) appear to blend into one another and to apply in a relative sense. Although a particular work usually has a distinct tone, structure, and character typology, it may embody aspects of other modes or visions as in romantic comedy, tragic irony, ironic comedy, and so on. Similarly, different therapies may operate predominantly from within one vision or another, at the same time potentially comprising aspects of other visions. Thus, we now recognize more clearly that there may be certain tragic and ironic elements in cognitive behavior therapy—along with its comic emphasis—and there appears to be an ever-increasing emphasis on the comic within the realm of psychoanalysis—its tragic, romantic, and ironic foci notwithstanding. Looking at the relative sense in which the visions apply may allow us to recognize some previously unnoticed points of overlap of psychoanalytic therapy and behavior therapy. Such an analysis allows for further consideration of the limits and possibilities of integration and a clearer delineation of which aspects of the therapies would need to be modified to allow for increased compatibility. What follows, then, is a comparison of psychoanalytic and behavioral therapies within each of the four reality visions.

THE TRAGIC VISION

Some of the central postulates of psychoanalytic *theory* place man in a basically unfortunate position. They suggest a view of peoples' "radical imperfectability" (Hyman, 1957) and of the limited possibilities in life (Rieff, 1959). Conflict is seen to be endemic in human affairs and cannot be eliminated but only confronted with a subdued hope of some alleviation. People as willing agents are seen as relatively helpless in the face of inner forces outside of their awareness and beyond their control. Thus, in Freudian theory, the relationship between the id and the ego is likened to that between horse and rider. Furthermore, a central discovery of Freudian developmental psychology—the Oedipus complex—implies that human development has an intrinsically tragic quality, being based on such unfortunate elements as unconscious rivalry, death wishes, relentless sexual urges, and reprisal. As Rieff (1959, p. 354) puts it:

> The unique crime of the tragic hero becomes an intention in every heart, and in the most ordinary of plots, the history of every family. . . . Misfortune . . .is the lot of every person.

In the spirit of tragedy, a person is locked in struggle with "inner forces of evil, and must win through to some private redemption and true-seeing by means of his own suffering" (Hyman, 1957, p. 169).

An operant approach that stresses environmental determinism or a social learning model positing reciprocal determinism between the environment and the person (Bandura, 1977b) are decidedly more optimistic about peoples' capacities to control their fate. A relative absence of interest in conflict and intention, even among cognitive behavior therapists who emphasize the importance of mediating internal events, precludes a tragic conception of human experience. The defining elements of tragedy include "purpose" (as witnessed in the shameful acts of the tragic hero), "passion" (suffering) and "perception" (self-knowledge) (Fergusson, quoted in Hyman, 1957, p. 170). May (1960), in discussing the Oedipus cycle and its relevance to psychotherapy, suggests that the essence of tragedy lies in the individual's self-consciousness of his or her fate and the struggle with it. An operant, extrapsychic determinism ignores inner purposes and pains and places no value on self-knowledge. Certainly no self-knowledge can come from the discovery that everything is based on external contingencies. Similarly, operant developmental psychology views fate in terms of a history of externally given reinforcements.

Although social learning theorists acknowledge the presence of an inner world, their emphasis on imitation and vicarious learning suggests a picture of a malleable, innocent, and perfectable infant if only skills are appropriately modeled. And the cognitive behavior therapists seem to imply a similar view in focusing on the correction of irrational cognitive constructions and attributions. If tragedy exists at all in these terms, it comes about through circumstance, not characterological flaws or biological inevitability for example, through the chance pairing of random stimuli and noxious unconditioned events, a history of inadequate or inappropriate reinforcement, or misguided mediational cognitions but not through the persistent operation of evil purposes. In this context, the controversy between the behavior therapists—both classical conditioners (Wolpe, 1958) and social learning theorists (Bandura, 1969)—and Freud (1909/1955) with regard to the etiology of Little Hans' phobia may be seen as a struggle between a basically comic and basically tragic view of life. Did Little Hans develop a phobia because of the chance pairing of stimuli, because his mother modeled and reinforced phobic attitudes, or as a displacement of castration fears associated with Oedipal "internal purposes"?

In addition to the tragic tone of some of the central postulates of psychoanalytic theory, psychoanalysis as *a treatment mode* appears to follow the structure of tragic drama and to deal with the tragic themes in the life of the analysand. Freud (1900/1965) himself likened psychoanalysis as a treatment to Sophocles' drama *Oedipus*:

> The action of the play consists in nothing other than the process of revealing, with cunning delays and ever-mounting excitement—a process that can be likened to the work of psycho-analysis—that Oedipus himself is the murderer of Laius. (p. 295)

Krook (1969) suggests that tragedy comprises four main elements: an act of shame—"the kind of act that men are constitutionally liable to commit" (p. 10); suffering and expiation in the hero that is met by the audience with pity and terror; knowledge; and a sense of affirmation or reaffirmation that is met by the audience with a sense of liberation from pain and suffering, or catharsis. Just as the tragic hero has usually committed shameful acts in reality, the analysand as tragic hero suffers from his or her unconsciously fantasied crimes (see Schafer, 1976, for a more detailed discussion of this parallel). He is helped to recognize and come to terms with these, thereby to have a sense of catharsis, achieve self-knowledge and personal resolution.

The sense of parallel between the structure of dramatic tragedy and the structure of psychoanalysis is enhanced when we consider the prototypical themes of tragedy and psychoanalysis. Frye (1967) distinguishes tragedies of "order"—typically involving murder of the ruler and revenge (e.g., *Hamlet* and *Julius Caesar*), tragedies of "passion" involving the separation of lovers and conflicts between duty and passion (e.g., *Romeo and Juliet*), and tragedies of "isolation" involving the removal of the hero from his social context (e.g., *King Lear*). Similarly, rivalry and competition and separation and loneliness are most likely to be dominant themes of psychoanalytic therapy.

Schafer (1976) suggests that during psychoanalysis patients must be helped to recognize themselves as tragic heroes in the sense that they are to move from a perception of their difficulties as essentially external and from a preoccupation with their symptoms to a full recognition of their situation and the limitations placed upon them by their formative experiences. This does not mean that analysands should be encouraged to overdramatize their situations or to despair but rather that they must be helped to confront their own suffering and conflicts directly. The analyst participates in a manner similar to the audience's participation with the hero in tragic drama. Just as the audience in tragedy responds with pity and terror based on an identification with the hero's plight, analysts participate empathically, based on resonance with similar tragic themes in their own lives, while at the same time recognizing the universal nature of the issues, conflicts, and anxieties. Note here an intersection of the tragic vision with introspective and subjective perspectives as well as with poetic and intuitive ways of knowing. The kind of self-knowledge to be required from a tragic vantage point demands a thoroughgoing internal focus. The comic vision, by contrast, with its emphasis on character habits and situational obstacles requires, as we shall see later, observation from an external perspective and coincides more closely with a demonstrative way of knowing and a rigorous scientific stance.

Where psychoanalysis draws inspiration from the world of dramatic tragedy, the behavioral approach is informed by the spirit and techniques of the experimental laboratory and the method of knowing of the natural sciences. Behavioral intervention thus ideally follows the format of a well-designed experiment or research project. Its spirit of efficiency and impartiality and its scientific climate are about as far as one can get from the climate of tragedy. Baselines are measured, goals are defined operationally as dependent variables, and techniques are introduced as independent variables. Excesses or deficits are modified and nonambiguously defined outcomes are measured. Whereas the psychoanalyst responds with empathic pity at the patient/tragic hero's excesses and deficits, the behavior therapist, although certainly not apathetic to the client's dilemma, introduces techniques to decrease or augment specific behaviors.

At the same time, there has been increasing emphasis in behavior therapy on the therapist–client relationship and on the importance of warmth, understanding, and a friendly attitude on the part of the therapist. But this attitude is probably better characterized as *sympathetic* rather than *empathic*. Wilson and Evans (1977) emphasize that behavior therapists are not merely technicians but that their attitude includes elements of persuasion, interpersonal attraction, and expectancy. This attitude facilitates practical cooperation on the part of the client. Behavior therapists do not use empathy in the same way as do psychoanalysts to understand the nuances of the client's experience and do not seem to respond on the basis of transient identification and recognition of their essential similarity to the client.

Both therapies are interested ultimately in facilitating increased rationality. Yet this is to be achieved quite differently. Where analysands are perceived as initially defended against the full recognition of their own irrationality and true personal dilemmas, behavior therapy clients are perceived as unrealistic, irrationally overreacting to situations to which they have been anxiously sensitized, or as habitually repeating overlearned, self-defeating patterns. The client is to be helped to feel better and/or to change the patterns—not to reach an inner reconciliation based on self-knowledge.

Despite these quite consistent differences within the tragic mode, there does appear to be at least a hint of the tragic spirit in Ellis's rational-emotive therapy. Ellis (1973) emphasizes human imperfectability and limitation and persistently exhorts his clients to accept their limitations, to stop catastrophizing about them, and to come to grips with the tragic elements in their lives by challenging their irrationality. The therapist's attitude is not marked, however, by empathic participation. The client is met instead with a combination of sympathy and ridicule—attitudes that are characteristic of the comic mode (Frye, 1957). And the thrust of this process is not to bring clients in touch with deeper needs and motives but rather to convince them that their performance and cognitions fail to approximate Ellisian standards of rationality.

The psychoanalytic approach to *therapeutic outcome* is marked, not unexpectedly, by a sense of tragic limitation: The successfully analyzed person remains vulnerable at times to neurotic response (Schafer, 1976); the permanence of gains is seen to depend on whether the analysand is spared "too searching a fate"; analysis is fundamentally interminable (Freud, 1937/1964); and the neurotic is helped to exchange neurotic misery for everyday unhappiness (Freud, 1895/1957). A "healthy person must have a capacity to suffer and be depressed" (Hartman, 1964, p. 6). A good therapeutic outcome within a tragic sense of life is a calm acceptance of a certain degree of despair.

Behavior therapists are not unaware of therapeutic recidivism. Nor do they necessarily claim unlimited success. In fact, they are interested in and address the possibility of relapse and may introduce follow-up measures to detect such eventualities. But, whereas reversals are seen by psychoanalysts as facts intrinsic to limited human possibilities, the behavior therapist tends to see these as reflective of current limitations of techniques. Increased effort in the direction of outcome research, identification of therapeutic variables and ingredients, more efficient interventions, and more precise assessment are perceived as likely to allow for singularly successful outcomes in the future. It would appear that underlying this particular outlook of behavior therapy is the central assumption of the comic mode: If only situational obstacles (technical ones in this instance) could be overcome through appropriate action, happy endings in the form of fully effective and efficient therapies are possible. This leads us to a consideration of the psychoanalytic and behavioral approaches within the comic mode. If the prospects of integration appear rather bleak following a description of issues from within the tragic mode, perhaps understandably they appear somewhat brighter when the comic aspects of these therapies are compared.

The Comic Vision

The comic vision is in many ways antithetical to the tragic: It emphasizes familiar, controllable, and predictable aspects of situations and people. Conflict is viewed as centered in situations, and it can be eliminated by effective manipulative action or via the power of positive thinking (Schafer, 1976). Note that the term *comic* is not used here pejoratively but in the sense of following the typical structure of dramatic comedy.

The tone, structure, and characters of dramatic comedy fit the tone, structure, and characters of behavioral theory, therapeutic process, and outcome expectation remarkably well. Comic drama emphasizes situational obstacles (in contradistinction to the tragic emphasis on characterological flaw) in much the same way as behavioral theory emphasizes (though not exclusively so) extrapsychic determinism. If there is recognition by behavior therapists of the limits placed on human potential by genetic endowment (Ellis, 1981), there seems to be an assumption tacitly held by many that if environmental contingencies are correctly managed and personal control and efficacy are brought to bear, then singularly positive outcomes are possible. For an extreme presentation of this view, consider Skinner's *Walden Two*.

If, in psychoanalysis the patient is envisioned as a tragic hero, in behavior therapy the client is perceived as the comic *character* portrayed by the dramatist. The comic character is typically presented as dominated by a habit (in Shakespearian terms, a "humour") rather than by shameful acts, mixed motives, or tragic flaws. We also have a remarkably close fit between the kind of knowledge acquired by comic characters in the course of the drama and the kinds of knowledge acquired by the client in behavior therapy: "This is not necessarily an introverted knowledge which is of little use to a comedy, but a sense of proportion and of social reality" (Frye, 1965, p. 79). For the word *comedy* in the preceding quote, insert *behavior therapist*, and the quotation reads like a prototypical description of the process and goals of behavior therapy.

Behavior therapy is an educational process, and it does result in increased knowledge for the client. Yet, this kind of knowledge cannot be regarded as self-knowledge in the tragic sense but applies to an increased pragmatic capacity to perform social roles more adequately.

Comic dramatists, like behavior therapists, are interested in their characters "from the outside." The audience of a comedy is exposed to the initially unfortunate social situation of the comic hero. Typically, the hero is a youth who unambivalently desires an attractive young lady but is met by situational obstacles (Frye, 1957). As an audience, we are not interested in the hero's character makeup or internal conflicts but in how this unfortunate situation is going to work itself out. In the face of the hero's prototypical role and identity confusions, the audience tends to respond with a mixture of sympathy and ridicule—very different from the pity and terror elicited in an audience by a tragedy. As mentioned in the section on the tragic vision, behavior therapists respond with a sense of sympathy to the client's situation. If they practice rational emotive therapy, they may possess a sense of ridicule toward the client's habitually irrational behavior and assumptions. Ellis's comic response to his comic character client, might be: "Why *must* you make a lot of money to be happy?" or "Why *must* you be loved by your son?"

The behavior therapist's attitude to *outcome* tends similarly to follow a comic vision. Compare the following view of a prominent eclectic behavior therapist with Hartmann's statement on the importance of the patient's capacity to tolerate depression: "The control or absence of unpleasant emotions, coupled with an increase in positive feelings is a most worthy goal" (Lazarus, 1976, p. 5).

The comic audience typically perceives the happy ending as desirable but not true (Frye, 1957). An orthodox Freudian analyst would have serious doubts about such singularly positive outcomes. From the Freudian point of view, comic structure, like the joke, the dream, and the slip of the tongue, follows the rules of wish fulfillment, not the reality principle.

> The action of comedy is intensely Freudian in shape. The erotic pleasure principle explodes underneath the social anxieties sitting on top of it and blows them sky high. But in comedy we see a victory of the pleasure principle which Freud warns us not to look for in everyday life. (Frye, 1965, p. 74)

Yet, despite its strong tragic overtones and suspicion of the comic vision, psychoanalysis as a treatment does have a basically comic intention: It aims "to clear the way towards sustained hopefulness, the experience of security and pleasure" (Schafer, 1976, p. 28). Perhaps outcome in comic drama is not exclusively wishful—some people live fairly happily much of the time! According to Frye (1965), comedies have three kinds of typical endings, all of which involve some aspect of *social* reconciliation and identity: The hero may be reconciled with and married to his lover, reconciled with social norms, or obtain increased clarity about his own social identity. Psychoanalytic therapists typically emphasize inner reconciliation over social reconciliation, but this need not mean that no value at all may be placed on social adjustment. Certainly, successful interpersonal relationships are the goal of behavioral and psychoanalytic therapies, albeit that success is differently defined by an analyst and behavior therapist. Analysts place value in a capacity to cope actively with situational obstacles. One suspects, in fact, that despite the tragic pessimism of Freudian theory and the tragic elements in the process of psychoanalytic treatment, psychoanalysts are often satisfied with improvements in coping skills, social reality testing, increased social assertiveness, and improved marriages, even if insight is incomplete and the patient has not attained deep reconciliation and self-knowledge.

A relative emphasis on comic goals seems, in fact, to characterize the neo-Freudians (Hyman, 1957), Alexander and French's (1946) brand of psychoanalytic therapy with its emphasis on the corrective emotional experience, the ego psychologists (e.g., Blanck & Blanck, 1974), and some object relations theorists (Guntrip, 1971). And there are voices within the psychoanalytic camp currently questioning the "idealization of insight" as the exclusive therapeutic ingredient (Appelbaum, 1981), even entertaining the possibility that supportive elements in therapy do not compromise outcomes (Horwitz, 1974).

It would thus appear that in the area of desired outcome, if not at the level of theory and therapeutic process, there is more overlap between psychoanalytic and behavior therapists than meets the eye, at least between neo-Freudian analysts and the cognitive behavior therapists. It is therefore within the comic mode that there appears to be some hope for integration or, at least, increased tolerance.

Psychoanalysis is, however, informed by romantic and ironic considerations that, for the most part, are foreign to behavior therapists. And it is only after a consideration of these visions that a balanced position about the possibilities of integration may be obtained.

The Romantic Vision

Like *comedy* and *tragedy*, the term *romantic* is rich in connotative meaning. It is often used in a pejorative sense to connote *unrealistic, impractical,* or *uncontrolled.* As with our usage of the word *comic*, no pejorative meaning is intended.

Beres (1965) suggests that Freud was exposed to and influenced by the romantic poets early in his career. The romantics' emphasis on exploring the unknown, the value they placed on the irrational and tolerance of uncertainty, their interest in early childhood, the dream and the unconscious (Beres, 1965), and an interest in what is concealed beneath superficial appearance (Trachtenburg, 1975–1976) are reflected in the basic postulates of Freudian *theory* as well as in Freud's mental set in approaching clinical material. The romantic vision is idealistic in perspective and dialectical in its mode of reasoning. It is the world as construed by the person, replete with its wish-fulfilling aspects, one in which meaning is emergent rather than given and available *ab initio.* Freud's discoveries appear to be derived from data obtained in a romantic spirit, by a poetic way of knowing, and then subjected to intense rational scrutiny (Beres, 1965).

A romantic attitude may, in fact, be an important part of the mental set of all good scientists, and in this sense, behavioral theorists assuredly approach their endeavor with quite as much adventurous spirit, curiosity, and interest in the unknown as do their analytic counterparts. At the same time, where psychoanalysis is interested in understanding and exploring the contradictory and uncertain aspects of human nature, behavior therapists are interested in prediction and control—in deliberately minimizing or eliminating the uncertain. And, they have not been, of course, at all interested in unconscious adventures or dream life.

Following Frye (1957), Schafer (1976) describes the essence of the romantic vision as constituting a series of adventures or quests, "a perilous, heroic, individualistic journey, an essentially lonely, drawn out, conflict ridden and difficult process . . . which ends after crucial struggles with exaltation" (p. 31). The mental set of the psychoanalyst as theoretician is influenced by the romantic spirit and, as such, psychoanalytic *therapeutic process* at times parallels the structure of the romantic quest, particularly when viewed from the point of view of the analysand. The analysand as romantic hero begins the analysis with a regressive wish for union with the analyst ("The romantic quest is marked by its extraordinarily persistent nostalgia, its search for some kind of imaginative golden age." [Frye, 1957, p. 186]). It proceeds through periods of "dragon-slaying" ("The antagonists of the quest are often sinister figures, giants, ogres . . . which clearly have parental origin" [p. 193]). In the initial phase of the analysis, analysands' representation of themselves and other people as either good or bad parallels the black-or-white qualities of the characters in the romantic adventure who are either for or against the hero. The analysand is not meant to persist with this kind of romantic object representation but to be helped through an inner journey in order to arrive at a more balanced, integrated, and realistic picture of him- or herself and others. Beres (1965), quoting Herford, suggests that romanticism's peculiar quality lies in this, that in "apparently detaching us from the real world, it seems to restore us to the reality at a higher point" (p. 408). This constitutes a rationale for the technique of free association and the intutive, passive-receptive mode of knowing!

Psychoanalytic therapists, operating in the romantic mode, hold an attitude of curiosity and openness to unexpected developments in the patient. Their persistently neutral and accepting attitude allows patients to test their good and bad object images against the analyst's behavior in the context of the transference (see Strachey, 1934).

Behavioral therapeutic process is much more consistently and directly pragmatic. Regressive detachment from the real world is never fostered. The client is encouraged to make specific adjustments in attitude and behavior in keeping with a basically normative view of the client's wishes and of consensual reality. In cognitive behavior therapy, the client's irrationalities are disputed; they are not explored or encouraged to emerge. The client's fantasy is only of interest in that it may be a key point of intervention allowing for specific behavior changes. Imagery may be utilized as part of covert conditioning procedures, the aim of which is to change behavior, not to effect a return to reality at a "higher level" of self-recognition.

Although the psychoanalytic process can be characterized as romantic and the behavioral process cannot, from the point of view of *desired outcome* behavior therapy and psychoanalysis are similar in their final rejection of the romantic in favor of the realistic. Both approaches encourage a rationally based adjustment resting on compromise with social demands even if for Freud this adjustment is intrinsically conflictual and for a behaviorist it is less ambivalently desirable. It is primarily the humanistically oriented therapists (e.g., Maslow, 1971; Rogers, 1961) who more consistently view life as a quest and who tend to emphasize such romantic goals as risk taking, the pursuit of a unique life-style, and the continuous search for self-realization. Might behavior therapy and psychoanalysis find a nexus by both of them becoming more humanistic?

The Ironic Vision

"No one in a romance, Don Quixote protests, ever asks who pays for the hero's accommodation" (Frye, 1957, p. 223). The ironic vision, by contrast, is characterized by a readiness to seek out contradictions, ambiguities, and paradoxes. "It aims at detachment . . . spotting the antithesis to any thesis" (Schafer, 1976, p. 51). Irony is interested in the "shifting ambiguities and complexities of an unidealized existence" (Frye, 1957, p. 223). Its basis is in the "independence of the way things are from the way we would like them to be" (Frye, 1967, p. 6). The attitude of detachment required when viewing events from the ironic standpoint links it with the realistic perspective—the external world of reality—and with the demonstrative way of reasoning.

Freud's *theoretical views* on the relation between instinct and civilization are basically ironic. The highest achievements of civilization are seen to be based on a sublimation of the most primitive urges (Freud, 1930/1961). The defense mechanisms of denial and reaction formation similarly hide contradictory motives. Freud's emphasis on sexuality appears to have a strongly ironic tone: "For Freud, sexuality was important not least rhetorically, as a 'humiliation of the highest possessions of civilization' " (Rieff, 1959, p. 148).

In psychoanalytic psychology, to borrow a phrase from Gilbert and Sullivan's *H.M.S. Pinafore,* "things are seldom what they seem: skim milk masquerades as cream." Selfishness is expressed as altruism, mendacity as honesty, and hostility as sugary kindness. Each aspect of a person's behavior may represent something else, be it a dream (latent vs. manifest content), a memory (which can be a screen for an earlier and more significant one), or a symptom (a displaced or distorted wish or drive). For the analyst, this kind of ambiguity and the possibilities for construing the multiple meanings it allows is intrinsic. No explanation is ever complete; analysis is intrinsically interminable. For the behavior therapist, such ambiguity is an unfortunate impediment to operationalization and to stipulation of the impact of one variable on another. Psychoanalytic theory is often criticized by behaviorists for being unnecessarily complex, contradictory, and essentially nonfalsifiable.

In the realm of *therapeutic process,* it is not surprising to find that the analytic therapist often takes a relatively inscrutable position of distance and detachment that is deemed necessary in order to spot the patient's contradictions. Consistent with this position is the fact that the analyst says little; it is precisely the technique of irony to say "as little, meaning as much as possible" (Frye, 1957, p. 40). Behavior therapists, on the other hand, tend to be more socially affable, less inscrutable, more transparent, and to accept clients' complaints and goals at face value (see Wachtel, 1977a, on normative assumptions). They speak to clients in nonambiguous language, encourage clarity about goals and ways in which they are to be measured, and assign clear-cut tasks to achieve clearly defined ends.

Somewhat at odds with the more typical literal-minded approach of behavior therapists is the currently popular usage of paradoxical intention by cognitively oriented behavioral therapists. This technique, in that it makes deliberate use of ambiguity and contradiction, is distinctly ironic in flavor and tone. It should be noted that this procedure is not derived from learning theory but from an existential approach to meaning and intention (Frankl, 1960), and it rests most comfortably within the framework of modern communications theory (Watzlawick, 1978). Behavior therapists use this technique because it works and, we suspect, because they basically enjoy its irony.

Behavior therapists, like analysts, are at times distant and detached. Their distance and detachment is designed to maximize procedural efficiency—a kind of distance required of scientists operating or designing complex machinery. This is not the same kind of distance required in order to perceive ambiguity of meaning and intention. The behavioral kind of distance probably involves something akin to isolation of affect; the analytic distance should maintain continued connection with feelings.

At the level of *desired outcome,* once again there seems to be more compatibility than would seem possible when viewing the level of theory or process and relationship. The ironic goals of psychoanalysis may be described as reducing the discrepancy between the ideal and the actual that can be obtained by modifying the ideal after recognizing its exaggerated or grandiose nature—that is, by reducing wants and becoming more resigned to one's limitations. The possibility of modifying one's behavior in order to more closely approximate one's ideals, a distinct logical alternative in this situation, is not as much an ironic as it is a comic possibility. Irony is characterized by resignation, comedy by action. The behavioral approach, in comic spirit, is more likely to encourage direct action in doing what one wants to, saying "no" when one means to, and assertively standing up to one's mother-in-law or boss. The psychoanalytic approach is more likely to emphasize an understanding of the childhood roots of one's difficulties with authority figures—over and above any change in behavior.

Behavior therapists do attend to their clients' unrealistic goals. Ellis, in particular, consistently attacks the discrepancy between the way things are and the way people would like them to be, insisting that people reduce their "must's" "should's" and "have to's" and accept things as they are. If Ellis's methods are quite dissimilar to the psychoanalysts', ironically enough, at the level of goals, there is more similarity than meets the eye at first glance!

We are left, then, with the question of integration: Is it desirable? Wherein is there overlap and wherein is there not? What continues to separate these approaches and, finally, what would each side have to give up in order to facilitate integration?

THE QUESTION OF INTEGRATION IN LIGHT OF THE VISIONS OF REALITY

In the realm of *theory,* there remains considerable discrepancy between psychoanalytic and behavioral therapies, particularly when viewed from within the tragic and ironic modes. Although behavior therapy is becoming increasingly cognitively oriented and is taking into account the inner world, its relative lack of interest in "intention" and in the conflictual nature of human motivation makes it an intrinsically nontragic point of view. At the same time, the neo-Freudians (e.g., Sullivan, Fromm, Horney) have largely eliminated Freud's tragic tone from theory (Hyman, 1957) and are, in the comic mode, more optimistic about peoples' relation to society and the possibility of well-being and self-fulfillment. Similarly, the ego psychologists (e.g., Blanck & Blanck, 1974) who emphasize the adaptive capacity of the ego, that is, its relative strength, are closer in some respects to the behavioral world view. It would appear that an emphasis on the interpersonal and the ego might provide a potential nexus for the two theories. This conclusion is essentially consistent with that of Wachtel (1977a).

Psychoanalytic *technique and process* remain dominated by tragic, romantic, and ironic elements. The central thrust follows a tragic structure: suffering, self-knowledge, and inner reconciliation. The content is characterized by a romantic interest in the unconscious, dreams, and childhood, and the style is characterized by a romantic attitude to uncertainty and unpredictability, mixed with an ironic sense of the need for detachment in the face of ambiguity and contradiction. Behavior therapy tends to follow an experimental structure, a comic interest in social skills and social reconciliation in a format and style marked by precision and specificity.

However, we find in writings on psychoanalytic therapy some movement away from the tragic position. Note the current interest in the "corrective experience" (e.g., Malan, 1976; Marmor, 1980), following Alexander and French (1946—recently reprinted in paperback in response to popular demand!), in the real (versus transference) relationship (e.g., Roland, 1967), and in the empathic provision of needed experiences for the sake of facilitating identity rather than insight (Kohut, 1977). There has been a recognition of the limitations of insight as an exclusive therapeutic ingredient and the analyst's tendency to overidealize it (Appelbaum, 1981), and a suggestion that the provision of support may not compromise analytic goals—a position derived from outcome research (Horwitz, 1974). Thus, we see, at least the beginnings of a movement that question some of the tragic aspects (insight related) of analytic therapeutic process in favor of what is comic, that is, corrective, ameliorative, and curative. This also can be viewed as a stepping stone to integration.

Despite the differences in specific nuances of *outcome criteria,* that is, the psychoanalytic therapist's tendency to focus on intrapsychic factors (inner reconciliation) and the behavior therapist's interest in extrapsychic social reconciliation as well as the analyst's emphasis on ability to tolerate depression and other negative affects versus the behavior therapist's expectation of more singularly positive outcomes, there is more agreement in this area than we initially granted. Behavior therapists and psychoanalytic therapists, in practice, are likely to agree that helping a patient to have positively toned human relationships, to function more productively and creatively at work, and to have a persistent sense of well-being are, in fact, positive and desirable. The willingness of the short-term psychodynamic therapists (e.g., Malan, 1976) to specify goals and measure outcomes objectively is another indicator of such a rapprochement.

How far are psychoanalytic therapy and behavior therapy likely to go in integrating the visions most characteristic of each other? Having pointed to some trends and possibilities for rapprochement, we will close this chapter by pointing to the limits and trade-offs involved in integration (Messer, 1983). Let us return to the example given earlier of the more classical behavioral and psychoanalytic approaches to stuttering. What if, after discovering through a psychodynamic assessment that a stutterer is conflicted about the expression of aggression, the therapist was to introduce graduated assertiveness training? By having the client try some new actions, the vicious cycle of inappropriate interpersonal behavior will have been entered with the potential of relieving the stuttering *and* dealing with the underlying fear of aggression that emerged in the psychodynamic phase of treatment. We believe this is what Wachtel, Rhoads, and others who advocate an integration of psychoanalytic and behavior therapies would propose. Certainly, there is much to commend such an approach.

Consider the following, however: In recommending action, psychoanalysts would have to temper their ironic vision by closing off avenues to further meaning and intention that a client's stuttering may conceal. Their therapeutic attitude of relative inscrutability and detachment that is necessary to spot contradiction and paradox and that allows transference to take place would be curtailed by involvement in the behavioral program. Similarly, they may complain that the romantic vision of psychoanalysis, implying a temporary regressive detachment of the client from reality with an ultimate return at a higher level of self-recognition, is compromised in favor of pragmatic changes in behavior. Thus, the likelihood of the stutterer coming to terms with the intensity and extensity of his or her rage and the conflict surrounding it—as a tragic vision demands—would be decreased. So too would emphasis on knowing from the inside, which would be replaced by a more external perspective and demonstrative way of reasoning. And the psychoanalytic therapist would have to adopt a more meliorative view of therapeutic outcomes as dictated by the comic vision. To some psychoanalytic therapists, such a shift would be agreeable; to others it would not.

Behavior therapists, from their side, would have to give up the appeal of clearly defined goals, specifiable stimulus conditions, and the elimination of a problem like stuttering in a focused and relatively uncomplicated way. The comic vision of familiar, controllable, and predictable aspects of situations and people would have to be tempered and a more tragic view accepted, including a recognition of "inner forces of evil" (Hyman, 1957) and the inevitability of suffering and pain. Introspection and subjectivity, poetic and intuitive ways of knowing, and a dialectical mode of reasoning consonant with the tragic and romantic visions would come more heavily into play. To some behavior therapists, the costs of such a shift in perspective will be affordable and worthwhile because of its resonance with their own values and a potential improvement on some criteria of therapeutic effectiveness. For others, the potential decrease of scientific exactness and its allied demonstrative way of reasoning and the loss of the parsimony of the comic vision and external perspective will constitute too high a price to pay for the promised gains of integration.

Acknowledgments

This chapter has benefited from the constructive criticism of several colleagues. Although they should not be held responsible for the points of view expressed, we want to acknowledge with appreciation the stimulation and challenge provided by Hal Arkowitz, Daniel Fishman, Muriel Fox, Sandra Harris, Nancy McWilliams, Donald Spence, Terence Wilson, and Robert Woolfolk.

AUTOBIOGRAPHICAL STATEMENT

For most of my professional career, I have taught at Rutgers University alongside prominent behaviorally oriented psychologists. As a psychoanalytic psychologist, I could hardly avoid being interested in and struck by the similarities and differences of psychoanalytic and behavior therapies and the related issue of their integration. At Rutgers, I am often called upon to defend the concepts, techniques, and scientific credibility of psychoanalysis and to explain how it differs from behavior therapy. Such was the concurrent and external impetus for me to reflect on the nature and value of these two therapies and my own theoretical and therapeutic allegiances.

Earlier educational influences also played their part. My initial training at McGill University was in experimental psychology with a heavy emphasis on demonstrative and scientific ways of knowing. Such an approach to psychology is most compatible with behavior therapy, and I was, in fact, very attracted to it. At the same time, my education and interest in the humanities prepared me for the more personalistic and psychodynamic emphases in Harvard's Department of Social Relations where I did my graduate work. I believe that my training in Jewish biblical commentary enhanced my appreciation of the tragic and ironic visions of reality and of the dialectical mode of knowing. Psychoanalysis, as readers of our chapter will learn, has much in common with the research methods of biblical, literary, and historical scholarship; it stresses poetic, intuitive, and dialectical styles of knowing and encompasses tragic and ironic visions. Because each of the modes of knowledge employed by psychoanalytic and behavior therapies has a certain appeal to me, each surely serves as a source of my dual interest in these two forms of therapy and in questions about their potential for rapprochement.

Were the influences on me—and on others interested in the integration debate—largely situational and educational, or were they built on a yet earlier base? To be true to a psychoanalytic orientation, the latter possibility must at least be considered. As Winokur and I argue, conducting psychoanalytic therapy requires a judicious blend of the poetic/intuitive and rational/analytic styles of knowing, whereas behavior therapy is more heavily invested in the rational/analytic mode alone. The poetic/intuitive mode is often labeled *tender-minded,* that is, feminine, and the rational/analytic, *tough-minded,* that is, masculine. Could it be, based on early sex-role identifications, that I and other psychoanalytic therapists prefer the mixture of stereotypical "masculine and feminine" modes, whereas the behavior therapist is more singularly comfortable with "masculine" modes? It may be that the particular mix of our visions of reality (tragic, comic, romantic, and ironic) is affected, likewise, by early experience and thus bears heavily on the kind of personality theory to which we ascribe and the psychotherapy we practice.

Stanley B. Messer, Ph. D.

My initial clinical training was in psychoanalytically oriented psychotherapy with a strong Rogerian overlay. This combination fit well with a humanistic attitude reflected in my study of English literature at the Hebrew University and of drawing and painting at the Art Students' League in New York City. After completing an M.A. in clinical psychology at the Hebrew University, I began working at its Student Counseling Service where I am now director of training. There I met behavior therapists whose emphasis on economy of procedure and claimed effectiveness of results struck in me a latent scientific chord and served as a challenge to undertake a few behaviorally oriented treatments. These attempts failed dismally, primarily because I consistently noticed the "wrong" kinds of things; that is, I was constantly tempted to deal interpretively with the transferential implications of the patient's attitude to the behavioral tasks.

Partly in the hope of extending my therapeutic repertoire to include some behavioral techniques, I entered the Psy.D. clinical program at the Rutgers University Graduate School of Applied and Professional Psychology. Ironically, while at Rutgers, I became more committed to the psychoanalytic point of view and more aware of why this was so. During this time, I participated in a seminar conducted by Stanley Messer in which we read recently published books by Wachtel and Schafer. The two of us then observed some prominent behavior therapists in action, which led to a collaboration in which we explored the limits to the integration of behavioral and psychoanalytic therapies (Messer & Winokur, 1980).

As I am about to begin full psychoanalytic training, I hope to have the opportunity to explore the childhood origins of the different visions of reality we discuss in our chapter. And, perhaps my personal preoccupation with the question of integration of psychoanalytic and behavior therapies will be resolved as a derivation of contradictory educational positions of my parents in my early life.

MEIR WINOKUR, PSY.D.

REFERENCES

Adler, M. J. *Dialectic.* New York: Harcourt, Brace, 1927.

Alexander, F., & French, T. M. *Psychoanalytic therapy: Principles and application.* New York: Ronald Press, 1946.

Appelbaum, S. A. *Effecting change in psychotherapy.* New York: Aronson, 1981.

Aronfreed, J. *Conduct and conscience.* New York: Academic Press, 1968.

Bakan, D. Clinical psychology and logic. *American Psychologist,* 1956, *11,* 655–662.

Balint, M. *The basic fault: Therapeutic aspects of regression.* London: Tavistock, 1968.

Bandura, A. *Principles of behavior modification.* New York: Holt, 1969.

Bandura, A. Self-efficacy: Toward a unifying theory of behavioral change. *Psychological Review,* 1977, *84,* 191–215. (a)

Bandura, A. *Social learning theory.* Englewood Cliffs, N.J.: Prentice-Hall, 1977. (b)

Beres, D. Psychoanalysis, science and romanticism. In M. Schur (Ed.), *Drives, affects, behavior: Essays in memory of Marie Bonaparte.* New York: International Universities Press, 1965.

Bettelheim, B. Freud and the soul. *The New Yorker,* March 1, 1982, pp. 52–93.

Bowers, K. S. "De-controlling" cognition and cognitive control. In M. J. Mahoney (Ed.), *Psychotherapy process: Current issues and future directions.* New York: Plenum Press, 1980.

Blanck, G., & Blanck, R. *Ego psychology: Theory and practice.* New York: Columbia University Press, 1974.

Breger, L. How psychoanalysis is a science and how it is not. *Journal of the American* Academy of Psychoanalysis, 1981, *9,* 261–275.

Brenner, C. Working alliance, therapeutic alliance, and transference. *Journal of the American Psycholoanalytic Association,* 1979, *27,* 137–158. (Supplement)

Chessick, R. D. Effects of the therapist's philosophical premises on psychotherapeutic process. *American Journal of Psychotherapy,* 1977, *31,* 252–264.

Ellis, A. *Humanistic psychotherapy: The rational–emotive approach.* New York: Julian, 1973.

Ellis, A. *The essence of rational psychotherapy: A comprehensive approach to treatment.* New York: Institute for Rational Living, 1970.

Ellis, A. Misrepresentation of behavior therapy by psychoanalysts. *American Psychologist,* 1981, *36,* 798–799.

Fay, A., & Lazarus, A. A. Psychoanalytic resistance and behavioral nonresponsiveness: A dialectical impasse. In P. Wachtel (Ed.), *Resistance: Psychodynamic and behavioral approaches.* New York: Plenum Press, 1982.

Fenichel, O. *The psychoanalytic theory of neurosis.* New York: W. W. Norton, 1945.

Fisher, S., & Greenberg, R. *The scientific credibility of Freud's theories and therapy.* New York: Basic Books, 1977.

Frankl, V. E. Paradoxical intention: A logotherapeutic. *American Journal of Psychotherapy,* 1960, *14,* 520–535.

Freud, S. The psychotherapy of hysteria. In J. Breuer & S. Freud, *Studies in hysteria.* New York: Basic Books, 1957. (Originally published, 1895.)

Freud, S. *The interpretation of dreams.* New York: Avon Books, 1965. (Originally published, 1900.)

Freud, S. Analysis of a phobia in a five-year-old boy. In J. Strachey (Ed.), *Standard edition of complete psychological works* (Vol. 10). London: Hogarth Press, 1955. (Originally published, 1909.)

Freud, S. The dissolution of the Oedipus complex. In J. Strachey (Ed.), *Standard edition of complete psychological works* (Vol. 19.). London: Hogarth Press, 1961. (Originally published, 1924.)

Freud, S. *Civilization and its discontents.* New York: W. W. Norton, 1961. (Originally published, 1930.)

Freud, S. Analysis terminable and interminable. In J. Strachey (Ed.), *Standard edition of the complete psychological works* (Vol. 23). London: Hogarth Press, 1964. (Originally published, 1937.)

Frye, N. *Anatomy of criticism.* New York: Athaneum, 1957.

Frye, N. *A natural perspective: The development of Shakesperian comedy and romance.* New York: Columbia University Press, 1965.

Frye, N. *Fools of time: Studies in Shakesperean tragedy.* Toronto: University of Toronto Press, 1967.

Geller, M. H. A practical guide to psychoanalytic psychotherapy. *Contemporary Psychology,* 1981, *26,* 357–358.

Goldfried, M. R. Anxiety reduction through cognitive-behavioral intervention. In P. C. Kendall & S. D. Hollen (Eds.), *Cognitive-behavioral intervention: Theory, research and procedures.* New York: Academic Press, 1979.

Goldfried, M. R. Resistance and clinical behavior therapy. In P. Wachtel (Ed.), *Resistance: Psychodynamic and behavioral approaches.* New York: Plenum Press, 1982.

Goldiamond, I. Fluent and nonfluent speech (stuttering): Analysis and operant techniques for control. In L. Krasner & L. P. Ullman (Eds.), *Research in behavior modification.* New York: Holt, Rinehart & Winston, 1965.

Greenson, R. That impossible profession. In K. A. Frank (Ed.), *The human dimension in psychoanalytic practice.* New York: Grune & Stratton, 1977.
Guntrip, H. *Psychoanalytic theory, therapy, and the self.* New York: Basic Books, 1971.
Hartmann, H. *Essays on ego psychology.* New York: International Universities Press, 1964.
Hawkins, D. R. A Freudian view. In M. Kramer (Ed.), *Dream psychology and the new biology of dreaming.* Springfield, Ill.: Charles C Thomas, 1969.
Holt, R. R. Freud's mechanistic and humanistic images of man. In R. R. Holt & E. Peterfreud (Eds.), *Psychoanalysis and contemporary science* (Vol. 1). New York: Macmillan, 1972.
Horwitz, L. *Clinical prediction in psychotherapy.* New York: Aronson, 1974.
Hyman, S. E. Psychoanalysis and the climate of tragedy. In B. Nelson (Ed.), *Freud and the twentieth century.* New York: Meridian Books, 1957.
Jones, J. W. *The texture of knowledge.* Washington, D.C.: University Press of America, 1981.
Kohut, H. *The restoration of the self.* New York: International Universities Press, 1977.
Krook, D. *Elements of tragedy.* New Haven: Yale University Press, 1969.
Langs, R. *The bipersonal field.* New York: Aronson, 1976.
Lazarus, A. A. *Multimodal behavior therapy.* New York: Springer, 1976.
Lazarus, A. A. *The practice of multimodal therapy.* New York: McGraw-Hill, 1981.
Levine, M. Investigative reporting as a research method. *American Psychologist,* 1980, *35,* 626–638.
Mahler, M. S. On the first three subphases of the separation-individuation process. *International Journal of Psychoanalysis,* 1972, *53,* 333–338.
Mahoney, M. J. *Cognition and behavior modification.* Cambridge, Mass.: Ballinger, 1974.
Mahoney, M. J. Psychotherapy and the structure of personal revolutions. In M. J. Mahoney (Ed.), *Psychotherapy process: Current issues and future directions.* New York: Plenum Press, 1980.
Malan, D. H. *The frontier of brief psychotherapy.* New York: Plenum Press, 1976.
Malcolm, J. *The impossible profession.* New York: Knopf, 1981.
Mark, C. B. A case study exploration into the relationship between the values of psychotherapists and their theoretical orientations (Doctoral dissertation, Rutgers—The State University, 1980). *Dissertation Abstracts International,* 1981, *41*(09), 3579B. (University Microfilms No. 8105201)
Marmor, J. Recent trends in psychotherapy. *The American Journal of Psychiatry,* 1980, *137:4,* 409–416.
Maslow, A. H. *The farther reaches of human nature.* New York: Viking Press, 1971.
May, R. The significance of symbolism. In R. May (Ed.), *Symbolism in religion and literature.* New York: Braziller, 1960.
Meichenbaum, D., & Gilmore, J. B. Resistance from a cognitive-behavioral perspective. In P. Wachtel (Ed.), *Resistance: Psychodynamic and behavioral approaches.* New York: Plenum Press, 1982.
Messer, S. B. Integrating psychoanalytic and behavior therapy: Limitations, possibilities, and trade-offs. *British Journal of Clinical Psychology,* 1983, *22,* 131–132.
Messer, S. B., & Schacht, T. E. A cognitive-dynamic theory of reflection-impulsivity. In J. Masling (Ed.), *Empirical studies of psychoanalytical theories* (Vol. 2). Hillsdale, N.J.: Analytic Press, in press.
Messer, S. B., & Winokur, M. Some limits to the integration of psychoanalytic and behavior therapy. *American Psychologist,* 1980, *35,* 818–827.
Messer, S. B., & Winokur, M. What about the question of integration? A reply to Apfelbaum and to Ellis. *American Psychologist,* 1981, *36,* 800–802.
Palmer, R. *Hermeneutics: Interpretation theory in Schleiermacher, Dilthey, Heidegger, and Gadamer.* Evanston, Ill.: Northwestern University Press, 1969.

Perold, E. *On the psychology of knowledge: Towards a truly psychological view.* Unpublished manuscript, July 1981. (Available from E. Periold, GSAPP, Rutgers University, P.O. Box 819, Piscataway, N.J. 08854).
Phillips, J. S. The active analyst and the intuitive behavior therapist. *Contemporary Psychology,* 1978, *23,* 131–132.
Polanyi, M. *Personal knowledge.* New York: Harper & Row, 1964.
Radnitzky, G. *Contemporary schools of metascience.* Chicago: Henry Regnery, 1973.
Reik, T. *Listening with the third ear.* New York: Farrar, Straus, 1949.
Ricoeur, P. The question of proof in Freud's psychoanalytic writings. *Journal of the American Psychoanalytic Association,* 1977, *25,* 835–871.
Rieff, P. *Freud: The mind of the moralist.* New York: Viking Press, 1959.
Rogers, C. *On becoming a person.* Boston: Houghton-Mifflin, 1961.
Roland, A. The reality of the psycho-analytic relationship and situation in the handling of transference resistance. *International Journal of Psychoanalysis,* 1967, *48,* 504–510.
Rychlak, J. F. *A philosophy of science for personality theory.* Boston: Houghton Mifflin, 1968.
Schafer, R. An overview of Heinz Hartmann's contributions to psychoanalysis. *International Journal of Psycho-analysis,* 1970, *51,* 425–446.
Schafer, R. *A new language for psychoanalysis.* New Haven: Yale University Press, 1976.
Sherwood, M. *The logic of explanation in psychoanalysis.* New York: Academic Press, 1969.
Steele, R. S. Psychoanalysis and hermeneutics. *International Review of Psychoanalysis,* 1979, *6,* 389–411.
Spence, D. *Narrative truth and historical truth.* New York: W. W. Norton, 1982. (a)
Spence, D. Narrative truth and theoretical truth. *Psychoanalytic Quarterly,* 1982, *51,* 43–69. (b)
Stein, H. F., & Kayzakian-Rowe, S. Hypertension, biofeedback, and the myth of the machine: A psychoanalytic–cultural exploration. *Psychoanalysis and Contemporary Thought,* 1978, *1,* 119–156.
Stern, K. *The flight from woman.* New York: Randy Press, 1965.
Stolorow, R. D., & Atwood, G. E. *Faces in a cloud.* New York: Aronson, 1979.
Stone, L. *The psychoanalytic situation.* New York: International Universities Press, 1961.
Strachey, J. The nature of the therapeutic action of psychoanalysis. *International Journal of Psychoanalysis,* 1934, *15* (2/3), 127–159.
Trachtenburg, S. The economy of comedy. *Psychoanalytic Review,* 1975–76, *62:4,* 557–578.
Wachtel, P. *Psychoanalysis and behavior therapy.* New York: Basic Books, 1977. (a)
Wachtel, P. Interaction cycles, unconscious processes, and the person-situation issue. In B. D. Magnusson & N. Endler (Eds.), *Personality at the crossroads.* New York: Lawrence Erlbaum, 1977. (b)
Waelder, R. The validation of psychoanalytic interpretations and theories. In Mujeebur-Rahman, Md. (Ed.), *The Freudian paradigm: Psychoanalysis and scientific thought.* Chicago: Nelson-Hall, 1977.
Watson, J. B. *Behavior: An introduction to comparative psychology.* New York: Holt, 1914.
Watzlawick, P. *The language of change: Elements of therapeutic communication.* New York: Basic Books, 1978.
Weimer, W. B. Psychotherapy and philosophy of science. In M. J. Mahoney (Ed.), *Psychotherapy process: Current issues and future directions.* New York: Plenum Press, 1980.
Wilson, G. T., & Evans, I. M. The therapist–client relationship in behavior therapy. In A. S. Gurman & A. M. Razin (Eds.), *The therapist's contribution to effective psychotherapy: An empirical approach.* New York: Pergamon, 1977.
Witkin, H. A., Dyk, R. B., Faterson, H. F., Goodenough, D. R., & Karp, S. A. *Psychological differentiation.* New York: Wiley, 1962.

Wolpe, J. *Psychotherapy by reciprocal inhibition.* Stanford: Stanford University Press, 1958.

Woolfolk, R. L., & Richardson, F. C. Behavior therapy and the ideology of modernity. *American Psychologist,* in press.

Yates, A. J. Behavior therapy: Past, present, future—imperfect? *Clinical Psychology Review,* 1981, *1,* 269–291.

Yates, A. J. Behavior therapy and psychodynamic psychotherapy: Basic conflict or reconciliation and integration? *British Journal of Clinical Psychology,* 1983, *22,* 107–125.

Zaidel, E. *Cerebral correlates of conscious experience.* Amsterdam: Elsevier, 1979.

Zeldow, P. B. Divergent approaches to milieu therapy. *Bulletin for the Menninger Clinic,* 1979, *43,* 217–232.

3

Tragedy, Irony, and Human Assistance

Commentary on Stanley B. Messer and Meir Winokur

PAUL L. WACHTEL

I would feel like a cad to be too critical of Messer and Winokur's chapter. It is, in so many respects, reasonable, fair minded, accurate—*and* it seems to move considerably away from the antiintegrationist position of their earlier paper and toward a cautious appreciation of the value of an integrative approach. Even their first paper, to be sure, was no one-sided anti-integrative tract but was more in the nature of a caution to whoever might rush too unheedfully into the thicket of problems that integration presents. Their present chapter also is such a caution, but I suspect that readers familiar with both will be struck by the more positive attitude toward integration that these two thoughtful writers express upon further reflection.

Yet, there are still a few places I can demur, in the service of assuring that my comments are not so blandly accepting of Messer and Winokur's new stance that they constitute a cure for insomnia. To begin with, I again want to object to the use of the term "comic." In my own chapter in this volume, I spelled out some of my objections to their use of this term in their first paper. Clearly, Messer and Winokur recognize the problem.

PAUL L. WACHTEL • Department of Psychology, City College of the City University of New York, New York, New York 10031.

However, recognizing it does not eliminate it. For their purpose, the term is fatally flawed. Messer and Winokur's disavowal of an implication of funny or nonserious is simply not able to dispel the connotations that the term will have for almost any reader. To present psychoanalysis as having a "tragic vision" (much less having a tragic vision *plus*) and at the same time to present behavior therapy's vision as comic seems to me inevitably to call forth schemata of profound versus superficial. That Messer and Winokur unwittingly stack the deck is evident even in their first paragraph where they tell us that psychoanalytic therapists "focus" on the inner world of experience, whereas behavior therapists are "preoccupied" with the outer world of consensual reality.

I leave to my behavioral colleagues to defend their turf as they will. My own concern here is to consider how such matters of connotation bear on the evaluation of an integrative approach. For there are ways in which—however fair and supportive they are for the most part—Messer and Winokur typify certain subtle biases and misperceptions regarding the nature of a dynamic-behavioral integration.

Messer and Winokur, for example, note that they "still find it hard to employ behavioral techniques such as systematic desensitization, assertiveness training, or biofeedback as Wachtel (1977a) would have dynamic therapists do." They seem to be—and in important respects are—fairly open in acknowledging the usefulness of these techniques "in the hands of others." But they are hesitant to do it themselves because of their commitment to "deepening of understanding."

The implication seems fairly clear that the use of such methods interferes with deep understanding. Thus, an acceptance of the use of such methods—whether by oneself or even by others—seems to require an acceptance of a more superficial understanding. Perhaps such methods are useful for more limited goals. Perhaps they can relieve distress in individuals too impatient (or impecunious) for the deeper but more delayed reworkings of the psychoanalytic method. But they ultimately represent a kind of compromise between practical exigencies and the loftier possibilities of the "pure gold" of analysis.

The argument, then, is but a variation of one that has been prominent within the psychoanalytic community, even apart from any issue of integrating methods from without, such as those of behavior therapy. It is a variant of the argument that has, by an odd linguistic convention distinguished *psychoanalysis* from *psychotherapy* (Wachtel in press.)

Implicit in Franz Alexander's experiments in psychotherapy was the assumption that it served Freud poorly to assume that his theoretical insights were not capable of yielding us a therapy more effective than the Model-T that Freud himself used early in this century. Though he waffled on the issue at times, in the face of enormous pressure from the psychoanalytic community, Alexander did (it seems to me) set out to *improve* upon psychoanalysis. Psychoanalytic therapy was to be not just a compromise, alloyed therapy for the masses—more accessible but less profound—but rather an attempt to utilize the basic principles of psychoanalytic theory more effectively, to achieve the goals of *analysis* more fully and efficiently rather than to water down those goals for a less elite clientele.

Alexander met with implacable resistance from the psychoanalytic community, which was committed to a view of the unique efficacy of the pure gold of analysis for those anointed who were "analyzable." The resistance was not always gross or overt. Typically, it was most effective when it did not appear to be resistance at all. Indeed, psychoanalytic psychotherapy (whether Alexander's version or that of other clinicians) was most effectively kept in its place when it was *endorsed*—endorsed, that is, on closer inspection, for patients not capable of the privations (psychic or monetary) required to achieve the even greater benefits that a full-scale analysis was assumed to provide.

Although in recent decades a number of important innovations have made a glacial advance into the sanctum of analysis proper, the distinction—and it remains, however subtly, an *invidious* distinction—between psychoanalysis and psychotherapy has remained. The more active and innovative variations of psychoanalytically guided therapeutic efforts have been effectively catalogued as compromises. This is, to some degree, what Messer and Winokur have done also—though, in this case, comparing psychoanalytic therapies more generally with integrations of psychoanalytic and other approaches. Such integrations also are, in a sense, controlled through endorsement, whereas "deep understanding" is reserved for more traditional approaches.

This is not to equate Messer and Winokur with the *arrière garde* that has dominated and debilitated organized psychoanalysis. Messer and Winokur's base is the university, not the psychoanalytic institute, and it shows in a far greater openness to new ideas and possibilities. One sees more change from their first to second paper on this topic than is seen in a decade of issues of the *Journal of the American Psychoanalytic Association.* My intention, therefore, is to pull out and magnify—in order to study under the microscope, as it were—much more subtle biases that have thus far shaped their reflections on the matters at hand.

Messer and Winokur value the patient's "coming to terms with the intensity and extensity of his or her rage." Their assumption is, it seems, that the rage is "there," come what may, and that the choice is to "come to terms with it" or not to (i.e., to deny or ignore it). This is true, despite their apparent recognition in the previous paragraph that an integrative approach would not in fact ignore the anger but rather attempt to alter the psychological conditions that produce it. The crucial question is whether the intensity and extensity of rage is a given, whether it is something that simply "is" and must be "come to terms with," or whether it results from the very efforts that the person makes to hide from it and hold it back. If one holds the latter view, as I do, one need not help the person to explore and experience the same degree of primitive rage that Messer and Winokur assume. Instead one helps him effectively to assert his rights and to accept that he feels as he does; as a consequence the "intensity and extensity of. . .rage" diminishes as the daily frustrations that fuel it subside. One still is committed to helping the person to experience fully the depth of his or her feelings. Those feelings themselves are seen not as the inevitable and unchangeable residue of the human tragedy but, to a larger degree, as the ironic consequence of our efforts to hide from ourselves (see in this regard Wachtel, 1977a, 1977b, 1981; Wile, 1981, 1982).

Thus, in an integrative approach, the ironic perspective may be said to replace the tragic to some degree. There are many things—from death to illness to accident—that we cannot control. But though humility and acceptance of the limits that frame human life are an essential backdrop for successful psychotherapy, in the foreground must be a conviction that "our fate lies not in our stars but in ourselves."

This recognition also can have a tragic note, as when what is stressed are "inner forces of evil." But it seems to me most forcefully—and most usefully—to point toward the *ironies* that underlie our problems, to an understanding of how our troubles are not inevitable and fated but are rather a consequence of our own choices and retreats. That the impulses we defend against are to so great a degree the product of those very defenses is the irony that lies at the heart of most neurotic distress and limitation. In emphasizing such a view, one unites to some degree the elements of tragedy and comedy: Both the happy ending and the tragic failure are possible results of the ironic trap. The aim of therapy is to make the former more likely than the latter.

At the core of the integrative approach I advocate is an emphasis on the vicious circles that account for so much of neurotic misery and on the means to intervene and reverse them. Such an emphasis is in no way antithetical to the quest for deep understanding or full experiencing. Indeed, one major purpose of active intervention techniques is to induce the person to take steps that will enable him or her to *experience* forbidden feelings, instead of just talking about them. Having taken active steps in his or her daily life, the patient is at a new vantage point where the previous balance of impulses and defenses is altered and where he or she is confronted with ideas, wishes, and affects that were previously submerged.

Such things happen, of course, in more classical approaches as well; but the experiencing is often muted, hedged by intellectualizing, and attained only after a great deal of time, suffering, and frustrating spinning of wheels. This is a consequence of the hesitance of psychoanalytic therapists to provide direction and to assist their patients more actively—a hesitance attributable, in significant part, to the perspective Messer and Winokur describe as *romantic*. Here is another of those words whose popular and technical meanings are so readily confounded. Does any red-blooded American want to disavow romance, to risk being perceived as a balding accountant? Yet much of the point of view subsumable under the rubric of the "romantic vision" is in fact the enemy of change and a roadblock on the path to a more vital and fulfilling life. I have discussed this in detail in a critique of Allen Wheelis's *How People Change* (1973), a marvelous little book whose keen insights about the difficulties of change are undermined by a romantic emphasis on the solitary, lonely struggle (Wachtel, 1977a, Chapter 12). More recently, I have been struck by the links between such a view of therapy and the governing imagery of a consumer capitalist culture (Wachtel, 1983). In psychotherapy (as in Ronald Reagan's America) it is time we learned that we respect people's humanity more when we reach out to help them than when we leave them to flounder on their own.

REFERENCES

Wachtel, P. L. *Psychoanalysis and behavior therapy: Toward an integration.* New York: Basic Books, 1977. (a)

Wachtel, P. L. Interaction cycles, unconscious processes, and the person–situation issue. In D. Magnusson & N. Endler (Eds.), *Personality at the crossroads: Issues in interactional psychology.* Hillsdale, N.J.: Lawrence Erlbaum Associates, 1977. (b)

Wachtel, P. L. Transference, schema, and assimilation: The relevance of Piaget to the psychoanalytic theory of transference. *The annual review of psychoanalysis* (Vol. 8). New York: International Universities Press, 1981.

Wachtel, P. L. *The poverty of affluence: A psychological portrait of the American way of life.* New York: Free Press, 1983. (a)

Wachtel, P. L. The philosophic and the therapeutic: Considerations regarding the role of psychoanalysis and other therapies. In R. Stern (Ed.), *Science and psychotherapy* (Vol. 4). New York: Haven Press, In press. (b)

Wheelis, A. *How people change.* New York: Harper & Row, 1973.

Wile, D. *Couples therapy: A nontraditional approach.* New York: Wiley, 1981.

Wile, D. *Kohut, Kernberg, and accusatory interpretations.* Paper presented at the annual meeting of the American Psychological Association, Washington, D.C., September 1982.

4

The Varieties of Integrative Experience

THOMAS E. SCHACHT

The resemblance of this chapter's title to that of William James's classic volume on religion is deliberate. This minor plagiarism was prompted, in part, by a reviewer's comments on the newly republished edition of James's *Principles of Psychology* (Adelson, 1982). By authoring this first (and only) comprehensive and integrated textbook of psychology, James became, in this reviewer's estimation, the final chronicler of the last time in history when one man could know everything in the field. Since then, most of us have engaged in a more or less intense struggle with a psychological elephant that simply cannot be grasped all at once. However, despite our progressive specialization and fragmentation, many psychologists retain a desire to return the field to a unified state. The integration of knowledge, although ever more elusive, remains a compelling ideal.

Most of the "unity" in clinical psychology today is of the de facto variety, in that historically most psychologists have not been trained to conceptualize their work in more than one framework. As Sigmund Koch (1964) described the situation of two decades ago: "What seems to have been imparted to the typical psychologist might be characterized as an ocean of awe surrounding a few islands of sloganized information" (p. 11). However, times have changed, and it is now common, even typical, for

THOMAS E. SCHACHT • Center for Psychotherapy Research and Department of Psychology, Vanderbilt University, Nashville, Tennessee 37240. This work was supported by the Vanderbilt Center for Psychotherapy Research and an NIMH Grant MH16247-01.

clinical training to encompass more than one theoretical perspective. Accordingly, the number of psychologists describing themselves as "eclectic" has shown a steady increase to present levels of about 50%, whereas the number professing allegiance to a single viewpoint has correspondingly decreased (Garfield, 1981; Garfield & Kurtz, 1976).

Psychology's proliferation of theoretical systems and empirical findings has, unfortunately, not been matched by a complementary advance in methods for bringing this diverse knowledge together. Our attempts to integrate often bog down at the level of simple juxtaposition of alternatives. In Piagetian terms, we assimilate but do not accommodate. The result is a virtual plethora of allegedly different therapies. Although optimists assert that "the conceptual unification of psychology can be a realistic level of aspiration" (Atkinson, 1981, p. 127), the actuality of integration rests on a horizon that often appears to recede in equal measure with our progress toward it.

This chapter is a set of variations on the theme of integrating knowledge. Behavior therapy and psychodynamic therapy happen to be the instruments on which the variations are played, but the conceptual music itself involves deeper issues that are related to much wider domains of study. With regard to the bringing together of the therapies, this music has been performed under a variety of titles and with many distinctive interpretations. Thus, we hear references to "compatibility," "synthesis," "congruence," "harmony," "merger," "consonance," "amalgamation," "combination," "fusion," "coalescence," "rapprochement," "convergence," "reconciliation," "détente," "common ground (elements, denominators)," "complementarity," "overlap," "bridging," "coalition," "unification," "blending," "intersection," "conjunction," "depolarization," "synergism," "mutual reinforcement," "potentiation," "alliance," "interdependence," "assimilation," "interface," and most generally, to "integration."

As this profusion of metaphors and descriptors indicates, the overall theme of integration means different things to different authors. The specific therapeutic elements deemed relevant to possible integration as well as the ways in which those elements are to be combined and compared vary in accordance with (often prereflective) schemata of what an integration is or ought to be. Virtually all existing literature on the integration of psychodynamic and behavioral therapies has focused on the immediate characteristics of the therapies *per se.* Although there is considerable range to these surface aspects (i.e., from narrow consideration of specific technical or theoretical points to very broad comparisons of implicit epistemological commitments and visions of reality), there has been almost no attention to the underlying form of these discussions, to questions of just what it means, abstractly, to integrate knowledge. These issues of form, as opposed to surface content, constitute a tacit framework on which various discussions of therapeutic integration, pro and con, may be compared.

The remainder of this chapter explicates some central aspects of this tacit framework. Three general domains are examined, as is indicated in the following groups of questions.

The first domain involves *units of analysis*—the basic question of what, exactly, is to be integrated. How are behavior therapy and psychodynamic therapy to be defined and which elements of each are to be selected for comparison as units of analysis? Where do we expect integration to occur—in theoretical propositions, in techniques, in philosophical and metapsychological ideas, or in relationships between these? To what extent may integration be understood in terms of reaching agreement on a set of shared central questions (to which we may not have even tentative current answers?). What principles of choice apply to the building up of a working group of elements?

The second domain is concerned with *models for the therapies' relationship.* This involves questions of how the selected elements of behavioral and psychodynamic approaches are to be compared. What general structures of meaning surround different attempts at integration (or attempts to argue that integration is impossible)? What yardsticks can one apply to a purported integration to determine whether it is genuine or successful? What are the relationships between different models of the integrative process?

The third domain involves *metatheoretical issues.* What issues in the psychology and philosophy of knowledge relate to the integration of behavioral and dynamic therapies? What do these issues imply for understanding both the history and the likely future of integration efforts? The remainder of this chapter examines each of these domains in turn.

UNITS OF ANALYSIS

Authors differ significantly when selecting units of analysis around which to formulate their discussions of therapeutic integration. There is discouragingly little uniformity on even the most basic aspects of this topic. Even the largest units of analysis (behavior therapy and psychodynamic therapy as global entities) are described so inconsistently and with reference to concepts and practices of such complexity and variety, that consensually acceptable definitions of either approach still elude us. Common reference to "schools," "models," "camps," "disciplines," "viewpoints," or "systems" implies a clarity and tangibility that, on close inspection, cannot be found. Rather than having clear-cut conceptual boundaries, behavior therapy and dynamic therapy are prototypical *fuzzy sets.*

Consequently, authors must frequently begin their discussions with a working definition of the subject matter. Some (e.g., Feather & Rhoads, 1972) rationalize their particular definitions on pragmatic grounds, using phrases like "for purposes of simplification" or "it is beyond the scope of this paper." However, many authors simply declare a definition without apparent consideration of how a limited or selective focus may be dwarfed by the unaddressed issues. Some authors (e.g., Marks & Gelder, 1966; Wachtel, 1977) openly acknowledge that behavior therapy and psychodynamic therapy are subject to multiple definitions, whereas others (e.g., Wolpe, 1981) run roughshod over such subtleties, seemingly unconvinced of the possible relevance of alternate viewpoints. Even studies employing expert therapists of both persuasions (who, one surmises, might hold adequate definitions of their own work) have been forced to employ "stipulated definitions" because of the difficulties involved in achieving a workable consensus (Sloane, Staples, Cristol, Yorkston, & Whipple, 1975).

All working definitions involve dividing the global domains of behavior therapy and psychodynamic therapy into smaller, more precisely specifiable units, including aspects of conceptual, theoretical, technical, and philosophical dimensions. When a number of similar units of analysis are treated together as a group or class, authors may refer to "levels" of analysis (cf. Goldfried, 1980), although the principles of grouping may themselves become problematic. Table 1 illustrates a variety of units of analysis drawn from a broad sampling of publications on therapeutic integration.

Note also that authors may differ in the extent to which particular units or elements are regarded as necessary and/or sufficient to their working definitions of behavioral and psychodynamic therapies. Thus, even if there is agreement on the nominal units of analysis, there may be disagreement with respect to the exact relationship of each unit to the overall definition and with regard to which units, if any, represent absolute essentials.

Historical considerations also enter the process of selecting units of analysis. Some authors primarily consider the more recent developments in the two therapies, whereas others range freely across the contemporary and the older literature as if there were no problem of comparability—as if each therapy were a fixed entity that, though evolving, possessed an unchanging core. The major danger here involves unexpunged anachronisms, psychology's perennial problem of transforming ephemeral historical documents into eternal historical monuments (Koch, 1964). An extreme of this problematic tendency (thankfully becoming infrequent) is demonstrated by authors who insist that all psychodynamic thinking must be understood as footnotes to Freud and that all behavioral therapies retain similar connections to Pavlov and Skinner.

Table 1. Examples of Units of Analysis on Which Behavioral and Dynamic Therapies Have Been Compared

Emotional arousal	Interpersonal behavior
Anxiety	Diagnostic methods
Empathy	Placebo processes
Interpretation	Role of the patient's past/history
Use of language and symbolism	Dreams
World views	Direct suggestion
Vision of reality	Reinforcement—overt and covert
Treatment goals	Relaxation
Activity level of patient and therapist	Environmental manipulation
Rapport building	Therapeutic relationship/role
Desensitization (underlying process)	Catharsis
Philosophical presuppositions	Modeling
Relation to learning theory	Identification
Cognition-insight	Relation to empirical science—canons of evidence
Role of the unconscious	Therapist's thought process—modes of knowing
Therapeutic time frame	Relapse—therapeutic recidivism
Meaning of symptoms and their removal	

In addition to serving as convenient simplifications, units of analysis also function as apperceptive backgrounds for making discriminations and combinations. Preexisting beliefs or attitudes may prompt selection of particularly consonant units of analysis, that, experientially, may almost "suggest themselves" to the researcher as seemingly self-evident dimensions of importance. Simultaneously, one's choice of analytic units may lead, almost reflexively, to seeing certain kinds of coherences and contradictions and to not seeing other kinds. A choice among analytic units may even represent a strategic rhetorical decision, based on one's prior views, pro or con, of the prospects for therapeutic integration.

To illustrate, consider Messer and Winokur's (1980; see also Chapter 3, this volume) important analysis of possible limits to the integration of behavioral and psychodynamic therapies. Their discussion relies on "perspectives" and "visions" of reality as units of analysis. For example, working from a philosophical stance that regards objectivity and subjectivity as incompatible opposites, Messer and Winokur argue that behavior therapy is relatively objective in its approach to psychological phenomena, whereas psychoanalysis, in contrast, involves more subjectivity. Because objectivity and subjectivity are incompatible opposites (at least within the philosophical rubric chosen by Messer and Winokur), it follows naturally that behavior therapy and psychodynamic therapy are likewise incompatible to the extent that they tend to be selectively identified with objectivity or subjectivity.

Messer and Winokur's argument is crisply drawn, and the overall line of reasoning seems compelling. However, if we attend to the question of units of analysis, we may note the availability of philosophical options other than the one they relied on. In particular, we may note the existence of thoughtful and persuasive claims that a dichotomy of subjectivity versus objectivity is a frequently false and illusion-promoting distinction (e.g., Bateson, 1979; Lakoff & Johnson, 1980; Pirsig, 1974). If such an alternate perspective had informed their selection of analytic units, then Messer and Winokur's argument might have evolved quite differently, especially regarding their estimate of the prospects for therapeutic integration.

The process of dividing therapeutic domains into units of analysis may be highly idiosyncratic. There are no limits, in principle, to the number of lines along which a domain of knowledge may be partitioned. Accordingly, there is also no general limit to the variety of different units of analysis that may be applied to questions of therapeutic integration. This capacity for pluralism creates a fundamental problem in deciding how to compare authors who employ different analytic units. How, for example, may conclusions be drawn from comparing two authors, one of whom focuses on technical issues (and is optimistic about prospects for integration), whereas the other attends primarily to epistemological and philosophical issues (and is pessimistic about integration)? Can we justify, or even imagine, a metaanalytic approach (cf. Smith & Glass, 1977) in which we compare ultimate conclusions regarding integration across multiple analytic units and methods?

Coping with multiple units of analysis may produce problems even when there is no comparison of arguments or viewpoints across authors. For example, Sloane's (1969) use of different analytic units leads him to lose track of his argument and fall into apparent self-contradiction. Thus, he states (p. 209): "It is chiefly in . . . *technical* aspects that the therapies differ." And then, two pages later he offers a different unit of analysis in the same role: "Clearly, the greatest barrier to the integration of present-day therapies lies in their differing *theoretical* assumptions" (emphasis mine).

Authors also differ on the question of which units of analysis (if any) should be regarded as more fundamental or important to issues of integration. Does compatibility in terms of technical therapeutic details like "establishing a positive relationship" carry more or less weight than compatibility in terms of "visions of reality"? One view echoes a conventional methodological wisdom by insisting that conceptual differences should be resolved by appeal to an empirical process (cf. Kazdin, Chapter 5, this volume). Unfortunately, the relationship of theory to data in psychotherapy is sufficiently loose that such empirical confrontations are exceedingly difficult to arrange (Weitzman, 1967). Because we have yet to complete the prerequisite task of imagining clearly testable models for therapeutic comparison, there is often very little to be empirical about.

Still another area of author variability involves use of the same word to denote different units of analysis. For example, consider the term "desensitization." Sloane *et al.* (1975) compare behavioral and dynamic therapies in units of analysis at the level of *technique*; thus, in their view, desensitization is a technical procedure assigned wholly to behavior therapy and explicitly excluded from psychodynamic therapy. However, other authors (e.g. Wachtel, 1977) also use "desensitization" to refer to an underlying psychological *process* that is shared by both therapies (rather than a technique characteristic of only one therapy). Only careful attention to differences in units of analysis that underlie the common terminology can forestall possible misinterpretation when comparing these authors.

The potential for pluralism in selection of analytic units is so great that even when a choice is restricted to a limited domain, the complexity of options may overwhelm efforts at systematic comparison. Consider, for example, a limited focus on philosophical presuppositions embodied in the two therapies. This limited focus severely constrains the range of pertinent analytic units by excluding comparisons of specific technical or theoretical points except as exemplars of a philosophical issue. Yet, even within this restricted range, the array of available choices is bewildering. Thus, in surveying recent literature that makes reference to philosophical presuppositions as units of analysis, I discovered 25 different "-ologies" and "-isms" that have been employed in comparisons of behavioral and dynamic therapies (Table 2).

Let me summarize the main points of this section.

1. Comparison of behavioral and dynamic therapies at a global level

Table 2. Philosophical Dimensions Employed as Units of Analysis in Comparisons of Behavioral and Dynamic Therapies

Centralism	Existentialism
Environmentalism	Empiricism
Objectivism	Humanism
Subjectivism	Teleology
Behaviorism	Reductionism
Positivism	Structuralism
Pragmatism	Epistemology
Operationism	Visions of reality
Metaphorism	Associationism
Extraspectionism	Rationalism
Introspectionism	Peripheralism
Phenomenology	Realism
	Idealism

is impractical. Working definitions, framed as precisely as possible, are required, and these involve division of the therapies into smaller units of analysis. It is these units of analysis and not the therapies as a whole that are compared in any discussion of prospects for integration. This line of reasoning implies the obsolescence of global "horse races" that pit crudely defined "dynamic therapy" against an equally global "behavior therapy" in some comparison of therapeutic process or outcome. Rather, future work should strive for precise specification of therapeutic operations and process/outcome measures (cf. Luborsky's 1982 recommendations regarding the use of procedural manuals to define various therapies operationally).

2. Apparent prospects for integration of the therapies are relative, variable, and context-dependent. There can be no absolute assessment of the question of integration apart from the context reflected in particular units of analysis. Choices regarding analytic units will shape one's perceptions and may prove to be critical determinants of the form and direction of relevant arguments.

3. Selection of analytic units is, in principle, a highly idiosyncratic process. Across authors there is wide variation in choice of units as well as variation in ideas about the relationship between particular units and the overall (global) therapies. This pluralism stands behind the central unresolved question of how to compare the arguments and conclusions of authors who approach the question of integration using different units of analysis.

MODELS FOR THE RELATIONSHIP OF BEHAVIORAL AND DYNAMIC THERAPIES

The particular units of analysis selected by a proponent of therapeutic integration do not spontaneously coalesce into a seamless whole. Likewise, those elements selected by an opponent of integration do not present their incompatibility in a self-evident manner. To be seen as compatible or not, any choice of elements must be arranged and organized and must be embedded in a framework of conceptual relationships. These relationships, which constitute the infrastructure of any given discussion of therapeutic integration, are the subject of this section. Six models are described. They are not presented as mutually exclusive: Thus, some authors, such as Wachtel (1977) and Goldfried (1982), employ more than one, although typically without explicit acknowledgment of a shift in conceptual underpinnings. The examples cited for each model represent particularly clear instances of the particular concept being described. Many authors other than those cited could be included under each model, but such an encyclopedic review is beyond the intent of this chapter, which is primarily to introduce basic concepts. In this regard, the six models do not exhaust the imaginable possibilities for relating behavioral and dynamic therapies. However, they do collectively represent a comprehensive summary of the major literature to date.

Model 1

Model 1 is a model of separatism in which behavior therapy and psychodynamic therapy are viewed as fundamentally incompatible and disparate (for the particular unit of analysis under consideration). There is no room for overlap, differences are stressed, and alleged commonalities are dismissed as superficial or illusory. Typically, those who endorse Model 1 cannot foresee even an approximate integration. There are frequently references to "paradigm shifts" or "emergent visions" as, in principle, the only possibilities for ever bringing the therapies closer together, and even these options may be viewed with some suspicion by authors who emphasize the value of preserving the "integrity" of each approach (cf. Franks, Chapter 8, this volume).

The rhetoric of Model 1 is replete with metaphors and images of conflict. It is behavior therapy "versus" dynamic therapy; there are "lines of battle" between the two therapeutic "camps." Authors who seek to refute this model often acknowledge this conflictual metaphor by writing in terms of "détente," "reconciliation," "rapprochement," or "alliance"—a language of peacemaking made necessary by the background of therapeutic apartheid. In addition to Franks, other examples of Model 1 may be found in Szasz (1967, quoted in Marmor & Woods, 1980) who describes behavior therapy and dynamic therapy as "rival systems of belief. . . . whose relative value is a matter of moral judgment" (p. 296) and in Lazarus (1981) and Bieber (1973).

Model 2

Perhaps an opposite extreme from Model 1, this second model involves various attempts to translate the concepts and/or language of behavior therapy into those of dynamic therapy and vice versa. In one type of translation, either behavior therapy or dynamic therapy is viewed as the "primary" language, a sort of mother tongue that can wholly encompass the ideas and observations of the other treatment. For example, consider Eysenck's (1960, quoted in Marmor & Woods, 1980) statement that "psychotherapy itself, when shorn of its inessential and irrevelant parts, can usefully be considered as a minor part of behavior therapy" (p. 295). A second type of translation involves attempting to express the concepts of *both* dynamic and behavioral therapies in the language of a third perspective, such as learning theory. This approach is common in the earliest literature on therapeutic integration (cf. French, 1933; Kubie, 1934; Shoben, 1948, 1949) as well as being characteristic of the more frequently cited authors (cf. Alexander, 1963; Breger & McGaugh, 1965; Dollard & Miller, 1950; Marmor, 1964; Shectman, 1975; Wolf, 1966).

All translation models are inherently reductionistic. If this reductionism yields theoretical parsimony without producing distortion or sacrificing explanatory power, then much is to be gained from it. However, such perfect translation may be impossible. Goldfried (1982) acknowledges this as primarily a problem of vocabulary differences and secondarily a problem of negative emotional conotations associated with a particular terminology. However, there are reasons to believe that difficulties with translation models go much deeper, that they reside in the basic nature of human symbolizing processes.

The major problem lies in the ambiguity inherent in all languages and, therefore, in any attempts to translate from one language system to another. Consider the argument of Bronowski (1978) who observes that no scientific language can be regarded as a clear and final exposition. He analogizes, pointing out that one "cannot say anything about a table or chair which does not leave [one] open to the challenge: 'Well, I'm using this chair as a table'" (p. 106). Arguments of this form abound in discussions of behavioral and psychodynamic therapies. Thus, a behavior therapist may suggest to a dynamically oriented colleague that she or he is using an interpretation as a reinforcer. Or a dynamic therapist may insist that a behavior therapist's reinforcements actually constitute a systematic manipulation of unconscious fantasies.

Koch (1964) argues that any translation efforts are doomed in principle. Thus, he states that "no natural language and no scientific one of any richness can be regarded as organized into logical levels such that all terms are reducible to or definable on a common definition base. We define words with equally ambiguous other words" (p. 26). He continues, asserting that the psychologist "who wishes to universalize the language community . . . will either be thwarted or will end up with an extraordinarily crass set of descriptive/systemic concepts and a degraded formulation of the psychological questions of interest" (p. 29).

In short, translation models risk producing empty constructs that fail to make effective observational and perceptual contact with the basic phenomena of interest. Such translation becomes a mere conceptual calisthenic, a demonstration of the tremendous human capacity to symbolize and imagine, to see something in terms of something else.

Model 3

This third model views behavior therapy and psychodynamic therapy as being complementary, in that each is suitable for dealing with separate problems in the same patient. Even acknowledgment of an *essential* separateness of the therapies does not produce irreconcilable conflict because each therapy is addressed to different aspects of the patient's condition. Thus, Marmor (1971) envisions behavior therapy and dynamic therapy as "options" that a therapist elects, depending upon the specific clinical problem and treatment goal. Brady (1968) likewise sees patient problems as the key factors in determining which treatment should be selected.

To elaborate, consider the hypothetical situation of a middle-aged executive (Mr. Smith) who seeks therapy because of a haunting sense that his life has become meaningless. These feelings have prompted intense and frightening fantasies of quitting his job, selling his possessions, and assuming the life of a simple vagabond. At the same time, Mr. Smith fears growing old and worries about becoming decrepit and dependent on others. The clinical history also reveals that this patient suffers from a crippling speech anxiety that has limited his career advancement and that may contribute, in part, to his present occupational dissatisfaction. A therapeutic prescription constructed according to Model 3 might offer an exploratory psychoanalytic therapy to deal with the existential and life-developmental issues expressed in Mr. Smith's prominent fantasies and fears, while simultaneously carrying out behavioral desensitization and assertiveness programs for the specific speech-anxiety problem.

The actual implementation of Model 3 has taken two forms. In the first instance, the behavioral and dynamic therapies are carried out sequentially or simultaneously by two separate therapists, each of whom is responsible for only one type of therapy addressed to separate ranges of problems (e.g., Levay, Weissberg, & Blaustein, 1976; Segraves & Smith, 1976). In the second instance, the two therapies are implemented by a single therapist (e.g., Gullick & Blanchard, 1973). This latter format is far less common, because, despite trends toward eclecticism, it is still very difficult to find therapists who are skilled in (or committed to) both types of therapies.

Model 4

The fourth model emphasizes the concept of synergistic effect. This is the idea that the two therapies will interact in the patient to produce a clinical result superior to that obtainable via either therapy alone.

The essential difference between Model 4 and Model 3 is that here the therapies are not restricted to operating on separate sets of problems. Rather, they both focus on the same problems, with a mutual potentiation of therapeutic effect. Each therapy retains its separate identity with the locus of integration within the patient. Lambley (1976, quoted in Marmor & Woods, 1980) offers a clear example of this model, referring explicitly to the "mutual interactions" of the therapies that permit a "more comprehensive approach to . . . therapeutic operation" (p. 334).

In the previously cited case of Mr. Smith, a Model 4 therapeutic prescription would emphasize the manner in which both the behavioral treatment for speech anxiety and the analytic treatment for existential and life-developmental problems would influence each other. The behavioral symptom reduction would be expected to produce corollary changes in self-image, fantasy life, and object relations, whereas the analytic treatment could be seen as freeing the patient's imagination from defensive operations that interfere with motivation to participate in behavioral treatment and that might limit Mr. Smith's ability to exploit his new assertiveness and speech skills in the service of independent self-actualizing activities. Each therapy would thus enhance the operation and outcome of the other.

Model 5

The locus of integration in Model 5 lies in emergent therapeutic techniques. This contrasts with Model 4, where the techniques of each therapy remain unchanged and where the locus of integration lies within their effects on the patient. The concept of emergence derives from general systems theory and refers to the occurrence of new properties in complex systems that could not have been predicted from simple knowledge of the system components. In the present case, dynamic and behavioral therapies combine to yield a novel hybrid approach. Feather and Rhoads' (1972) "psychodynamic behavior therapy" most clearly exemplifies this model. Their therapy marries the behavioral procedures of systematic desensitization to the psychodynamic concern with repressed impulses and unconscious fantasies. The result is a therapy that desensitizes patients to underlying, dynamically inferred impulses and fantasies rather than simply to presenting overt symptoms.

Returning to the case of Mr. Smith, a Model 5 therapist might observe a pattern of consistent difficulties with authority figures, which was dynamically involved in both his career problems (Oedipal fears of competitiveness and achievement), his speech anxiety (castration fears), and his fantasies of escaping to a carefree vagabond existence (wish to regress to a nonconflictual pre-Oedipal state, perhaps involving an imagined symbiotic harmony with the environment). The Model 5 therapist, upon noting these dynamic underpinnings, might then proceed to desensitize Mr. Smith to such things as fantasies of assertively confronting his father over the latter's ambitions for and disappointment with his son. In this way, the dynamic process and the behavioral treatment method are welded together into a new form.

As a general systems concept, the notion of emergent technique is inherently nonspecific regarding particular psychological theories. Consequently, the idea of emergence may be subject to various forms of intellectual abuse. In particular, because behavior therapy and psychodynamic therapy claim broad generality and explanatory power, virtually *any* technique from *any* therapy can be interpreted and rationalized (using the concept of emergence) in terms of either approach.

For example, even a manifestly nonpsychological treatment such as pharmacotherapy can be understood in terms of psychodynamic and behavioral effects (cf. Sarwer-Foner, 1980). Thus, a psychodynamic practitioner may view drugs as agents that reduce inner drive pressures, thereby freeing the resources of the ego for more adaptive work. Likewise, a behavior therapist may understand drugs as permitting more effective counterconditioning by promoting a physiologically relaxed state.

These analyses could, in principle, logically lead to the conclusion that drug therapy represents an emergent technique that results from the integration of behavioral and dynamic therapies. Ordinarily, of course, such a conception would seem highly improbable. We do not typically conceive of drug therapy as an emergent technique but rather view it as an approach entirely in its own right. By what principles, then, can we distinguish between emergent ideas that represent a genuine integration of behavioral and dynamic approaches and nonemergent techniques that are nevertheless subject to interpretation and explanation in terms of behavioral and dynamic concepts? What seems crucial is whether the originators of a given technique were explicitly inspired in their initial conception by deliberate analogies to behavioral and psychodynamic ideas. If the analogy is serendipitous, the associated technique is not regarded as emergent (as with drug therapy). Alternately, if the analogy is intentional, the technique is seen as an example of integration and is labeled *emergent* (as with Feather and Rhoads's treatment approach).

Model 6

Integration of dynamic and behavioral therapies at this level presents the most formidable intellectual challenge. The loci of integration in Model 6 involve various abstractions or metapsychologies, including ideas of theoretical synthesis (e.g., Birk & Brinkley-Birk, 1974; Liotti & Reda, 1981) and hopes for emergent models of human beings (cf. Mahoney, Chapter 10, this volume). Such global models of man are often expressed in terms of a central metaphor, such as "man as information-processing machine" or "man as the locus of existential agency." Wachtel's (1977, Chapter 2, this volume) merging of the interpersonal and intrapsychic into an arena for theoretical synthesis is perhaps the best-known integration effort that falls under the rubric of Model 6.

Those who are pessimistic about integration (cf. Model 1) also frequently focus their arguments at this level. Thus, Messer and Winokur (1980, Chapter 3, this volume), Lazarus (1981), and Shectman (1975) all claim that behavior therapy and psychodynamic therapy may be fundamentally incompatible because of basic differences in their models of human beings and/or reality.

It is important to note that integration in terms of Models 2–5 may occur without regard to whether or not the therapies appear compatible in terms of Model 6. Integration or compatibility at this abstract level does not constrain integration in other modes, unless one places all six models in a hierarchy and postulates that technical integration without corresponding abstract integration is a spurious solution. Model 6 thus represents one kind of integration among multiple possibilities; it is not necessarily superordinate but is simply more abstract.

METATHEORETIC ISSUES

The Fallacy of Common Elements

Many discussions of therapeutic integration center on a search for common elements shared by both behavioral and psychodynamic therapies (cf. Frank, 1976; Goldfried, 1980; Strupp, 1977). The justification for this search involves a belief that finding such common elements constitutes evidence that bears positively on the question of integration. Some authors provide tables or lists of common elements, with the implication that a larger list demonstrates a greater degree of integration (e.g., Marks & Gelder, 1966; Marmor, 1971). There is thus a tacit cumulative assumption to the search for common elements—as if each common element possessed a "quantum of integration," with the current total of such quanta reflecting the aggregate prospects for integration of the therapies. Despite frequent use of common elements as evidence for integration, there are no compelling reasons to accept such arguments. Indeed, cogent lines of reasoning suggest that simply finding common elements may be a seductively dangerous basis for drawing conclusions about therapeutic integration.

One problem with arguments based on finding common elements is their often implicit use of predicate logic that, of course, is inherently fallacious. The following example illustrates:

1. My mother is a woman.
2. The Virgin Mary is a woman.
3. Therefore, my mother is the Virgin Mary.

This chain of reasoning appears ridiculous instantly. Yet, logically parallel arguments have been invoked in discussions of common elements in behavioral and psychodynamic therapies. Thus, regarding the oft-cited common element of "learning":

1. Behavior therapy is a learning process.
2. Psychodynamic therapy is a learning process.
3. Therefore, behavior therapy is (integral with) psychodynamic therapy.

Even if the search for common elements escapes the trap of predicate logic, there is still the problem of contextualization (Goffman, 1974), which is also referred to by Lazarus (1981) as the problem of phenotypic versus genotypic similarities. This perspective stresses the general notion that any given element acquires significance only within a structure of meanings and a system of functional relations. Thus. salt in one's soup is quite different from salt in one's gas tank. There is a common element (salt), but the vast differences in context destroy any possibilities for easy and straightforward extrapolation or inference from one case to the other.

Likewise, the finding of common elements in behavioral and dynamic therapies is of uncertain significance unless these elements are also connected in a common system of functional relations or in a common structure of meaning. Thus, the activation of unconscious fantasies in the context of a behavioral therapy (cf. Mendelsohn & Silverman, Chapter 9, this volume) need not have much in common with the elicitation of such fantasies in a psychoanalysis: The contexts are different. Or, a process resembling desensitization that occurs in dynamic therapy may phenotypically resemble something that occurs in behavior therapy but that may be considerably different on a genotypic level.

Concept of the Prototype

Ultimately, a reliance on common elements as the basis for claiming integration forces confrontation of a more fundamental issue involving the essential nature of the terms *behavioral* and *psychodynamic.* Conceptually, these global labels refer to categories. As such, there are two broadly different ways of understanding them. In the first (traditional) view, a category is bounded and well defined by explicit rules for inclusion or exclusion of specific elements as members of the category. These rules specify features that are individually necessary and jointly sufficient for category membership: Everything in the universe may thus be placed either inside or outside the category without equivocation.

Recent theorizing and research in cognitive psychology (e.g., Rosch, 1977; Rosch,Mervis, Gray, Johnson, & Boyer-Braem, 1976) offers the concept of a "prototype" as an alternate means for constituting a category. Unlike the clearly delineated boundaries of a traditional category, a prototype is "fuzzy." All of the properties of a prototype characterize at least some members of the category, but no property (or group of properties short of the whole) is either sufficient or necessary for membership in the category. This conception of the prototype resembles an earlier notion, that of the "open concept" (Pap, 1953, cited in Meehl, 1973).

If behavior therapy and psychodynamic therapy are regarded as traditional categories with clear boundaries and a well-defined set of necessary and sufficient conditions for category membership, then finding common elements implies relatively unambiguous support for integration. A substantial sharing of elements is an absolute prerequisite, in this view, to an integration of the categories of behavior therapy and psychodynamic therapy.

On the other hand, if behavior therapy and psychodynamic therapy are regarded as prototypes, then finding common elements bears a less certain relationship to prospects for integration. Because the relations of individual elements to a prototypic whole are variable,* even a quantitatively substantial sharing of elements may not support a conclusion of essential similarity or integration of the therapies. Although it is intuitively appealing to assume that finding a "large" number of common elements would improve an argument for integration, this is simply not the case. As previously noted, there is no limit to the number of ways in which a domain of knowledge can be partitioned. Hence, there is no limit to the number of elements that are potentially common to dynamic and behavioral therapies. Ultimately, the issue of common elements must rest on the assertion of common functional relationships: The issue cannot be reduced to a simple cumulative counting up of instances of apparent commonality.

* Lakoff and Johnson (1980, Chapter 19) offer an instructive discussion of the potential for variability in prototype categories. Even particular purposes may enter into the classification process. Lakoff and Johnson offer, as an example, the observation that whereas, for purposes of insurance, a moped is not categorized as a motorcycle, it becomes categorized as one for purposes of bridge tolls.

Knowledge as Unitary, Pluralistic, or?

Integration is both etymologically and conceptually related to ideas of oneness. It implies a reduction of multiplicity into a unitary form. All efforts to integrate psychodynamic and behavioral therapies signify attempts, however piecemeal, to transform currently perceived multiplicities into a unified perspective.

Beginning, perhaps with the ancient Greeks' search for the Immortal Principle, the unification of knowledge has been a consistent theme in Western thought (Pirsig, 1974). The philosopher–historian Foucault (1972) observes that modern scholasticism makes it a virtual "duty" to seek underlying principles of cohesion when one is faced with apparent contradiction, irregularity, or incompatibility. The effects of the search for unity may be traced through the broadest cultural manifestations (e.g., historical shifts toward monotheistic religious forms) as well as through narrower and more personal contexts (e.g., an individual's representational world in which the "good" and the "healthy" are defined in terms of wholeness and integration of one's self [cf. Greenwald, 1980; Kernberg, 1976]). In the case of science, researchers are constrained by principles of parsimony not to multiply distinctions or contradictions: Indeed, it is commonly believed that the core purpose of the scientific method is to select a single truth from among many hypothetical truths.

However, there is not unanimity on the subject of unification. Cogent voices claim that Occam's razor would have multiple blades, that the search for unity is a fool's quest. Royce (1970) asserts flatly that psychology is "unready" for "grand unifying theories"; he argues his point by tracing a history of failed efforts, each based on overgeneralizations and inadequate data. Shaw (1972), writing under the title "Towards Continued Disunity in Psychology" expresses disbelief in even the potential worth of integration efforts. Koch (1964) steps beyond the doubting stances of Royce and Shaw and argues that psychology *cannot avoid* heterogeneity of knowledge. He endorses outright abandonment of philosophical presuppositions that prompt an "absurd quest for conceptual homogeneity and unbridled generality" (p. 33). An example of a scholar, most extremely opposed to the search for unity is Feyerabend (1970) who actually offers an outline for what he calls an "anarchic theory of knowledge."

The heart of this ancient* controversy is captured elegantly by Bronowski (1978) who asks:

> Are we creating the concepts out of which we make science, or are they hidden there all the time? Now this is a tremendous intellectual bifurcation. And also

* See, for example, the ancient Greek distinction between *essence* and *appearance* or Emmanuel Kant's concept of *a priori* categories.

> a fairly emotional one . . . the world is . . . pretty well divided into people who would like to think that our analysis of nature is a personal and highly imaginative creation and those who would like to think we are merely discovering what is there. (pp. 54–55)

Those who believe that we are simply "discovering what is there" typically regard the integration or unity of knowledge as a given, *a priori* state of affairs (e.g., Bateson, 1979; Bronowski, 1978; Staats, 1981). There is a belief that the world is "totally connected," that "there are no events in the universe which are not tied to every other event in the universe" (Bronowski, 1978, p. 58). This belief affirms but one, ultimate, actuality: The various disciplines and epistemologies must all be finally reflective of this single unitary reality. Differences in the superficial conceptual expression of that reality may exist and may even seem irreconcilable, but they are all necessarily part of the same interconnected totality. A belief in knowledge as unitary stands behind assertions that "strong inference" methods (Platt, 1964) and other self-corrective methods of science will lead to automatic refinement and eventual convergence of theories.

In contrast, those who believe that knowledge is ultimately an imaginative creation (a position not necessarily inconsistent with an empirical orientation!) typically regard our understanding of reality as fundamentally pluralistic. In Royce's (1982) words, our knowledge is inescapably "multimethodological, multivariate, multiepistemic, multi-world-view, multiparadigmatic, multitheoretic, and multi-disciplinary" (p. 259). Koch (1981) concurs, observing that "paradigms, theories, models (or whatever is one's label for conceptual ordering devices) can never prove pre-emptive or preclusive of alternate organizations" (p. 268). The clearest instances of pluralistic knowledge orientations appear in mathematics where the formalities of axiomatic presupposition literally create new worlds of meaning. Thus, for example, we have Euclidean and non-Euclidean geometries, each of which instantiates its own universe through the creative device of positing its own set of fundamental axioms. An especially explicit example of pluralistic reality orientation occurs in psychology with the work of Hillman (1975). Hillmann argues that the inconsistent manifestations of a personality actually represent multiple selves living in multiple realities and not simply different faces of a single self. In sum, the pluralistic view holds that unities or integrations are simply convenient and perhaps heuristic resting places for thought, created rather than discovered, that punctuate but do not define the flow of an infinite *multi*verse (rather than *uni*verse).

These two views of reality have profound implications for the integration of behavioral and psychodynamic therapies. The knowledge-as-unitary perspective prompts the common arguments that there are "hidden similarities" between the two therapies. Likewise, common assertions that behavior therapists "unwittingly" employ transference and unconscious fantasy manipulations (cf. Mendelsohn & Silverman, Chapter 9, this volume), whereas dynamic therapists inadvertently use principles of systematic reinforcement, extinction, or desensitization, also rest on the assumption that knowledge is unitary and that we are simply blinded to this fact by surface variability.

Thus, proponents of the knowledge-as-unitary view hold that contradictions between behavioral and dynamic therapies are ultimately illusory. Efforts are directed at resolving and dissipating these seeming differences in order that the *a priori* unity, the hidden resemblances, may be revealed. Claims that behavioral and dynamic therapies are irreconcilable seem nonsensical, in this view, because nothing is ultimately irreconcilable in a unitary reality. In short, the task here is not to discover whether integration is possible but, rather, to specify the details of how it can best be uncovered.

Alternately, a view of reality and knowledge as pluralistic finds immediate support in the manifest surface diversity of behavioral and dynamic therapies. In contrast to the reality-as-unitary position, which views contradictions as ultimately illusory, the pluralistic position cherishes contradictions as spurs to the creation of knowledge and as antidotes to the suffocating intellectual effects of an *a priori* assumption of unity. The pluralistic view, like the Freudian unconscious, easily accommodates stable contradictions that do not press for resolution. Thus, unlike the reality-as-unitary position, which can only support the view that behavioral and dynamic therapies are compatible, the pluralistic position may accommodate any possible stance on questions of integration. It is possible to claim under the pluralistic rubric that the therapies are fundamentally incompatible. However, it is also possible to claim that, among the multiple conceivable realities, there exists one or more in which dynamic and behavioral therapies are not contradictory. This latter argument may be implicit in assertions that an integration will require the emergence of a third, more encompassing paradigm (cf. Mahoney, Chapter 10, this volume; Wachtel, 1977).

It is also possible to step outside the dichotomous framework of "unitary" versus "pluralistic" into a third perspective (indicated by the question mark in the title of this section). This third option is a neutral one that withholds assumptions about the nature of reality and views contradictions as something to be simply described, characterized, and localized, without attempt to discover evidence or viewpoints with which inconsistencies may be either dissipated or confirmed. From this neutral perspective, the unitary and the pluralistic positions both may be valued, and together may transform the process of knowledge seeking into a heuristic dialectic between leveling (unitary) and sharpening (pluralistic). We have an investment in unity, but we also have an investment in multiplicity and contradiction, else what is there to unify?

From this neutral perspective, an ultimate therapeutic integration would be tragic. It would sap psychology of its intellectual vitality by removing the multiplicity that fuels the knowledge-generating process. Likewise, if the search for integration were abandoned, a surrender to unlimited multiplicity would also bring knowledge generation to a halt. Here, the question of whether therapeutic integration is possible becomes no more or less than the question of whether behavior therapists and psychodynamic therapists can continue a dialogue, knowing that integration is a *process* and not a *product,* and that therefore no final or ultimate answer is attainable or even appropriate. Integration is thus, in one sense, welcome and inevitable; and in another (totalistic) sense, it is undesirable.

CONCLUSIONS

In the preface to his 1977 book *Psychoanalysis and Behavior Therapy: Toward an Integration,* Paul Wachtel said: "Psychology has been obsessed with answers. This book is concerned mainly with questions." I have argued here, in much the same spirit, that meaningful inquiry into possibilities for therapeutic integration requires prior attention to three classes of auxiliary questions: (a) What, exactly, is being integrated (units of analysis)? (b) How are the units interrelated (models for the relationship of the therapies)? and (c) What philosophical issues condition our overall view of integration?

Examination of the existing literature on therapeutic integration shows a wide variation in the way these questions are implicitly or explicitly answered. This variation confuses the scholarly dialogue and confounds disagreement over substantive issues with disagreement over how best to approach the subject. We risk concluding that the therapies are incompatible when, in fact, we have only demonstrated our ability to structure the questions of integration in divergent ways.

Still, one might ask about a supreme integration, one that somehow manages to encompass all possible units of analysis and all possible models of relationship; one that supersedes apparent philosophical divergence with an alternate, superordinate metaphilosophy. In response to such a rhetorical question, I can only offer a personal vision, expressed in the following conjectures.

First, I believe there is no single best pathway to an integration. Over time, we should expect to see multiple mini-integrations (i.e., integrations of circumscribed aspects of each therapeutic domain), and we must resist undisciplined extrapolation from these necessarily simple cases to the complex whole. The issues of integration will not yield to easy analysis, and we should expect and tolerate uncertainty and ambiguity for an indefinite period. There will be inevitable dead ends and pseudoissues along the way that are accompanied by the perennial danger of premature closure.

Second, I believe that a meaningful integration will involve more than a simple "fading of blinders": It will be an active, imaginative, creative process that takes advantage of all resources for thought. We need empirical data, rational analysis, *and* emergent metaphors. I disagree with Franks's (Chapter 8, this volume) placement of these sources of knowledge in a hierarchic arrangement with rationality at the top and the "notional" (metaphoric) at the bottom. Much can be gained from viewing these epistemological choices as coequals (cf. Royce, 1970).

Third, I believe the best initial hope for integration may lie outside the realm of scholarship. I expect that the seed crystals of integration may grow first in the preintellectual awareness of therapists who have a practical working knowledge of both approaches.* Book learning is not enough! Assimilation of the crucial subtleties of each approach requires face-to-face contact with acknowledged masters. Consequently, the major long-term task of integration becomes an administrative and political one—that of arranging training programs and practice environments that permit or even require the juxtaposition of both therapies in a single therapist. Paraphrasing Koch (1964), to expect someone untrained in the subtle discriminations and sensitivities of both therapies to make a substantial contribution to their integration is as grotesque as supposing that an illiterate might contribute to the psychology of language.

Finally, our approach to therapeutic integration (and to the advancement of therapeutic knowledge generally) might be facilitated if we avoided the terms *behavior therapy* and *psychodynamic therapy*. We commonly acknowledge that these words have few, if any, consensus referents; that each subsumes enormous multiplicities, some of which may even be internally contradictory. Yet, there seems to be strong resistance to dumping the use of these global labels as unproductive. Perhaps, as Goldfried (1980) suggests, without these terms we would not know which conventions to attend

* I owe this conviction to the ideas of mathematician Henri Poincaré who made a similar point regarding the role of the subliminal self in mathematical invention ("Mathematical Creation," reprinted in *The World Of Mathematics*. New York: Simon & Schuster, 1956, pp. 2041–2050).

or which journals to read. Such inconveniences would be trivial if, by abandoning this language, we could move our observations and discussions closer to the specificity of their phenomenal occurrence, leaving behind some excess freight of loose extended families of abstract concepts. I imagine a situation in which, whenever someone wished to say behavior therapy or psychodynamic therapy, he or she would be encouraged to paraphrase the remarks in a simpler language, less fortified with jargon, obscure abstractions, and reifications. We might be tongue-tied for a while, but in the long run I believe the exercise would sharpen our thinking about therapy and about prospects for therapeutic integration.* Indeed, from such a perspective we might even conclude that the question "Is integration possible?" represents a pseudoissue and that other questions, some yet unasked, will advance us farther toward the ultimate goal of understanding what makes therapy work.

AUTOBIOGRAPHICAL STATMENT

In the world as I imagine it, most clinicians concerned with the integration of behavioral and psychodynamic therapies have learned the two approaches one at a time. A solid grounding in one form of therapy provides, I expect, a comforting base for excursions into alien therapeutic territory.

My own professional education, in contrast, did not permit such a developmental course. The required first-year curriculum at Rutgers Graduate School of Applied and Professional Psychology placed an introduction to psychoanalytic theory (taught by a card-carrying Freudian analyst) side by side with a parallel course in behavior therapy (taught by no less an authority than Cyril Franks). Consequently, I was dealing with issues of therapeutic integration almost before I knew there was supposed to be some incompatibility between the two approaches.

Subsequent experiences were equally catholic. Later course work at Rutgers included classes and intensive clinical supervision in long- and short-term dynamic therapies, in behavioral therapies, and in interpersonal approaches—all offered and received in an atmosphere of remarkable openness, tolerance, and cooperation that obviated any inclination to form rigid allegiance to one or another perspective. This going back and forth between behavioral and dynamic influences continued after graduate school. A clinical internship and postdoctoral residency at the University of Oregon Medical School leaned heavily in the behavioral direction, whereas my present position at the Vanderbilt Center for Psychotherapy Research focuses on the study of time-limited dynamic treatments.

* Reviewers of earlier drafts of this chapter split about evenly on the question of whether such an exercise is possible. My own belief is that it is worth trying, keeping in mind that being stripped of one's jargon can be an extremely uncomfortable experience.

The collective effect of this diverse education has been somewhat unsettling. There have been occasions when the pull of contrasting ideas has left me feeling a bit like a decompensated multiple personality. The ideas of this chapter are, in a sense, a personal diary, the accumulated notes of a wandering traveler. They represent the current state of my efforts to digest an exceptionally eclectic education. I share these reflections optimistically, with the expectation that others on a similar path may find them useful.

THOMAS E. SCHACHT, PSY.D.

REFERENCES

Adelson, J. Still vital after all these years. *Psychology Today,* 1982, *16*(4), 52–59.

Alexander, F. The dynamics of psychotherapy in the light of learning theory. *American Journal of Psychiatry,* 1963, *120,* 440–448.

Atkinson, J. W. Studying personality in the context of an advanced motivational psychology. *American Psychologist,* 1981, *36*(2), 117–128.

Bateson, G. *Mind and nature: A necessary unity.* New York: E. P. Dutton, 1979.

Bieber, I. On behavior therapy: A critique. *Journal of the American Academy of Psychoanalysis,* 1973, *1,* 39–52.

Birk, L., & Brinkley-Birk, A. Psychoanalysis and behavior therapy. *American Journal of Psychiatry,* 1974, *131,* 499–510.

Brady, J. P. Psychotherapy by a combined behavioral and dynamic approach. *Comprehensive Psychiatry.* 1968, *9,* 536–543.

Breger, L., & McGaugh, J. L. Critique and reformulation of 'learning theory' approaches to psychotherapy and neurosis. *Psychological Bulletin,* 1965, *63,* 338–358.

Bronowski, J. *The origins of knowledge and imagination.* New Haven: Yale University Press, 1978.

Dollard, J., & Miller, N. E. *Personality and psychotherapy.* New York: McGraw-Hill, 1950.

Eysenck, H. J. *Behaviour therapy and the neuroses.* Oxford: Pergamon, 1960.

Feather, B. W., & Rhoads, J. M. Psychodynamic behavior therapy—I. Theory and rationale. *Archives of General Psychiatry,* 1972, *26,* 496–502.

Feyerabend, P. Against method: An outline of an anarchic theory of knowledge. In M. Radner & S. Winokur (Eds.), *Minnesota studies in the philosophy of science* (Vol. 4). Minneapolis: University of Minnesota Press, 1970.

Frank, J. D. Restoration of morale and behavior change. In A. Burton (Ed.), *What makes behavior change possible?* New York: Brunner/Mazel, 1976.

French, T. M. Interrelations between psychoanalysis and the experimental work of Pavlov. *American Journal of Psychiatry,* 1933, *12,* 1165—1203.

Foucault, M. *The archaeology of knowledge.* New York: Pantheon, 1972.

Garfield, S. L. Psychotherapy: A 40 year appraisal. *American Psychologist,* 1981, *36*(2), 174–183.

Garfield, S. L., & Kurtz, R. Clinical psychologists in the 1970's. *American Psychologist,* 1976, *31*(1), 1–9.

Goffman, E. *Frame analysis: An essay on the organization of experience.* Cambridge: Harvard University Press, 1974.

Goldfried, M. R. Toward the delineation of therapeutic change principles. *American Psychologist,* 1980, *35,* 991–999.

Goldfried, M. R. (Ed.). *Converging trends in psychotherapy.* New York: Springer, 1982.

Greenwald, A. G. The totalitarian ego: Fabrication and revision of personal history. *American Psychologist,* 1980, *35*(7), 603–618.
Gullick, E. L., & Blanchard, E. B. The use of psychotherapy and behavior therapy in the treatment of an obsessional disorder—An experimental case study. *Journal of Nervous and Mental Disease,* 1973, *156,* 427–431.
Hillman, J. *Re-visioning psychology.* New York: Harper & Row, 1975.
Kernberg, O. *Object-relations theory and clinical psychoanalysis.* New York: Aronson, 1976.
Koch, S. Psychology and emerging conceptions of knowledge as unitary. In T. W. Wann (Ed.), *Behaviorism and phenomenology: Contrasting bases for modern psychology.* Chicago: University of Chicago Press, 1964.
Koch, S. The nature and limits of psychological knowledge: Lessons of a century qua "science". *American Psychologist,* 1981, *36*(3), 257–269.
Kubie, L. S. Relation of the conditioned reflex to psychoanalytic technic. *Archives of Neurology and Psychiatry,* 1934, *32,* 137–1142.
Lambley, P. The use of assertive training and psychodynamic insight in the treatment of migraine headache. *Journal of Nervous and Mental Disease,* 1976, *163,* 61–64.
Lakoff, G., & Johnson, M. *Metaphors we live by.* Chicago: University of Chicago Press, 1980.
Lazarus, A. A. In support of technical eclecticism. *Psychological Reports,* 1967, *21,* 415–416.
Lazarus, A. A. Has behavior therapy outlived its usefulness? *American Psychologist,* 1977, *32,* 550–554.
Lazarus, A. A. *The practice of multimodal therapy.* New York: McGraw-Hill, 1981.
Levay, N., Weissberg, J. H., & Blaustein, A. B. Concurrent sex therapy and psychoanalytic psychotherapy by separate therapists: Effectiveness and implications. *Psychiatry,* 1976, *39,* 355–363.
Liotti, G., & Reda, M. Some epistemological remarks on behavior therapy, cognitive therapy, and psychoanalysis. *Cognitive Therapy and Research,* 1981, *5,* 231–236.
Luborsky, L. *Evaluation of manual-guided therapies by rated tape sessions.* Paper presented at the Society for Psychotherapy Research, Jeffersonville, Vt., 1982.
Marks, J. M., & Gelder, M. G. Common ground between behavior therapy and psychodynamic methods. *British Journal of Medical Psychology,* 1966, *39,* 11–23.
Marmor, J. Psychoanalytic therapy and theories of learning. *Science and Psychoanalysis,* 1964, *7,* 265–279.
Marmor, J. Dynamic psychotherapy and behavior therapy: Are they irreconcilable? *Archives of General Psychiatry,* 1971, *24,* 22–28.
Marmor, J., & Woods, S. M. (Eds.). *The interface between the psychodynamic and behavioral therapies.* New York: Plenum Press, 1980.
Meehl, P. E. Some methodological reflections on the difficulties of psychoanalytic research. In *Psychological Issues,* Monograph 30, Vol. VIII(2). New York: International Universities Press, 1973.
Messer, S. B., & Winokur, M. Some limits to the integration of psychoanalytic and behavior therapy. *American Psychologist,* 1980, *35*(9), 818–827.
Pap, A. Reduction sentences and open concepts. *Methodos,* 1953, *5,* 3–30.
Pirsig, R. M. *Zen and the art of motorcycle maintenance.* New York: Morrow, 1974.
Poincaré, H. Mathematical creation. In J. R. Newman (Ed.), *The world of mathematics.* New York: Simon & Schuster, 1956.
Rosch, E. Human categorization. In N. Warren (Ed.), *Advances in cross-cultural psychology* (Vol. 1) New York: Academic Press, 1977.
Rosch, E., Mervis, C. B., Gray, W. D., Johnson, D. M., & Boyer-Braem, P. Basic objects in natural categories. *Cognitive Psychology,* 1976, *8,* 382–439.
Royce, J. R. The present situation in theoretical psychology. In J. R. Royce (Ed.), Toward

unification in psychology: The 1st Banff Conference on Theoretical Psychology. Toronto: University of Toronto Press, 1970.

Royce, J. R. Philosophic issues, Division 24, and the future. *American Psychologist*, 1982, *37*(3), 258–266.

Sarwer-Foner, G. J. Combined psychotherapy and pharmacotherapy. In T. P. Karasu & L. Bellak (Eds.), Specialized techniques in individual psychotherapy. New York: Brunner/Mazel, 1980.

Segraves, R., & Smith, R. C. Concurrent psychotherapy and behavior therapy: Treatment of psychoneurotic outpatients. *Archives of General Psychiatry*, 1976, *33*, 756–763.

Shaw, R. Towards continued disunity in psychology. *Contemporary Psychology*, 1972, *17*, 75–76.

Shectman, F. A. Operant conditioning and psychoanalysis: Contrasts, similarities, and some thoughts about integration. *American Journal of Psycotherapy*. 1975, *29*, 72–78.

Shoben, E. J. A learning theory interpretation of psychotherapy. *Harvard Educational Review*, 1948, *18*, 129–145.

Shoben, E. J. Psychotherapy as a problem in learning theory. *Psychological Bulletin*, 1949, *46*, 366–392.

Sloane, R. B. The converging paths of behavior therapy and psychotherapy. *American Journal of Psychiatry*, 1969, *125*, 877–885.

Sloane, R. B., Staples, F. R., Cristol, A. H., Yorkston, N. J., & Whipple, K. *Psychotherapy versus behavior therapy*. Cambridge: Harvard University Press, 1975.

Smith, M. L., & Glass, G. V. Meta-analysis of psychotherapy outcome studies. *American Psychologist*, 1977, *32*, 752–760.

Staats, A. W. Paradigmatic behaviorism, unified theory, unified theory construction methods, and the zeitgeist of separatism. *American Psychologist*, 1981, *36*(3), 239–256.

Strupp, H. H. A reformulation of the dynamics of the therapist's contribution. In A. S. Gurman & A. M. Razin (Eds.), *Effective psychotherapy: A handbook of research*. New York: Pergamon, 1977.

Szasz, T. S. Behavior therapy and psychoanalysis. *Medical Opinion Review*, 1967, *2*, 24–29.

Wachtel, P. *Psychoanalysis and behavior therapy: Toward an integration*. New York: Basic Books, 1977.

Weitzman, B. Behavior therapy and psychotherapy. *Psychological Review*, 1967, *74*, 300–317.

Wolf, E. Learning theory and psychoanalysis. *British Journal of Medical Psychology*, *1966*, *39*, 1–10.

Wolpe, J. Behavior therapy versus psychoanalysis: Therapeutic and social implications. *American Psychologist*, 1981, *36*(2), 159–164.

4

Integration, Emergence, and the Structure of Scientific Progress

Commentary on Thomas E. Schacht

MICHAEL J. MAHONEY

I enjoyed reading Schacht's chapter and commentaries on our diverse approaches to the issue of integration among the psychotherapies. As someone not infrequently seduced by what Lewis Thomas (1979) calls "transcendental metaworry," I also found myself fascinated with Schacht's analysis of metatheoretical issues and the problems of communication—let alone "unit analysis"—when competing paradigms and perspectives are being considered.

I shall begin my commentary by concurring with Schacht that one of the serious impediments to an adequate analysis of "convergence" and/or "integration" lies in the naive assumption of equivalence common to many "uniformity myths" (Kiesler, 1966). In the case of psychoanalysis and behaviorism, Schacht has lamented that some authors seem to deal only with the more recent developments in these two areas:

> [Some writers] range freely across the contemporary and the older literature as if there were no problem of comparability—as if each therapy were a fixed entity that, though evolving, possessed an unchanging core. The major danger here involves unexpunged anachronisms, psychology's perennial problem of transforming ephemeral historical documents into eternal historical monuments

MICHAEL J. MAHONEY • Department of Psychology, Pennsylvania State University, University Park, Pennsylvania 16802.

> (Koch, 1964). An extreme of this problematic tendency (thankfully becoming infrequent) is demonstrated by authors who insist that all psychodynamic thinking must be understood as footnotes to Freud and that all behavioral therapies retain similar connections to Pavlov and Skinner. (p.110)

The problem of defining a paradigm and pointing to an instance of it is one that Schacht is well aware of and is one that remains a major task for the sociology and psychology of science (Lakatos & Musgrave, 1970; Weimer, 1979). Whatever else they may be, however, it seems increasingly clear that neither theories nor therapies are "fixed entities" at all. Evolution and development have become so apparent in the last two decades of psychotherapy research that it would require a fairly rigid and parochial myopia to overlook the major and minor changes in which we are participant observers. I also concur with Thomas Kuhn in his (1977) defense of the unchanging and more conservative aspects of structure as offering valuable contributions to the overall development of science.

This point could be extended by noting that the meaning of technical terms within a paradigm may change over time as the paradigm matures. It would not be difficult to document, for example, how some of the most seminal concepts in early psychoanalysis and behaviorism have been modified and refined—often by their own creators—as experience and inquiry have dictated. I am not quite as pessimistic as Schacht seems to be about the possibility of genuine communication at the "unit level," but I must confess to having no tangible lexicon for practical applications. Goldfried's (1980) invitation to use the language of cognitive psychology may be a step in a neutral and progressive direction (although the state of the lexicon in that field is not quite as clean or crystalline as one might desire). Moreover, there is a growing consensus on the issue referred to earlier—namely, that it is simply impossible to select units of analysis and questions or commentaries comprised of their compound without incurring extensive and enduring battles with a host of ambiguities. The ambiguities, in my opinion, stem from the impossibility of translating incompatible deep structures into surface structure particulars that are supposed to be compatible. Surface structure content—whether it is analyzed at the level of stream of consciousness, psychotherapy process, or wherever—must always be a reflection of (and therefore constrained by) the abstract processes in the human nervous system that constitute its core-ordering activities.

I believe that this is again a point of agreement—or at least convergence—between my own views and those of Schacht. In outlining the six models that he sees as describing a relationship between behavioral and dynamic therapies, he notes that the "translation problem" is a pervasive one in any discussion of this topic. Going beyond Goldfried's (1980) acknowledgment of inevitable vocabulary differences and occasional negative emotional connotations, Schacht goes on to contend:

> There are reasons to believe that difficulties with translation models go much deeper, that they reside in the basic nature of human symbolizing processes.
> The major problem lies in the ambiguity inherent in all languages and, therefore, in any attempts to translate from one language system to another. (p. 116)

> In short, translation models risk producing empty constructs that fail to make effective observational and perceptual contact with the basic phenomena of interest. Such translation becomes a mere conceptual calisthenic, a demonstration of the tremendous human capacity to symbolize and imagine, to see something in terms of something else. (p. 116)

Translation models are, of course, only one of those proposed as describing the aforementioned relationship. The other five are the separatism model (which views the two perspectives as fundamentally incompatible and disparate), the complementarity model (which views each perspective as suitable for distinct but complementary functions), the synergistic model (which contends that each perspective and therapy can "enhance the operation and outcome of the other"), the emergence model (which points to the development of new properties), and finally, the metatheoretical model (which might be more appropriately described as an approach rather than a model). I found Schacht's classificatory system quite intriguing and heuristic. My hunch is that he would agree that these classifications, like most others, are "tentative" and nonexclusive.

As a student of process, I find it difficult to resist the temptation to note briefly the (unconscious?) progression implied in the sequencing of these models. The separatism model is presented first and—because it views the two perspectives as fundamentally incompatible—there is little to be hoped for in the way of either integration or exchange. Both paradigms retain their insular identities, and the competition continues. Model 2 is explicitly labeled as a "polar opposite" of Model 1 in that it subjugates the "concepts and/or language" of one perspective to those of the other. Because one of the perspectives must be viewed as "primary" in this model, there are also limited opportunities for the kind of mutualistic exchange considered essential for conceptual development. Model 3 (complementarity) returns to an egalitarian relationship in which separateness is seen as essential *and* heuristic. It is here for the first time that there is any genuine "working together," and even this involves a very cautious coordination of therapeutic effort. It is also noteworthy that in this most primitive form of exchange, the client becomes the crucible for the chemistry involved. Little or no benefits accrue to the conceptual scaffolding and technical expertise of the estranged contributors.

In the fourth model (synergistic), we see the beginnings of mutualistic exchange. The client remains a crucible here, but the two therapies "are not restricted to operating on separate sets of problems. Rather, they both focus on the same problems with a mutual potentiation of therapeutic effect." There is, again, a protection of each therapy's precious identity, but there is some hope that the forced interaction in service of a joint goal may lead to a facilitative and welcome effect for the client involved. It should be noted that in Models 3 and 4, the dividends from using conjoint approaches to therapy are received by the client (and vicariously, one would hope, by the contributing therapists). It is only when we move to Model 5, however, that "emergent" therapeutic techniques are anticipated. This is a point that Schacht appropriately notes. He then goes on to discuss some of the more esoteric issues around "genuine integration" and the demarcation between emergent and nonemergent techniques. Finally, in Model 6, we reach the level that "presents the most formidable intellectual challenge." It is here, in the ethereal abstractions of "metapsychologies" that a more global model of human nature is expected to develop. Although Schacht does not consider Model 6 to be "necessarily superordinate" over the other five, he concedes that it is "simply more abstract" and then goes on to devote the final section of his chapter to "metatheoretic issues."

This rhetorical progression from insular "separatism" toward metatheoretical analysis is, to my reading, a harmonic one that points us in the direction of examining our abstractions. Although I concur with Schacht's concern about the naiveté of equating "common elements" with logical warrant for integration, I think it is also important to recognize and commend attempts to move to the level of principles. As reflected in my biographical statement (Chapter 10, this volume), much of my own interest in the issue of convergence has stemmed from my belief that some forms of robustness may be detected *across* ostensibly divergent perspectives. This search for the "invariance within the variance" is similar to the strategy espoused by Goldfried (1980) when he notes:

> It has been suggested that there exists a "therapeutic underground," which may rarely appear in the literature, but which nonetheless reflects some common observations among well-seasoned clinicians as to what tends to be effective. If this indeed is the case, then such commonalities are likely to shed light on some very significant principles of change as they have managed to emerge in spite of the theoretical biases inherent in each of our varying orientations.

I believe that there are, of course, numerous ways to search for the "metaprinciples of change," but I think that this remains one of the more productive.

Introduction of the concept of a "prototype" as an "open concept" and contrasting its heuristic potential with that of the more confining boundaries of our traditional categories is an excellent prelude to the affirmation of *process* over *product* in the prioritization of our research endeavors. The concept of a prototype is not unlike that of a "schema," at least as the latter has been used by some theorists. Ironically, after pointing out the differential effects of considering behaviorism and psychoanalysis as either categories or prototypes, we are left to decide for ourselves as to which category [*sic*] to assign them. It is, indeed, most appropriate that the relevance of our psychological "edging processes"—the processes that create and modify the "boundaries" of our experiencing—should be so aptly illustrated in the context of its own discussion!

The final section of Schacht's chapter is devoted to the nature of knowledge and, in particular, to whether knowledge would be more adequately conceptualized as a unitary or pluralistic endeavor (or, in commendable openness, he allows the possibility that it is neither and/or both of these). Having strewn my own net on these waters before, I shall try to be brief in my present commentary (Mahoney, 1976, 1979, in press). Let me begin by saying that I could not agree more heartily with my colleague's having brought this issue to the forefront. We must persevere in harvesting our growing recognition that human knowing processes lie at the very foundation of our science and that a refinement of our understanding of them will necessarily move us on to a more adequate understanding of developmental psychopathology, the maintenance of self-limiting and antisocial patterns, and—most importantly—what we can (and cannot) hope to do in facilitating the use of that knowledge in psychotherapy, parenting, and other forms of education. The idea of separate realities and an infinite "*multi*verse" is one that emphasizes the need for our understanding more about the development and maintenance of personal meaning systems ("personal realities"). To ask whether knowledge is unitary or pluralistic, however, is to somehow separate knowledge from the knower, and this is perhaps why my own tentative "bet" is placed on the wisdom inherent in teleonomic growth. It is, I believe, in this sense that Schacht is quite accurate in suggesting that integration may be "welcome and evitable" while simultaneously being "undesirable."

Before I stray a bit from the structure of the chapter, let me say that I find myself in substantial agreement with its general direction and conclusion:

> The issues of integration will not yield to easy analysis, and we should expect and tolerate uncertainty and ambiguity for an indefinite period. There will be inevitable dead ends and pseudoissues along the way that are accompanied by the perennial danger of premature closure. (p. 127)

I also concur that the "seed crystals of integration may grow first in the preintellectual awareness of therapists." Although I do not think we need to confine this to therapists who have been trained in the two competing perspectives, I share Schacht's concern about the limitations of modern rationalization. Our next generation of models are not likely to emanate from the sterile deductions of a "ratiocentric" analysis. And, it is on this point that an increasing number of us seem to be nodding in agreement regarding the "illusion of technique" (Barrett, 1967) and the inherent limitations of all symbolic maps that presume to capture the elusive territory of experience. A related point here is the distinction between "contexts of discovery" and "contexts of evaluation" in scientific inquiry (Weimer, 1979). To philosophers, sociologists, and psychologists of science, the subjective aspects of learning and its evaluation are becoming increasingly inescapable. Although ratiocentric methods still dominate the current policies regarding hypothesis testing and theory evaluation, it is probably just as saturated with subjectivity as is the other side of inquiry (i.e., the context of discovery).

I shall conclude by reiterating my respect for the issues and themes that Schacht has brought into focus. Because my current conceptual home seems to hover somewhere around Models 5 and 6 in his system, it should not be surprising that I would close with some further genuflection toward emergence and metatheoretical analysis. For me, the unilateral pursuit of either unification or anarchy reflects a more profound failure to appreciate the complex dynamics of information exchange in an open system. In matters like these, I often find myself taking things slowly, minimizing foreclosure on possible paths of movement, and hoping/trusting that what will come out of all this will be far more lasting than the rhetoric.

REFERENCES

Barrett, W. *The illusion of technique.* New York: Doubleday, 1967.

Goldfried, M. R. Toward the delineation of therapeutic change principles. *American Psychologist,* 1980, *35,* 991–999.

Kiesler, D. J. Some myths of psychotherapy research and the search for a paradigm. *Psychological Bulletin,* 1966, *65,* 110–136.

Kuhn, T. S. *The essential tension: Selected studies in scientific tradition and change.* Chicago: University of Chicago Press, 1977.

Lakatos, I., & Musgrave, A. (Eds.). *Criticism and the growth of knowledge.* Cambridge: Cambridge University Press, 1970.

Mahoney, M. J. *Scientist as subject: The psychological imperative.* Cambridge: Ballinger, 1976.

Mahoney, M. J. Psychology of the scientist: An evaluative review. *Social Studies of Science,* 1979, *9,* 349–375.

Mahoney, M. J. Scientific publication and epistemic progress. *American Psychologist,* in press.

Thomas, L. *The Medusa and the snail.* New York: Viking Press, 1979.

Weimer, W. B. *Notes on the methodology of scientific research.* Hillsdale, N. J.: Erlbaum, 1979.

5

Integration of Psychodynamic and Behavioral Psychotherapies

Conceptual versus Empirical Syntheses

ALAN E. KAZDIN

Integrationism refers to the combination of alternative views or conceptual positions into a unified whole. In the context of clinical psychology, several areas can be identified in which alternative and seemingly conflicting conceptual positions are undergoing integration. Efforts toward integration might be viewed as a pervasive ecumenical spirit or heightened scholarship among professionals whose views have been in opposition. However, underlying the spirit of compromise and openness is the stark realization that simple answers to major questions and narrow conceptual positions do not begin to explain current evidence in many areas of research. The complexity of the findings in many areas within clinical psychology have helped foster an increased receptivity to integrationism and eclecticism.

The larger movement toward integrationism in clinical psychology can be illustrated in different areas of research. In the area of personality theory, as one example, several different views on the nature, organization, and

---

ALAN E. KAZDIN • Western Psychiatric Institute and Clinic, University of Pittsburgh School of Medicine, Pittsburgh, Pennsylvania 15261. Completion of this chapter was supported in part by a Research Scientist Development Award (MH 00353) and a grant (MH 35408) provided by the National Institute of Mental Health.

structure of personality and behavior have been proposed. Two opposing types of models are *trait theory* and *situationism* (Endler & Magnusson, 1976b). Trait theory accounts for consistencies in behavior by posing dispositions (traits) within individuals. Specific theories differ greatly in the nature, constellation, and types of traits but share in the view that overriding response dispositions account for performance across situations and over time. Alternatively, situational views have proposed that performance is accounted for primarily by environmental influences and contingencies of reinforcement rather than by influences within the individual. Situational views have been especially useful in accounting for the seeming inconsistencies in performance that persons evince across situations. Both trait and situational views, as general models of behavior, have their own sources of supporting evidence, but neither position adequately handles both the consistencies and inconsistencies in performance across situations and over time.

Trait and situational views, at seeming odds for many years, have been the focus of integrational efforts. Interactional models of personality have developed that look at the contribution of the person, the situation, and their interaction (Endler & Magnusson, 1976b; Pervin, 1977). Interactionism, sometimes referred to as a *situation-response model,* encompasses the merits of trait and situational theories by emphasizing the importance of the combined and reciprocal influences of person and situation variables. Behavior is viewed as a continuous interaction between the person and situations he or she encounters. The benefits of an interactional approach have been frequently demonstrated in studies showing that the interaction of person and situation variables provides a better account of performance than either trait or situation influences alone (Endler & Magnusson, 1976a). Interactionism in personality theory is an especially interesting example of integrationism because the convergence of trait and situational views has stimulated new areas of research.

The move toward integrationism has been of special interest in the area of psychotherapy. Different signs of integrationism can be discerned, depending on the level of analysis. For example, within behavior therapy, cognitive and behavioral views of maladaptive behavior and behavior change have often been in conflict. Yet, recently, views have been integrated in different ways (see Kendall & Hollon, 1979). Proponents of cognitive views, such as Bandura (1977b), have suggested that some of the more effective ways of altering cognitions is by focusing directly on overt behavior. Thus, cognitive ends are considered to be altered in part through behavioral means. Alternatively, cognitively based interventions (e.g., training in problem-solving skills) have been combined directly with manipulations of overt behavior (e.g., through reinforcement and punishment contingencies) to merge into cognitive-behavioral interventions.

In the area of psychotherapy, integrationism has recently referred to broad-based attempts to bring together disparate theoretical positions. Psychodynamic and behavioral views usually have been the major focus of integration (e.g., Goldfried, 1982; Marmor & Woods, 1980; Wachtel, 1977; Woody, 1971), in part because they represent the seemingly most discrepant and incompatible positions. However, other combinations have been proposed as well, such as behavioral and humanistic, or client-centered, views (e.g., Martin, 1972; Thoresen, 1973; Wandersman, Poppen, & Ricks, 1976) or psychodynamic and cognitive, or gestalt, views (Appelbaum, 1976; Sarason, 1979).

Integration of alternative views of psychotherapy can be achieved in different but somewhat related ways. First, different views or theories can be combined into a relatively unified position. Different views (e.g., psychodynamic and behavioral) or procedures might be combined, as for example, those that are reflected in the work of Wachtel (1977) and Feather and Rhoads (1972a, 1972b). Second, different theories and treatment procedures can be integrated by proposing a new superordinate theoretical framework or unifying construct that subsumes (or ignores) seemingly competing conceptual positions. In this form of integration, different treatment techniques (e.g., modeling, flooding, verbal psychotherapy) might be integrated, insofar as they are explained by a singular theoretical construct, as for example, those that are reflected in the work on self-efficacy by Bandura (1977a). Finally, integration might be achieved by seeking common elements from different treatment approaches. This form of integration focuses on strategies or principles of change that are evident in different treatments and is illustrated in the work of Goldfried (1980) and Frank (1973). These different ways of integrating alternative psychotherapies are not necessarily independent. For example, seeking common elements closely resembles seeking superordinate constructs. Certainly, the former is likely to lead to the latter.

This chapter focuses on the integration of psychodynamic and behavioral views of psychotherapy. The initial portion of the chapter will focus on the issues and obstacles associated with the attempt to combine psychodynamic and behavioral views. Other types of integration are discussed later.

The central thesis of the chapter is that integrationism as a general movement represents a highly significant development in psychotherapy. However, it may be the general movement that is worth promoting rather than the specific attempt to integrate psychodynamic and behavioral views. At this point, individual positions suffer from loose concepts and weak empirical bases, problems that are not resolved and perhaps may even be exacerbated by their combination. The overall goal is establishing an empirically based and theoretically viable account of therapy. Premature integration of specific positions that are not well supported on their own may greatly impede progress.

INTEGRATIONISM IN PSYCHOTHERAPY

The advisability, goals, and utility of adopting an integrationist approach toward therapy can be appreciated by looking at the impetus for the current movement. The contemporary historical context can also suggest whether particular forms of integration are more likely than others to satisfy the goals that are being sought.

Impetus for Integrationism

The history of integrationism involves more than the elaboration of past efforts to merge or identify bridges between competing conceptual views of psychopathology and psychotherapy (e.g., Alexander, 1963; French, 1933; Kubie, 1934). There is also a contemporary history and zeitgeist that are difficult to identify fully. The current influences must await the perspective that history, written in the future, will provide. Past efforts at integration have been reviewed elsewhere (Goldfried, 1982b; Goldfried & Padawer, 1982). For present purposes, it is useful to highlight some of the current influences that provide the impetus for seeking broad-based views of psychotherapy.

First, a major impetus for integrationism is recognition of the limitations associated with any singular or narrowly based treatment approach. The limitations can be illustrated with examination of diverse approaches. However, behavior therapy provides a useful illustration, in part, because of its recency as a movement and because of the strength of the claims that have been made on its behalf. Early in the history of behavior therapy, claims were made that behavioral techniques produced greater change than other techniques, especially those based on psychodynamic tenets. Also, specific techniques such as systematic desensitization were posited as extremely effective, even if they were restricted in the range of problems to which they might be applied. The claims made for "behavior therapy" as a general approach, of course, are difficult to interpret because the evidence only applies to specific procedures for select problems. There is no particular technique called "behavior therapy" for which evidence can be adduced. Also, when one examines specific techniques, advances have been made in some areas, but the jury is still out for many others (Kazdin & Wilson, 1978). Even for well-investigated techniques such as systematic desensitization, increased evidence has required increased humility in the claims that can be made (Emmelkamp, 1979). In short, the evidence for the clinical effectiveness of behavioral techniques is not that clear in many problem areas. For other techniques as well, claims about the clinical effectiveness are difficult to support. However, the case for behavior therapy may be especially dramatic, in part because of the claims for effectiveness and the extensive outcome research that has been conducted to test these claims.

Second, and related to the first point, is that comparisons of alternative treatment techniques, especially from opposing conceptual views, have failed to demonstrate the clear superiority of one technique over another. Conclusions reached from individual outcome studies (e.g., Sloane, Staples, Cristol, Yorkston, & Whipple, 1975) or reviews of the literature (e.g., Bergin & Lambert, 1978; Luborsky, Singer, & Luborsky, 1975) have indicated that different treatments produce change but are not differentially effective. More recently, meta-analyses have evaluated large numbers of outcome studies (e.g., Shapiro & Shapiro, 1981; Smith & Glass, 1977; Smith, Glass, & Miller, 1980). The results vary slightly from each other, but the overall conclusions are that different treatments tend to produce change and that they are not very different in the effects they produce. Although disagreements of the verdicts of meta-analysis remain (Kazdin & Wilson, 1978; Rachman & Wilson, 1980), it is fair to state that no set of techniques or general approach has an agreed-upon basis for flaunting its superiority. Ambiguity on the superiority of any particular approach certainly has provided the climate for integrationism.

Third, therapeutic approaches and techniques have proliferated greatly over the last several years. Although, at any given time, it is difficult to pinpoint the precise number of techniques in use, surveys have revealed tremendous growth. In the early 1960s, approximately 60 different types of psychotherapies were identified (Garfield, 1982). By the mid-1970s, over 130 techniques were delineated (National Institute of Mental Health, 1975). By the late 1970s, growth continued to encompass over 250 techniques (Herink, 1980). Of course, the emergence of new techniques has not been associated with the discarding of old techniques based on their lack of evidence (Frank, 1982). The large number of techniques point to the need to reach some common ground. Because no single general approach with a strong empirical base can be argued, an integration of many different views represents a viable if not essential option.

Fourth, increased attention has been accorded the fact that techniques that depart greatly in theory share many similarities in practice. Observations of treatment sessions and analyses of process variables such as therapist warmth, empathy, and other characteristics reveal great similarities among outpatient treatments, whether they are psychodynamic or behavioral (see Klein, Dittman, Parloff, & Gill, 1969; Sloane *et al.*, 1975). Also, the therapeutic relationship, long acknowledged as critical in traditional forms of insight-oriented psychotherapies, has been shown to be critical in various behavioral procedures as well (e.g., Alexander, Barton, Schiavo, & Parsons, 1976; Ford, 1978). Agreement on the importance of several common features among diverse therapies suggests the viability of a broadly based account of treatment.

Fifth, within particular areas of work, conceptual views have expanded. As already noted, within behavior therapy, concepts from cognitive psychology have broadened the conceptual bases of clinical problems and their treatment (Mahoney, 1974; Meichenbaum, 1977). Cognitive-behavioral therapy is now discussed as a broadened approach within behavioral research (Kendall & Hollon, 1979). The expansion of conceptual frameworks within previously restricted camps invites an even broader integrationism. Moreover, cognitive behavior therapy is closer to psychodynamic views than are noncognitively based behavioral positions (Messer & Winokur, 1980).

The preceding characteristics of the field by no means exhaust the sources of impetus for the contemporary movement toward integrationism (see Goldfried, 1982a, 1982b). The aforementioned points and others that might be listed all reflect the "growing discontent" (Goldfried, 1980) and "lack of satisfaction" (Garfield, 1982) with narrow views and approaches to the nature of therapy. The pervasive rejection of singular positions has also been attested to by surveys suggesting that the majority of clinical psychologists embrace eclecticism in their views of treatment (Garfield & Kurtz, 1976; Kelly, Goldberg, Fiske, & Kilkowski, 1978; Smith, 1982).

The general context for the current movement toward integrationism is important to mention independently of any particular attempt at integration. Scholars connected with current efforts have frequently discussed the integration of psychodynamic and behavioral positions (e.g., Marmor & Woods, 1980; Wachtel, 1977). However, the significance of integrationism may not be in the attempt to achieve this particular union but rather the larger interest in advancing the field beyond narrow views.

Obstacles

Although the current climate may support integration, there may be serious limitations if the field moves prematurely in advancing any particular or specific version. Consider, as a point of reference, the interest in combining psychodynamic and behavioral views. At first glance, psychodynamic and behavioral views might be seen as the least likely candidates for integration, especially by proponents already identified with one of these two general approaches.

Psychodynamic views of clinical disorders are characterized primarily by reliance upon intrapsychic factors. Therapeutic change is attained by focusing on intrapsychic factors that are considered to underlie behavior. The treatment process is considered to be somewhat removed from the presenting problem, which is altered through such processes and therapeutic maneuvers as interpretation, resolution of transference, and elaboration of the meaning and subjective reality of the client (Messer & Winokur, 1980). Behavioral views usually focus more directly on the reported presenting problem at the level of current behavior or at the immediate antecedents of that behavior. Treatment is designed to intervene directly on the overt problems and relies heavily on active rehearsal, practice, and overt enactments to achieve therapeutic change. Important changes have been made in orthodox psychodynamic and behavioral positions. In behavioral views, the significance of factors that underlie overt behavior, as already noted, have been accorded increased importance. In psychoanalytic theory over the years, greater attention has been devoted to the role of environmental influences, the closed energy and hydraulic model has been challenged, and reformulations have appeared to emphasize overt behavior (see Wachtel, 1982).

Despite movement toward less extreme positions, integration of psychodynamic and behavioral approaches still has major obstacles. First, conceptual obstacles limit the prospect of reaching a uniform or cohesively integrated position. There is no single psychodynamic or behavioral view that could serve as a basis to provide a uniform position. Within each orientation, several different and often competing theories can be identified to explain clinical problems and therapeutic techniques. For example, within behavioral viewpoints, positions vary in the extent to which they rely on environmental determinants or intervening variables to explain clinical problems and treatment techniques. At more specific levels of analysis, the incompatibility of views within the behavioral approach are quite evident. For example, among views that rely on intervening variables, different variables (e.g., anxiety, cognitions) can be readily identified. When specific clinical problems are examined, the range of theories and techniques that fall under the rubric of *behavioral approaches* is large. For example, for the treatment of depression, alternative views focus on environmental events, cognitive processes, and learning experiences (see Rehm, 1981). There is no single set of principles or constructs that could serve as the basis for developing a unified conceptual position.

The conceptual diversity within psychodynamic and behavioral approaches might initially be seen as an advantage rather than as an obstacle to integration. The diversity provides greater opportunity from which to select theoretical constructs for an integrated hybrid. Yet, because of the disharmony and incompatibility that exists within individual theoretical camps, any final hybrid would be very narrow and not at all integrative in any broad sense. Perhaps narrow portions or subviews of psychodynamic or behavioral positions could be integrated. Any larger integration, however, presupposes a homogeneity of the individual positions that does not exist.

Second, between general psychodynamic and behavioral orientations, the absence of a common language to refer to personality and behavior makes integration difficult. Of course the differences in language *per se* are not critical; yet, the terms reflect different levels of analysis of personality and behavior and presuppositions about the nature of psychopathology and its etiological basis. For example, the notion of a "symptom" in psychodynamic views does not translate simply to "overt behavior," as discussed in behavioral views. The terms differ in connotative meaning even if the denotative referent is the same presenting problem. The connotative meanings embrace a larger theory about the *nature* of the presenting problem.

Even where referents in the therapeutic process are similar, they still may be used slightly differently. For example, proponents of psychodynamic or behavioral positions may refer to the therapeutic relationship as important (DeVoge & Beck, 1978). However, they may be referring to disparate aspects of the relationship in treatment. In psychodynamic views, the relationship is relied upon, in part, because of its significance as a medium for elaborating important aspects of the client's problem and experience. In behavioral treatment, the relationship is more typically viewed as an important basis for developing a working interaction on which other procedures can be superimposed.

Third, and related to the second point, is the fact that the criteria considered to be relevant for evaluating their respective treatments differ between psychodynamic and behavioral orientations. With psychodynamic therapies, success in treatment, insofar as success is a relevant term, is more likely to be measured in terms of altering or elaborating the client's subjective experience, general coping responses, and ability to handle life. To be sure, direct changes in overt behavior are important, but such changes are not given primacy. Indeed, focus on overt behavior change may deprive the client of larger, more global, and even more important changes in personality (Messer & Winokur, 1980). In contrast, behavioral approaches tend to emphasize the primacy of behavior change. Subjective experience may be critical as well. However, reorganization of experience and one's views of the world at a more global level are usually of less direct interest.

When such differences in outcome criteria exist in the different approaches, it is tempting to state that the different criteria are complementary rather than incompatible. Although such a view reflects an admirable ecumenical spirit, it also naively neglects the thrust of the individual positions. Neither approach states that one sort of outcome is the only type of change that occurs. Yet, the approaches differ in the types of changes that are sought and that are regarded as fundamental and primary. Statements that diverse measures complement each other ignore the fundamental assumptive conflict in the different approaches.

Direct comparisons of alternative treatments from opposing orientations may be inappropriate because the constituent interventions would be expected to produce fundamentally different outcomes. Integration of psychodynamic and behavioral views, although possible at the conceptual level, would be very difficult to evaluate empirically. Empirical tests of the benefits of such an integration presuppose agreement on the appropriate outcome criteria. At present, such agreement does not exist.

Fourth and perhaps of underestimated significance is that evidence for theoretical concepts within particular approaches are insufficiently well established for them to be joined with constructs from yet another approach. Within a particular orientation, many questions remain about the nature of clinical problems, how they emerge and are maintained, and how they should be ameliorated. The empirical foundations within a particular approach are relatively weak and would not provide a strong base for a larger theoretical superstructure. For example, data on how neurotic anxiety develops, either from a psychodynamic or behavioral perspective, are not yet available, although the number of theories within and between the approaches is manifold. Although alternative explanations might be integrated at the conceptual level, they usually have little in the way of adequate empirical data to suggest that they account for the problem.

SYMPTOM SUBSTITUTION: A CASE STUDY OF CONCEPTUAL CLASH AND EMPIRICAL INTEGRATION

The preceding discussion suggests several difficulties with the integration of psychodynamic and behavioral views. The lack of empirical data on major concepts within each approach represents a significant obstacle for a meaningful integration. The problem is not merely the paucity of data. The added problem is that concepts limit the types of data that are even sought. Thus, concepts from individual approaches may prematurely foster narrow views of the nature of clinical disorders and misrepresent the empirical phenomena the concepts are designed to explain. The conceptual difficulties of attempting and integration of psychodynamic and behavioral views and the problems of insufficient evidence for the constituent positions can be illustrated concretely by examining the notion of *symptom substitution*. Symptom substitution has served as a focal point in the conceptual clashes of psychodynamic and behavioral views and also in an area where integration has interesting prospects.

Symptom substitution has referred to the possibility that successful elimination of a particular problem or "symptom" without treating the underlying cause may result in the appearance of a new (substitute) symptom. Interest in symptom substitution has stemmed primarily from the importance the notion has been accorded by proponents of behavior modification (Kazdin, 1979a). As behavior modification emerged in the late 1950s and early 1960s, symptom substitution was raised as a critical area where differences between psychodynamic and behavioral positions were especially clear (e.g., Eysenck, 1959; Ullmann & Krasner, 1965; Yates, 1958). Strong claims were made by proponents of behavior modification that a psychodynamic view would predict symptom substitution following treatment that failed to consider the client's underlying (intrapsychic) problem.

Alternative Views of Symptomatic Treatment

The psychodynamic view of symptomatic treatment has served as the basis for predicting symptom substitution. The view generally has been that overt behavioral problems stem from underlying intrapsychic forces. Treatment of the overt behaviors without treating the underlying problem would produce only transient effects. The underlying forces would either result in the reemergence of the original symptoms (relapse) or in the emergence of a new problem (substitute symptom). The new symptom, as it were, serves as a substitute for expression of the original underlying problem.

Proponents of behavior modification have emphasized that symptom substitution would not be likely to result from treatment of overt behaviors (symptoms). Indeed, early views in the field suggested that the "symptom," rather than some underlying putative conflict, is the problem (Eysenck, 1960). In fact, treatment of overt behavior was more likely to result in improvements in other areas of functioning. The beneficial effects predicted by behavioral treatments were considered to result from *generalization*. Either because the nontreated behaviors were similar to the target problem or because they followed from the target problem (e.g., increased social interaction following successful treatment of stuttering), broad improvements following treatment of overt behavior might be expected.

Over the years, the extreme and simplified views of psychodynamic and behavioral positions have greatly modified. To begin with, the fact that neither orthodox nor modified psychodynamic views necessarily predict symptom substitution has now been widely acknowledged. Symptoms that initially emerge as an expression of underlying conflict or psychic energy may become functionally autonomous of the original cause (see Freud, 1936; Weitzman, 1967). Because the underlying psychic cause may no longer play a role in symptom maintenance, symptoms may be treated successfully without new symptoms emerging (Bookbinder, 1962; Rapaport, 1959; Weitzman, 1967). Also, many proponents of behavior modification have acknowledged that under some circumstances new problems might readily emerge after behavioral treatment (Bandura, 1969; Cahoon, 1968; Yates, 1970). Indeed, reports of behavior therapy outcomes have occasionally suggested the appearance of new problems following symptomatic treatment (Blanchard & Hersen, 1976; Crisp, 1966; Foa & Steketee, 1977; Hand & Lamontagne, 1976; Stoudenmire, 1973). Thus, even though the notion of "symptoms" was rejected by proponents of behavior modification, the phenomenon to which symptom substitution referred has been acknowledged as a possibility and an occasional reality.

The notion of generalized beneficial effects resulting from behavioral treatment also received support. Several studies indicated that focusing on specific areas within treatment, such as circumscribed fear reactions, were associated with broader changes as well (e.g., Baker, 1969; Boersma, Den Hengst, Dekker, & Emmelkamp, 1976; Donner, 1970; Paul, 1967, 1968; Solyom, Heseltine, McClure, Ledwidge, & Kenny, 1971). Thus, generalization was shown to be a possible consequence of behavioral ("symptomatic") treatment.

Difficulties in Evaluating Symptom Substitution and Generalization

Assuming for a moment that changes following treatment are consistent with the notions of symptom substitution (emergence of new problems) and generalization (spread of beneficial effects to nontarget symptoms), combination of the different conceptual views might be appealing. An integrationist approach might embrace upon notions and seek the conceptual harmony that has been illusive on the matter of symptomatic treatment. Yet, there are several conceptual and methodological problems with both symptom substitution and generalization that are not in any way resolved by their integration.

With symptom substitution, several difficulties can be readily identified. First, it is unclear for most psychological problems what is a symptom as opposed to an underlying problem. With physical diseases, the distinction between the underlying problem (e.g., bacterial infection) and the overt symptom (e.g., runny nose) often can be independently verified. Also, a causal relationship can be demonstrated by showing that treatment of the underlying infection ameliorates the symptom and not vice versa. Independent methods of distinguishing symptoms from their putative underlying causes are not available in the same way with psychological disorders. Thus, supporting the view that there are symptoms and underlying problems is difficult, to say the least.

Second, when a new problem emerges after treatment, it is difficult to determine if it is a substitute symptom. New problems may have emerged anyway, whether or not symptomatic treatment or any treatment had been provided. The problem may have been present all along but only became more evident after treatment. Third, how and when symptom substitution is manifest make verification of the notion extremely difficult. Diverse changes in affect, cognition, or overt behavior following treatment all might qualify as symptom substitution. Which change will occur cannot be predicted in advance. Also, the substitute symptom might emerge immediately or years after treatment (Bookbinder, 1962). These and other problems have made the notion of symptom substitution difficult to support empirically (see Kazdin, 1982).

Generalization as a concept to explain the nature of changes following treatment is not much better off than symptom substitution. Generalization is a technical term derived from the psychology of learning that has been extended to treatment outcome. In the context referred to here, generalization refers to changes in one behavior leading to or being associated with changes in other behaviors. Generalization is a function of the resemblance or common response elements of the target and nontarget behaviors. The extent of generalization should be a function of some gradient of similarity across the target and nontarget behaviors. In studies showing the spread of beneficial effects of treatment (e.g., Paul, 1967, 1968), there is no evidence that the degree or types of changes in areas not focused on directly bear any similarity to the target problem.

If behaviors improve that are not topographically similar to the target behavior, one could say that their meaning or underlying cognitive processes unites them in some way. Thus, generalization may result from the spread of effects at the cognitive level that connects behaviors that bear little topographical resemblance. However, no clear evidence exists in the context of psychotherapy outcome that concomitant changes associated with treatment are connected to the target behavior to make generalization a meaningful notion.

Some evidence, as noted previously, exists both for the emergence of new problems and for the spread of beneficial effects following treatment (see Kazdin, 1982). Thus, the phenomena to which symptom substitution and generalization might refer are not devoid of referents. Yet, the respective notions are heavily laden with assumptions and conceptual ambiguities that are difficult to resolve empirically. Attempts to integrate the different concepts would provide an illusory advance, because, separately, the notions have major sources of ambiguity and little direct empirical support.

An Empirical Rapprochement

Symptom substitution and generalization are not mere descriptions of phenomena following treatment, but they also implicitly specify the mechanisms through which such changes occur. Although evidence might be cited to support the general empirical phenomena to which the notions refer, evidence is not available that suggests that the mechanisms implicit in the notions are operative. Indeed, difficulties with each of the concepts have largely ensured their failure to achieve empirical scrutiny.

Rather than considering integration of the different views at the conceptual level, one might look more closely at the empirical phenomena to which each notion refers. The general phenomenon is that change in one aspect of personality or behavior may be associated with other changes, some of which may be viewed as negative (as implied by "symptom substitution") and others that may be viewed as positive (as implied by "generalization"). Recent research in the context of treatment has suggested that alteration of one area of behavior is likely to be associated with multiple changes in other areas (see Kazdin, 1982; Voeltz & Evans, 1982). Essentially, responses tend to covary. *Responses* here can be defined broadly to include affect, cognitions, overt behavior, and other levels of analysis of personality and behavior. *Response covariation* encompasses diverse assessment methods, including self-report, direct observation, psychophysiology, and so on.

To date, the most direct evidence for response covariation has emanated from child behavior therapy. A few examples from diverse clinical applications with children have conveyed the breadth and types of changes following treatment of specific target behaviors. As one case in point, Becker, Turner, and Sajwaj (1978) decreased vomiting in a 3-year-old girl who had a history of rumination. When regurgitation decreased, crying also decreased, and smiling and spontaneous social interaction increased. In addition to these positive changes, stereotypic play with objects and head slapping also increased. Sajwaj, Twardosz, and Burke (1972) found that increasing attentiveness of a preschool retarded child also led to increases in initiation of conversations and cooperativeness. Yet, disruptive behaviors, at other times of the day than when the program was conducted, increased as well.

The reasons why multiple changes occur following treatment of particular behaviors are unclear. The basis for such changes has been partially elaborated by Wahler and his colleagues who have examined the organization of the behavior of deviant children who are treated in different settings (see Wahler, Berland, & Coe, 1979). Wahler found that behaviors tend to be organized into clusters that consist of a variety of responses that systematically covary.

Wahler (1975) observed children over an extended period (approximately 3 years) who were referred for treatment because of disruptive behaviors. Observations were made of several behaviors at home and at school to determine the correlations among different classes of responses. As an illustration, for one child, working on assignments at school was positively correlated with engaging in self-stimulatory behaviors and negatively correlated with fiddling with objects, staring into space, and not interacting with others. The interrelations among the behaviors could not be accounted for simply by the fact that the behaviors were incompatible with working. For this same child at home, several other behaviors were intercorrelated. Specifically, sustained play with toys was inversely associated with compliance with adult instructions, social interaction with adults, and self-stimulation.

In general, Wahler has found stable clusters of behaviors that can be identified in the repertoires of individual children. Moreover, when interventions are implemented to alter particular behaviors, concomitant changes are evident in other behaviors. For example, in the Wahler (1975) study, interventions that altered specific problem behaviors at school affected other behaviors with which the target behaviors were correlated. Also, changes at school were associated with changes in different behaviors at home. Multiple changes were evident, some of which might be viewed as desirable, and others as undesirable. For example, for one child, decreases in the problem behavior at school were associated with increases in peer interaction at home but also with increases in oppositional behavior at school. Thus, both desirable and undesirable changes were evident.

The work on response covariation has shown that the breadth of treatment effects encompasses a variety of behaviors. To some extent, the types of concomitant changes that are likely to occur with treatment can be predicted by pretreatment assessment of the response cluster of which the target behavior is a part. For example, Wahler and Fox (1980a) found that solitary play and oppositional behavior were inversely correlated among four children with conduct problems. Knowledge that these responses were negatively correlated suggested that alteration of one response might be inversely associated with changes in the other response. Indeed, positive reinforcement for solitary play led to systematic and marked reductions in oppositional behavior (Wahler & Fox, 1980a, 1980b). In general, responses that tend to correlate positively with the target behavior are likely to increase, and responses that correlate negatively with the target behavior are likely to decrease following treatment. However, the relationship is not invariable (see Kara & Wahler, 1977).

The notion of response covariation and its supporting evidence have important implications for the discussion of symptom substitution and generalization and for the larger issues of integration of psychodynamic and behavioral views. The evidence for response covariation raises basic theoretical questions about the organization of personality and behavior and the nature of therapeutic change. Existing notions seem of little assistance in explaining the emergent data on response covariation. Symptom substitution is of little help, because it emphasizes the appearance of new responses following symptomatic treatment. Yet, response covariation refers to clusters of behavior that currently exist in the individual's response repertoire. Several behaviors coexist and change together—a phenomenon that is not exactly the direct focus of symptom substitution. The changes are not necessarily the emergence of new problems; some of the changes are improvements in positive or desirable behaviors. Also, the behaviors that form a cluster are not obviously related or interconnected by particular psychodynamic themes. Indeed, current evidence suggests a marked situational specificity to clusters of behavior, so that particular sets of behaviors may be interconnected differently in different situations. Generalization also is not very useful in explaining current evidence on response covariation. *Generalization* refers to changes of one aspect of behavior spreading to other behaviors that are similar or share some of the same response elements. Yet, responses that tend to cluster and covary systematically bear no obvious topographical resemblance.

General Comments

Symptom substitution and generalization represent an area where psychodynamic and behavioral views merge in some way. The views do not necessarily make incompatible predictions about the concomitant changes that are associated with treatment. Neither psychodynamic nor behavioral views argue that one type of change or another necessarily follows a particular type of treatment. Both symptom substitution and generalization point to the breadth of changes that may result from treatment. The concepts raise important points about integration of the larger conceptual approaches from which they are derived.

As an explanation of concomitant changes of psychotherapy, both symptom substitution and generalization are used very loosely. Examination of the individual concepts raises several problems in terms of their verifiability and/or empirical support. A major difficulty for considering their integration is that each concept tries at once to *describe* an empirical phenomenon (e.g., one type of change following treatment) and also to *explain* the theoretical basis for the change. Existing data suggest increases in problematic behaviors as well as decreases in nontarget behaviors following treatment. Thus, the descriptive feature of symptom substitution and generalization, by stretching the concepts slightly, might be argued as being partially supported. However, an entirely separate matter is establishing the basis for such changes. If such changes are evident, it is not completely clear that the models and explanations embraced by symptom substitution or generalization provide the most parsimonious accounts. In the absence of basic information about the nature of therapeutic change, arguing for particular explanations of these changes is premature. Further, arguing that the explanations offered by two unsupported general positions—psychodynamic and behavioral views—somehow provides an increment of knowledge or is useful in some other substantive way does not follow.

A much more detailed empirical base is needed to describe the etiology, nature, and prognosis of clinical problems and their amelioration. Theory might well be useful to guide this research. However, it is difficult to argue that unsupported theoretical notions, which are difficult to verify in their own right, should be integrated. The recent demonstrations of response covariation are instructive insofar as they reveal complex empirical phenomena that loosely relate to other notions, such as symptom substitution and generalization. However, neither of these concepts provides clear insights about the organization of behavior and the basis for particular response covariations that have been found. The concepts are too limited because they have not evolved to handle empirical data on the complex patterns of behavior change.

INTEGRATION OF PSYCHOTHERAPIES

Levels of Analysis

Integration of alternative psychotherapies can be attempted at different levels of analysis (Goldfried, 1980). The advantages and disadvantages and feasibility of integration efforts are likely to vary greatly as a function of these different levels.

Conceptual Integration

Many concepts of psychodynamic and behavioral positions might be relatively easily integrated at a theoretical or abstract level. The higher the level of abstraction, the greater are the similarities that might be drawn between seemingly incompatible notions. At the abstract level, individual concepts from one view can be expanded to embrace a related concept from a different view. The net effect is to relate phenomena and concepts that otherwise might seem conceptually incompatible. For example, one could extend the concepts of avoidance conditioning to encompass phobic behavior, as is discussed in behavioral views, and resistance and selective forgetting, as is discussed in psychodynamic views.

Attempts to seek conceptual bridges for behavioral and psychodynamic views are by no means new. The most elaborate attempt, by Dollard and Miller (1950), is frequently seen as the major achievement along these lines. The work is noteworthy, perhaps, as well for contemporary reasons because it may illustrate the pitfalls or fate of integration at the conceptual level.

When integration remains at the conceptual level, the primary accomplishment is to extend the meaning or application of general concepts beyond the phenomena they were proposed to explain. The extension *per se* is not objectionable. However, the danger is that the exercise remains at the conceptual level and has few implications for research or practice. Many of the concepts used to explain personality and behavior within narrow conceptual views already are loose and difficult to subject to empirical tests. When the meaning of such concepts is extended, their utility may be diminished further. Integration at the conceptual level may lead to a sense of harmony among proponents of otherwise opposing views. Yet, it is unclear what has been achieved beyond a conceptual truce, with respect to empirical implications or predictions about the phenomena of interest.

Procedural Integration

At the other extreme, integrationism in psychotherapy might focus on the common procedures or actual techniques among different therapies. In practice, many techniques are similar. For example, in outpatient psychotherapy for adults, many different techniques are likely to utilize statements that foster client expression of feelings, or therapists may provide selective attention to encourage a more positive and constructive outlook. Also, many of the influences referred to as nonspecific treatment factors, such as attending sessions, discussing one's problems with a therapist, and so on might be referred to as common characteristics or procedures of alternative treatments and serve as the basis for integration.

Integration at the level of specific procedures is unlikely to be very productive. Relatively few procedures are common among the very large number of techniques that currently exist (Herink, 1980). An analysis of different techniques probably would lead to a clustering of many procedures. For example, at the procedural level, one cluster might include those techniques that emphasize imagery (e.g., desensitization, flooding, covert conditioning) or behavioral rehearsal (role playing, psychodrama). Alternatively, techniques might cluster on the basis of those that focus on evocation of client feelings and subjective experience (e.g., psychodynamic, client-centered treatments) versus those that provide direct advice or active practice (e.g., various behavioral therapies). No matter how the clustering was accomplished, it would become clear quickly that there is a great overlap among the clusters. Techniques include multiple procedures, and the overlap among alternative clusters could be large. By looking for techniques that are procedurally similar, one would only reduce a large set of current techniques to a smaller number of clusters of techniques. The result would not be an integration of alternative positions as much as a grouping of techniques. The grouping of techniques might be useful for some purposes (see Shapiro & Shapiro, 1981; Smith *et al.*, 1980). However, integration at the procedural level might not achieve the broader purposes of the movement.

Strategy Integration

Another level of integration is the focus on the strategies or principles of different therapies (Goldfried, 1980). *Strategy,* as discussed here, refers to what therapy is accomplishing or altering at a level once removed from the specific procedures. Essentially, diverse therapies may produce similar effects because they have impact on similar mechanisms of change. The procedures of different therapies may be integrated by assuming that they all have some common end or process that they accomplish or invoke.

The advantage of this level of analysis is that it seeks or proposes higher order concepts that transcend particular procedures, a first requirement for developing an integrative approach that handles the diversity of treatment techniques. Also, this level of integration avoids many of the problems associated with unwieldy and assumption-laden concepts that the theoretical positions of alternative techniques embrace. Because several current integration attempts are primarily directed at this level, alternative efforts are highlighted separately in the discussion that follows.

Current Efforts to Integrate Alternative Treatments

The previous discussion has focused on major issues associated with the attempt to integrate psychodynamic and behavioral positions by combining concepts from each approach. Yet, integration can be attempted at different levels of analysis. Three efforts at content integration that appear to be particularly promising focus primarily at the level that is intermediate between abstract concepts and procedures. It is at this level that commonalities can be found that may generate research.

Demoralization Hypothesis

The view that alternative therapies may include several common principles has been consistently advocated by Frank (1961, 1973). The commonalities across different forms of therapy might be reflected both in what the clients bring to different treatments and what they receive once they arrive. Frank (1982) has suggested that patients seek therapy not only for their specific symptoms but also because of their demoralization. "Demoralization" refers to a state of mind characterized by subjective incompetence, poor self-esteem, alienation, hopelessness, and helplessness. The demoralized person, either through a lack of skills or confusion of goals, becomes unable to master situations or experiences stress with which he or she cannot cope. Symptoms such as anxiety, depression, and loneliness may result from demoralization. However, despite the different symptoms that patients may bring to treatment, demoralization is a common theme.

Treatments are considered by Frank to be effective because of their characteristics that help ameliorate patient demoralization. Independently of their idiosyncratic procedures, alternative techniques share the following general ingredients. The treatments provide

1. an emotionally charged and confiding relationship with a person identified as a helping agent;
2. a setting in which patients' expectancies for help and confidence in the therapist's role as a healer are strengthened;
3. a rationale or conceptual scheme that plausibly explains the symptoms and prescribes a procedure for their resolution; and
4. a set of procedures in which both the patient and therapist engage that they believe to be the means of restoring the patient.

Frank believes that the rationale to explain the patient's problems (the myth) and the procedures in which therapist and patient engage (the ritual) are critical to combating patient demoralization. The myth and ritual provide new learning experiences, evoke expectancies for help, provide opportunities for rehearsal and practice, and strengthen the therapeutic relationship.

From the standpoint of integration, Frank's (1982) view provides obviously important research leads. He reviews his own program of research that has produced results consistent with his views and that has helped consolidate his views of the role of patient expectancies for change. Also, existing research for different treatments is consistent with the general model. For example, the role of the therapeutic relationship continues to be recognized as a common and critical ingredient among different techniques (DeVoge & Beck, 1978; Kazdin, 1979a). More direct tests of the model could be provided. For example, common client reactions may be evoked by the myths (rationales) or rituals (procedures) of alternative techniques. Indeed, these characteristics of treatment can be varied to determine their differential impacts on client expectations of improvement. Alternatively, client involvement in the treatment might be varied within a given treatment technique to determine if it has impact on client expectancies for change or therapeutic outcome. Some of the research on the common ingredients might need to be evaluated under highly controlled laboratory conditions (analogue research) because of ethical constraints in meeting the needs of patients who seek treatment. Yet, manipulation of aspects of the rationale or procedures might be a matter of degree and hence possible to study in clinical applications of treatment.

Self-Efficacy

Another avenue for integration of psychotherapies intermediate between procedures and existing conceptual orientations can be achieved by proposing a mechanism of change common among alternative techniques. "Self-efficacy theory," proposed by Bandura (1977a), illustrates this type of integration. Self-efficacy was originally proposed in the context of analyzing change in the treatment of fear and avoidance. It has been extended as well to many areas of research, including diverse clinical problems and academic performance (DeClemente, 1981; Kazdin, 1979b; Keyser & Barling, 1981).

"Self-efficacy" refers to a person's expectation that he or she can successfully perform behaviors that will lead to a certain outcome. The expectations of whether one can perform the behavior is distinct from the expectation that a given behavior leads to a certain outcome. A person may believe that particular behaviors will result in a particular outcome (outcome expectancy) but not believe that he or she can successfully perform the behaviors (efficacy expectation). Bandura's notion of self-efficacy is part of a larger social learning, cognitively based conceptual framework of behavior change (see Bandura, 1977b). For present purposes, self-efficacy is isolated here from the larger framework because it has been advanced as the mechanism to explain behavior changes resulting from different treatments. Self-efficacy is the final common pathway through which different treatments are considered to produce change.

Expectations of mastery are proposed to influence a person's initiation and persistence of coping behavior and the situations in which they enter. High-self-efficacy persons are more likely to persist or provide greater effort. Those who succeed are likely to have self-efficacy further enhanced. Low-self-efficacy persons are more likely to evince persistence; those who cease to cope or who try unsuccessfully are likely to have their low-efficacy expectations further supported.

Bandura and his associates have completed several investigations to evaluate the role of self-efficacy in behavior change (e.g., Bandura, Adams, & Byer, 1977; Bandura, Adams, Hardy, & Howells, 1980). The research has focused on showing that the extent to which therapeutic change is achieved across different techniques is a function of changes in self-efficacy and that techniques are differentially effective because they vary in their success in altering self-efficacy.

The research has primarily studied volunteer clients who fear harmless snakes, but the research has been extended to persons with fears of open spaces, darkness, elevators, and heights (Bandura *et al.*, 1980; Biran & Wilson, 1981). Many behavior therapy techniques have been studied, including live, covert, and participant modeling, desensitization, guided exposure, and cognitive restructuring. Self-efficacy has been proposed to explain existing findings that techniques relying on overt performance (e.g., participant modeling, *in vivo* desensitization) are more effective in the outcomes they produce than are techniques based on vicarious experiences (e.g., symbolic modeling), persuasion (e.g., interpretative treatments), or emotional arousal (e.g., attribution) (see Bandura, 1977a).

Self-efficacy represents an important advance to integrate alternative techniques for different reasons. First, the notion has been couched in terms that permit empirical investigation. The measurement of self-efficacy was described when the notion was first introduced. Thus, self-efficacy is not another abstract construct awaiting operationalization. Second, multiple studies have already been completed that attest to the relationship between self-efficacy and behavior change. Of course, self-efficacy theory or research has not proceeded without criticism. Both the conceptual framework and methodological problems raised by its assessment have been noted (Kirsch, 1980; Rachman, 1978). Also, the research has been restricted to a relatively narrow set of treatments within behavior therapy and to volunteer clients seen under laboratory conditions. Investigators vary in the extent to which they see this as a relevent issue in evaluation of the underlying mechanisms of therapeutic change. However, the critical issue for present purposes is the fact that self-efficacy represents a researchable construct designed to describe a common mechanism for changes achieved by alternative treatments.

Common Strategies of Clinical Change

Commonalities among alternative techniques have been sought without regard to such specific notions as demoralization or self-efficacy. Recently, several investigators have sought a rapprochement among seemingly competing conceptual views on the nature of clinical problems and therapeutic change. The rapprochement, referred to here as *integrationism,* has been elaborated by Goldfried (1980, 1982b) who has advocated identifying a common set of clinical strategies or principles of behavior change among diverse therapeutic approaches. The strategies include experiences provided in treatment above the level of specific procedures. Different techniques may implement the strategies differently, but the overall goal is achieved nonetheless. Similarities in the strategies of different therapies include

1. initially inducing client expectancies that treatment will be helpful;
2. providing a therapeutic relationship in which clients can participate;
3. encouraging corrective experiences; and
4. providing clients with the opportunity to reality test and to obtain an external perspective on their problems.

The movement toward integrationism must be distinguished from simple *eclecticism.* An eclectic approach recognizes the virtues of different approaches or techniques and tries to sample from them as needed to effect therapeutic change. Thus, an eclectic therapist might adopt and combine desensitization, insight-oriented psychotherapy, and rational-emotive therapy as needed. Eclecticism tends to draw from several different approaches, recognizing their separate integrity. Also, eclecticism can consist of an infinite number of variations, depending on which combinations of available techniques clinicians choose (Garfield, 1982; Garfield & Kurtz, 1976). Integrationism is eclectic in the sense of its openness to diverse approaches, but it looks at a higher level of abstraction to cull common threads among different treatments.

From the standpoint of treatment evaluation, integrationism has the potential for identifying processes and procedures that transcend individual techniques. The processes and procedures can become the focus of research. For example, a common procedure among diverse techniques is the use of extratreatment practice in which the client is encouraged to engage in therapeutically relevant activities to augment therapeutic change. For example, Alexander and French (1946) recommend that psychodynamic therapies require patients to perform in everyday situations those activities that they previously were unable to perform. Other conceptual approaches in varying degrees have advocated similar types of activities (e.g., Ellis,

1962; Fenichel, 1941; Haley, 1963; Herzberg, 1945; Salter, 1949). A recent survey indicated that approximately 60% of all outpatient treatment studies of behavior therapy incorporate extratherapy practice for such diverse problems as phobias, obsessive-compulsive disorders, depression, sexual dysfunctions, marital discord, and others (see Shelton & Levy, 1981a, 1981b). Extratreatment practice might be one of the common clinical strategies that spans many different treatments and that is worth investigating (see Kazdin & Mascitelli, 1982a, 1982b).

An integrationist approach provides an important initial analysis of commonalities among alternative treatments. The strategies identified in this fashion need to be followed up with theory and research. An integrationist program of outcome research would take a potentially momentous turn away from existing research that tends to focus on individual techniques and their comparison with other techniques that are rivals for therapeutic superiority.

General Comments

The preceding discussion highlights three attempts to seek a common ground among alternative treatments. The different views are by no means imcompatible nor are they exhaustive. Related attempts to seek commonalities have been identified with such other concepts as "nonspecific treatment factors," "placebo effects," and others. As has already been noted, attempts to seek commonalities among different techniques are by no means new. Yet, recent efforts have emerged at a time when research in psychotherapy is particularly active. The area of psychotherapy has never suffered from nonempirical extremes such as armchair theorizing or anecdotal accounts of processes and outcomes of particular treatments. What is new in some of the current proposals is that they are accompanied by recognition of the need to develop new lines of research and to make empirical advances rather than merely to promote conceptual harmony among alternative schools of thought.

CONCLUSIONS

Advances in psychotherapy have been slow, a fact often attributed to the inherent complexity of treatment and the multiplicity of clinical problems to which treatments are directed. Recent progress has stemmed in part from the acknowledgment that answers are not likely to come from singular, narrowly conceived theoretical views. Integrationism as a general movement can be viewed as an affirmative approach to develop bridges among conceptual positions and to cull those common features that seem essential from diverse techniques as they are practiced.

The type of integration that is attempted to advance the field needs to be considered carefully. Integration of existing conceptual orientations, such as psychodynamic and behavioral views, may be of questionable value. Existing concepts within each of these general approaches often are far removed from empirical phenomena and are saddled with meaning and assumptions that may not be useful to adopt. The notions of "symptom substitution" and "generalization," proposed to describe as well as explain aspects of therapeutic change from psychodynamic and behavioral positions, respectively, were discussed to illustrate the point. It is illusory to assume that individual concepts from different positions that are difficult to verify and have little empirical basis somehow overcome their disadvantages or lead to greater insights when they are combined.

Integration can be achieved without attempting to combine different conceptual positions, each of which has its own problems. An especially promising approach is the attempt to identify strategies or principles of behavior change that are free from ties to particular schools of thought or conceptual positions. The basis for this level of integration is examination of psychotherapies as they are implemented in practice rather than looking at the abstract concepts that are used to account for how therapy is executed. Of course, drawing from different psychotherapies to generate a singular integrative approach is not without problems.

A major initial problem will be deciding on a language to describe the phenomena of therapy that are free from current conceptual positions. The task is to *describe* the concepts so they can be investigated without suggesting at this point implicit explanations of the phenomena as well. For example, the concept of "response covariation," which was discussed earlier, illustrates an empirical formulation of notions embedded in symptom substitution and generalization. The concept is useful because it is primarily descriptive at this time and does not presuppose or limit the basis for the empirical relationships that have been demonstrated.* Certainly, when the phenomenon is more well elaborated in research, theoretical formulations would be quite welcome to synthesize the data. However, attempts at integration need to maintain the distinction, to the extent possible, between

* One might argue that "response covariation" is hardly free from conceptual underpinnings. "Covariation" is relatively neutral because it reflects empirical relationships that would be consistent with several different views. However, "response" could be argued as entailing a behavioral view that focuses on a specific level of analysis and units of behavior that have no clear counterpart beyond a behavioral formulation. As noted earlier, response can be defined broadly to reflect affect, cognitions, behavior, and other levels of performance that can be measured. Indeed, response can be viewed methodologically as molar or molecular aspects of personality or behavior as they are assessed.

a description of the phenomena of psychotherapy and their putative theoretical bases.

Several authors have suggested the use of concepts from cognitive psychology as a common way of referring to phenomena of different psychotherapies (Goldfried, 1982b; Ryle, 1978; Sarason, 1979). The advantage is that such concepts are likely to be the most acceptable (or least objectionable) to proponents of psychodynamic and behavioral positions. The concepts deal with meaning of events, underlying processes, and ways of structuring and interpreting experience. They can encompass affect, perception, and behavior. Consequently, cognitive processes and their referents probably provide the place where the gap between psychodynamic and behavioral views is the least wide (Messer & Winokur, 1980). However, the concepts embrace a particular (even if heterogeneous) approach and an implicit view of the primary features of clinical problems and level of therapeutic change. Cognitive processes may be irresistibility tempting because they capitalize on and reflect the wave of enthusiasm in psychology regarding the primacy of cognitions. The danger for integrationism in psychotherapy is that cognitive psychology has its own assumptions and referents that could limit what is extracted and focused on in psychotherapy. The problem that is likely to emerge from adapting a language of cognitive psychology is that the meanings of terms, when applied to the phenomena of clinical disorders and psychotherapy, would greatly depart from their experimental referents. We would not only inherit some of the ambiguities associated with diverse terms within their own experimental research paradigms but also have the problem of trying to explain complex phenomena for which the concepts were never designed (cf. Breger & McGaugh, 1965). A cognitive approach toward therapy needs to be promulgated and researched in its own right because of the advances it has already provided. However, as a common language to address diverse therapies, there are predictable problems and limitations with such an approach.

The significance of integrationism as a movement at this point in time may not derive from the attempt to unify particular substantive positions such as psychodynamic and behavioral views. Rather, the significance lies in the increased openness of professionals to alternative views of psychotherapy. The openness reflects a critical admission that no one type of treatment or school of thought provides the answers to the outstanding questions of treatment. The first sign of an impending advance may be to cease viewing singular theoretical formulations and orientations as panaceas for clinical work. To proceed further, the next step will require describing or delineating the common features of alternative approaches that are relatively free from narrow conceptual underpinnings.

An interesting parallel might be drawn to other areas of clinical research that also have been overly laden with theoretical assumptions that have restricted rather than advanced progress. For example, in the classification of mental disorders in psychiatry, a major advance of the *Diagnostic and Statistical Manual of Mental Disorders* (DSM-III, American Psychiatric Association, 1980) was developing a system in which disorders could be delineated descriptively based on presenting symptoms. Assumptions of the etiology of the disorder and the theoretical models that account for disorders have been largely abandoned in the current diagnostic system. Once clear descriptive syndromes can be delineated in empirical research, theories that explain the basis of various disorders will be more appropriate. However, the first step is delineating the phenomena of interest. Therapy research can profit from a step away from abstract views about what should happen, according to one theory or another.

Perhaps the major implication of integrationism as a movement is the hope for research on the phenomena that transcend particular therapies. An integrationist approach aimed at generating a new type of research, rather than at promoting conceptual harmony, heightens the prospect for genuine advances. But the principal goal must be kept in mind. Efforts toward integrationism must be evaluated on the basis of their empirical yield rather than on the compatibility of the different views that are achieved. If the empirical yield is viewed as the ultimate criterion, no doubt many existing theoretical notions will be discarded, and others will be retained or modified. Ultimately, integrationism is likely to lead to a new position that does not lobby for conceptual harmony but for heightened empiricism.

AUTOBIOGRAPHICAL STATEMENT

In my view, the objectives of psychotherapy research, as quite distinct from the means by which these are obtained, are relatively straightforward. The objectives include the development of an empirically based set of interventions that produce clinically significant therapeutic change and the formulation and evaluation of alternative theories that account for the development, maintenance, and alleviation of clinical disorders. These objectives are important to state to convey my own position regarding the current movement toward integration of alternative therapeutic approaches and the background factors that account for that position.

My interest in integration is not as an end or exercise in itself but only insofar as it may concretely advance the aforementioned objectives. Different forms of integration may vary in how or whether the objectives are advanced. Integration may consist of combining specific theoretical views or treatment procedures (e.g., psychoanalysis and behavioral approaches). Such a combination might lead to greater theoretical and empirical advances than the individual constituent approaches. I rather doubt that, but the result remains to be seen. The difficulty with an integration based on specific combinations of alternative views is that the likely result is yet another specific position with its spokespersons, adherents, professional groups, journals, and other signs of specialization. Integration in this form is likely to follow the path of other, more narrowly conceived movements and perhaps not uniquely contribute to the objectives of psychotherapy research that were noted previously.

Alternatively, the general movement toward integration of alternative views may contribute greatly to the objectives of psychotherapy research. Such a movement may mark the abandonment of the view that individual conceptual positions are likely to provide definitive answers for many research and clinical questions. Also, the resulting orientation would consist of an increased openness to diverse positions. The first step toward broad-based research in psychotherapy may be the explicit acknowledgment that singular views or orientations are in fact, if not necessarily, limited.

Integrationism as a movement, to me, is only significant insofar as it, in fact, leads to improved research and theory. The signs of such improvement would be evident if more effective treatments were identified, if existing techniques were matched better to certain sorts of patients or clients, and if the development of specific clinical problems was clarified, to mention a few. It is premature to judge efforts toward integration on such criteria. However, for me, these criteria are important to keep in mind at the outset so that departure from the prime directive can be detected early.

I look to integrationism with optimism and skepticism. One might ask what events in my background would account for such a stance. The major impetus for my orientation with respect to therapy research can be traced to my graduate training at Northwestern University. Although the usual substantive courses were taught, the graduate program was very heavily weighted with courses in methodology, design, and statistics. The purposes, problems, and prospects for scientific research were detailed in many different ways. The impact on many persons who completed the program, including me, was a keen interest in methodology and design. Naturally, I had developed substantive areas of interest such as behavior modification. However, this was somewhat secondary to, if not derivative from, the interest in research design. Indeed, it is often the case still today that I am more interested in the methodological issues raised by the means of answering questions scientifically than I am in the substantive answers themselves.

My interest in the objectives of psychotherapy research and treatment research methodolgy raises great hopes for the impact of integrationism. Research might well be improved by looking anew at therapy without some of the constraints and presuppositions of current schools. Broader constructs than those of the past may well be identified, and commonalities among alternative treatments may finally be researched rather than merely discussed. The risk involved in openly welcoming integration efforts, as I see it, is relatively small—namely, disappointment. Psychotherapy has been discussed and explained in dramatically different ways over the last 50 years. Integrationism might merely have an impact on how therapy is described and discussed. However, the promise of new types of empirical research is encouraging. The new research may resolve some of the substantive impasses caused by arguing from singular positions. To someone like me, integrationism, at best, may handle only the substantive issues regarding therapy and its effects. Major problems remain regarding fundamental questions about how treatment should be evaluated, the criteria that should be used and their prioritization, and so on. In many ways, further progress will require gains in these areas, which may or may not be influenced by entertaining new combinations of substantive positions about psychotherapy.

ALAN E. KAZDIN, PH.D.

REFERENCES

Alexander, F. The dynamics of psychotherapy in light of learning theory. *American Journal of Psychiatry*, 1963, *120*, 440–448.

Alexander, F., & French, R. M. *Psychoanalytic therapy: Principles and applications.* New York: Ronald, 1946.

Alexander, J. F., Barton, C., Schiavo, R. S., & Parsons, B. V. Systems-behavioral intervention with families of delinquents: Therapist characteristics, family behavior, and outcome. *Journal of Consulting and Clinical Psychology*, 1976, *44*, 656–664.

American Psychiatric Association. *Diagnostic and statistical manual of mental disorders* (3rd ed.). Washington, D.C.: American Psychiatric Association, 1980.

Appelbaum, S. A. A psychoanalyst looks at gestalt therapy. In C. Hatcher & P. Himmelstein (Eds.), *The handbook of gestalt therapy*. New York: Aronson, 1976.

Baker, B. L. Symptom treatment and symptom substitution. *Journal of Abnormal Psychology*, 1969, *74*, 42–49.

Bandura, A. *Principles of behavior modification*. New York: Holt, Rinehart & Winston, 1969.

Bandura, A. Self-efficacy: Toward a unifying theory of behavioral change. *Psychological Review*, 1977, *84*, 191–215. (a)

Bandura, A. *Social learning theory*. Englewood Cliffs, N.J.: Prentice-Hall, 1977. (b)

Bandura, A., Adams, N. E., & Beyer, J. Cognitive processes mediating behavioral change. *Journal of Personality and Social Psychology*, 1977 *35*, 125–139.

Bandura, A., Adams, N. E., Hardy, A. B., & Howells, G. N. Tests of generality of self-efficacy theory. *Cognitive Therapy and Research*, 1980, *4*, 39–66.

Becker, J. V., Turner, S. M., & Sajwaj, T. E. Multiple behavioral effects of the use of lemon juice with a ruminating toddler-age child. *Behavior Modification*, 1978, *2*, 267–278.

Bergin, A. E., & Lambert, M. J. The evaluation of therapeutic outcomes. In S. L. Garfield & A. E. Bergin (Eds.), *Handbook of psychotherapy and behavior change: An empirical analysis* (2nd ed.). New York: Wiley, 1978.

Biran, M., & Wilson, G. T. Treatment of phobic disorders using cognitive and exposure methods: A self-efficacy analysis. *Journal of Consulting and Clinical Psychology*, 1981, *49*, 886–899.

Blanchard, E. B., & Hersen, M. Behavioral treatment of hysterical neurosis: Symptom substitution and symptom return. *Psychiatry*, 1976, *39*, 118–129.

Boersma, K., Den Hengst, S., Dekker, J., & Emmelkamp, P. M. G. Exposure and response prevention in the natural environment: A comparison with obsessive-compulsive patients. *Behaviour Research and Therapy*, 1976, *14*, 19–24.

Bookbinder, L. J. Simple conditioning versus the dynamic approach to symptoms and symptom substitution: A reply to Yates. *Psychological Reports*, 1962, *10*, 71–77.
Breger, L., & McGaugh, J. L. Critique and reformulation of "learning theory" approaches to psychotherapy and neurosis. *Psychological Bulletin*, 1965, *63*, 338–358.
Cahoon, D. D. Symptom substitution and the behavior therapies: Reappraisal. *Psychological Bulletin*, 1968, *69*, 149–156.
Crisp, A. H. "Transference," "symptom emergence," and "social repercussion" in behaviour therapy. *British Journal of Medical Psychology*, 1966, *39*, 179–196.
DeClemente, C. C. Self-efficacy and smoking cessation maintenance: A preliminary report. *Cognitive Therapy and Research*, 1981, *5*, 175–187.
DeVoge, J. T., & Beck, S. The therapist–client relationship in behavior therapy. In M. Hersen, R. M. Eisler, & P. M. Miller (Eds.), *Progress in behavior modification* (Vol. 6). New York: Academic Press, 1978.
Dollard, J., & Miller, N. E. *Personality and psychotherapy*. New York: McGraw-Hill, 1950.
Donner, L. Automated group desensitization—A follow-up report. *Behaviour Research and Therapy*, 1970, *8*, 241–247.
Ellis, A. *Reason and emotion in psychotherapy*. New York: Lyle Stuart Press, 1962.
Emmelkamp, P. M. G. The behavioral study of clinical phobias. In M. Hersen, R. M. Eisler, & P. M. Miller (Eds.), *Progress in behavior modification* (Vol. 8). New York: Academic Press, 1979.
Endler, N. S., & Magnusson, D. (Eds.). *Interactional psychology and personality*. Washington, D.C.: Hemisphere, 1976. (a)
Endler, N. S., & Magnusson, D. Toward an interactional psychology of personality. *Psychological Bulletin*, 1976, *83*, 956–974. (b)
Eysenck, H. J. Learning theory and behaviour therapy. *Journal of Mental Science*, 1959, *105*, 61–75.
Eysenck, H. J. (Ed.). *Behavior therapy and the neuroses*. New York: Pergamon, 1960.
Feather, B. W., & Rhoads, J. M. Psychodynamic behavior therapy. I. Theory and rationale. *Archives of General Psychiatry*, 1972, *26*, 496–502 (a).
Feather, B. W., & Rhoads, J. M. Psychodynamic behavior therapy. II. Clinical aspects. *Archives of General Psychiatry*, 1972, *26*, 503–511 (b).
Fenichel, O. *Problems of psychoanalytic technique*. Albany, N.Y.: *Psychoanalytic Quarterly*, 1941.
Foa, E. B., & Steketee, G. Emergent fears during treatment of three obsessive compulsives: Symptom substitution or deconditioning? *Journal of Behavior Therapy and Experimental Psychiatry*, 1977, *8*, 353–358.
Ford, J. D. Therapeutic relationship in behavior therapy: An empirical analysis. *Journal of Consulting and Clinical Psychology*, 1978, *46*, 1302–1314.
Frank, J. D. *Persuasion and healing*. Baltimore: Johns Hopkins University Press, 1961.
Frank, J. D. *Persuasion and healing: A comparative study of psychotherapy* (2nd ed.). Baltimore: Johns Hopkins University Press, 1973.
Frank, J. D. Therapeutic components shared by all psychotherapies. In J. H. Harvey & M. M. Parks (Eds.), *Psychotherapy research and behavior change* (Vol. 1). The master lecture series. Washington, D.C.: American Psychological Association, 1982.
French, T. M. Interrelations between psychoanalysis and the experimental work of Pavlov. *American Journal of Psychiatry*, 1933, *89*, 1165–1203.
Freud, S. *The problem of anxiety*. New York: Norton, 1936.
Garfield, S. L. Eclecticism and integration in psychotherapy. *Behavior Therapy*, 1982, *13*, 610–623.
Garfield, S. L., & Kurtz, R. Clinical psychologists in the 1970s. *American Psychologist*, 1976, *31*, 1–9.

Goldfried, M. R. Toward the delineation of therapeutic change principles. *American Psychologist*, 1980, *35*, 991–999.
Goldfried, M. R. (Ed.). *Converging themes in psychotherapy: Trends in psychodynamic, humanistic, and behavioral practice.* New York: Springer, 1982. (a)
Goldfried, M. R. On the history of therapeutic integration. *Behavior Therapy*, 1982, *13*, 572–593. (b)
Goldfried, M. R., & Padawer, W. Current status and future directions in psychotherapy. In M. R. Goldfried (Ed.), *Converging themes in psychotherapy: Trends in psychodynamic, humanistic, and behavioral practice.* New York: Springer, 1982.
Haley, J. *Strategies of psychotherapy.* New York: Grune & Stratton, 1963.
Hand, I., & Lamontagne, Y. The exacerbation of interpersonal problems after rapid phobia removal. *Psychotherapy: Theory, Research and Practice*, 1976, *13*, 405–411.
Herink, R. (Ed.). *The psychotherapy handbook.* New York: New American Library, 1980.
Herzberg, A. *Active psychotherapy.* New York: Grune & Stratton, 1945.
Kara, A., & Wahler, R. B. Organizational features of a young child's behaviors. *Journal of Experimental Child Psychology*, 1977, *24*, 24–39.
Kazdin, A. E. Fictions, factions, and functions of behavior therapy. *Behavior Therapy*, 1979, *10*, 629–654. (a)
Kazdin, A. E. Imagery elaboration and self-efficacy in the covert modeling treatment of assertive behavior. *Journal of Consulting and Clinical Psychology*, 1979, *47*, 725–733. (b)
Kazdin, A. E. Symptom substitution, generalization, and response covariation: Implications for psychotherapy outcome. *Psychological Bulletin*, 1982, *91*, 349–365.
Kazdin, A. E., & Mascitelli, S. Behavioral rehearsal, self-instructions, and homework practice in developing assertiveness. *Behavior Therapy*, 1982, *13*, 346–350. (a)
Kazdin, A. E., & Mascitelli, S. Covert and overt rehearsal and homework practice in developing assertiveness. *Journal of Consulting and Clinical Psychology*, 1982, *59*, 250–258. (b)
Kazdin, A. E., & Wilson, G. T. *Evaluation of behavior therapy: Issues, evidence, and research strategies.* Cambridge, Mass.: Ballinger, 1978.
Kelly, E. L., Goldberg, L. R., Fiske, D. W., & Kilkowski, J. M. Twenty-five years later: A follow-up study of the graduate students in clinical psychology assessed in the VA selection research project. *American Psychologist*, 1978, *33*, 746–755.
Kendall, P. C., & Hollon, S. D. (Eds.). *Cognitive-behavioral interventions: Theory, research, and procedures.* New York: Academic Press, 1979.
Keyser, V., & Barling, J. Determinants of children's self-efficacy beliefs in an academic environment. *Cognitive Therapy and Research*, 1981, *5*, 29–40.
Kirsch, I. "Microanalytic" analyses of efficacy expectations as predictors of performance. *Cognitive Therapy and Research*, 1980, *4*, 259–262.
Klien, M. H., Dittman, A. T., Parloff, M. B., & Gill, M. M. Behavior therapy: Observations and reflections. *Journal of Consulting and Clinical Psychology*, 1969, *33*, 259–266.
Kubie, L. S. Relation of the conditioned reflex to psychoanalytic technic. *Archives of Neurology and Psychiatry*, 1934, *32*, 1137–1142.
Luborsky, L., Singer, B., & Luborsky, L. Comparative studies of psychotherapies: Is it true that "everyone has won and all must have prizes"? *Archives of General Psychiatry*, 1975, *32*, 995–1008.
Mahoney, M. J. *Cognition and behavior modification.* Cambridge, Mass.: Ballinger, 1974.
Marmor, J., & Woods, S. M. (Eds.). *The interface between psychodynamic and behavioral therapies.* New York: Plenum Press, 1980.
Martin, D. B. *Learning-based client-centered therapy.* Monterey, Calif.: Brooks/Cole, 1972.
Meichenbaum, D. *Cognitive-behavior modification: An integrative approach.* New York: Plenum Press, 1977.

Messer, S. B., & Winokur, M. Some limits to the integration of psychoanalysis and behavior therapy. *American Psychologist*, 1980, *35*, 818–827.

National Institute of Mental Health, Report of the Research Task Force. *Research in the service of mental health*. DHEW Publication (No. 75-236). Rockville, Md.: DHEW, 1975.

Paul, G. L. Insight vs. desensitization in psychotherapy two years after termination. *Journal of Consulting Psychology*, 1967, *31*, 333–348.

Paul, G. L. Two-year follow-up of systematic desensitization in therapy groups. *Journal of Abnormal Psychology*, 1968, *73*, 119–130.

Pervin, L. The representative design of person–situation research. In D. Magnusson & N. S. Endler (Eds.), *Personality at the crossroads: Current issues in interactional psychology*. Hillsdale, N.J.: Erlbaum, 1977.

Rachman, S. J. (Ed.). Perceived self-efficacy: Analyses of Bandura's theory of behavioural change. *Advances in Behaviour Research and Therapy*, 1978, *1*, 137–269.

Rachman, S. J., & Wilson, G. T. *The effects of psychological therapy* (2nd ed.). Oxford: Pergamon, 1980.

Rapaport, D. The structure of psychoanalytic theory: A systematizing attempt. In S. Koch (Ed.), *Psychology: A study of a science* (Vol. 1). New York: McGraw-Hill, 1959.

Rehm, L. P. (Ed.). *Behavior therapy for depression: Present status and future directions*. New York: Academic Press, 1981.

Ryle, A. A common language for the psychotherapies? *British Journal of Psychiatry*, 1978, *132*, 585–594.

Sajwaj, T., Twardosz, S., & Burke, M. Side effects of extinction procedures in a remedial preschool. *Journal of Applied Behavior Analysis*, 1972, *5*, 163–175.

Salter, A. *Conditioned reflex therapy*. New York: Straus & Young, 1949.

Sarason, I. G. Three lacunae of cognitive therapy. *Cognitive Therapy and Research*, 1979, *3*, 223–235.

Shapiro, D. A., & Shapiro, D. *Meta-analysis of comparative studies: A replication and refinement*. Paper presented at annual meeting of the Society of Psychotherapy Research, Aspen, Colorado, June 1981

Shelton, J. L., & Levy, R. L. (Eds.). *Behavioral assignments and treatment compliance: A handbook of clinical strategies*. Champaign, Ill.: Research Press, 1981. (a)

Shelton, J. L., & Levy, R. L. A survey of the reported use of assigned homework activities in contemporary behavior therapy literature. *The Behavior Therapist*, 1981, *4*(4), 13–14. (b)

Sloane, R. B., Staples, F. R., Cristol, A. H., Yorkston, N. J., & Whipple, K. *Psychotherapy versus behavior therapy*. Cambridge: Harvard University Press, 1975.

Smith, D. Trends in counseling and psychotherapy. *American Psychologist*, 1982, *37*, 802–809.

Smith, M. L., & Glass, G. V. Meta-analysis of psychotherapy outcome studies. *American Psychologist*, 1977, *32*, 752–760.

Smith, M. L., Glass, G. V., & Miller, T. I. *The benefits of psychotherapy*. Baltimore: Johns Hopkins University Press, 1980.

Solyom, L., Heseltine, G. F. D., McClure, D. J., Ledwidge, B., & Kenny, F. A comparative study of aversion relief and systematic desensitization in the treatment of phobias. *British Journal of Psychiatry*, 1971, *119*, 299–303.

Stoudenmire, J. Behavioral treatment of voyeurism and possible symptom substitution. *Psychotherapy: Theory, Research and Practice*, 1973, *10*, 328–330.

Thoresen, C. E. Behavioral humanism. In C. E. Thoresen (Ed.), *Behavior modification in education*. Chicago: University of Chicago Press, 1973.

Ullmann, L. P., & Krasner, L. (Eds.). *Case studies in behavior modification*. New York: Holt, Rinehart & Winston, 1965.

Voeltz, L. M., & Evans, I. M. The assessment of behavioral interrelationships in child behavior therapy. *Behavioral Assessment*, 1982, *4*, 131–165.

Wachtel, P. L. *Psychoanalysis and behavior therapy: Toward an integration.* New York: Basic Books, 1977.

Wachtel, P. L. What can dynamic therapies contribute to behavior therapy? *Behavior Therapy,* 1982, *13,* 594–609.

Wadnersman, A., Poppen, P., & Ricks, D. (Eds.). *Humanism and behaviorism: Dialogue and growth.* Oxford: Pergamon, 1976.

Wahler, R. G. Some structural aspects of deviant child behavior. *Journal of Applied Behavior Analysis,* 1975, *8,* 27–42.

Wahler, R. G., & Fox, J. J. Solitary toy play and time out: A family treatment package for children with aggressive and oppositional behavior. *Journal of Applied Behavior Analysis,* 1980, *13,* 23–39. (a)

Wahler, R. G., & Fox, J. J. *Response structure in deviant child–parent relationships: Implications for family therapy.* Paper presented to the Nebraska Symposium on Motivation, University of Nebraska, Lincoln, October 1980. (b)

Wahler, R. G., Berland, R. M., & Coe, T. D. Generalization processes in child behavior change. In B. B. Lahey & A. E. Kazdin (Eds.), *Advances in clinical child psychology* (Vol. 2). New York: Plenum Press, 1979.

Weitzman, B. Behavior therapy and psychotherapy. *Psychological Review,* 1967, *74,* 300–317.

Woody, R. H. *Psychobehavioral counseling and therapy: Integrating behavioral and insight techniques.* New York: Appleton-Century-Crofts, 1971.

Yates, A. J. Symptoms and symptom substitution. *Psychological Review,* 1958, *65,* 371–374.

5

Psychoanalytic Constructs and Empirical Research

Commentary on Alan E. Kazdin

ERIC MENDELSOHN and LLOYD H. SILVERMAN

Alan Kazdin's chapter is a clearly written and thought-provoking contribution to the study of the integration issue. We agree with his emphasis on empirical study and join in his call for research designed to identify processes and strategies common to the various schools of therapy. As does Kazdin, we also consider it necessary to define the "level" at which integration is being considered and view integrations on the levels of broad theory, concepts, strategies, and methods as differing from each other conceptually and methodologically. Further, we agree that integration on the level of strategy holds considerable promise for generating useful research. Having stated our general positive response to Kazdin's position, we will, in the remainder of this comment, take up a number of issues raised by his discussion that, in our opinion, merit elaboration or reconsideration.

ERIC MENDELSOHN • The New York Hospital-Cornell Medical Center, Westchester Division, White Plains, New York 10605. LLOYD H. SILVERMAN • New York Veterans Administration Regional Office, New York, New York 10001 and Department of Psychology, New York University, New York, New York 10003.

EMPIRICISM

The first issue concerns the effects of approaching the study of psychoanalysis (or the integration of the behavior therapies and psychoanalysis) empirically. When phenomena of concern to psychoanalysts are subjected to controlled experimental study (rather than examined in depth via the single-case method), it is likely that certain features of psychoanalysis will be emphasized whereas others are not. Controlled experiments, whether they are geared to the discovery of common strategies and processes among the psychotherapies, as Kazdin proposes, or to the elucidation of psychodynamic relationships as we discuss in our chapter, will tend to focus on objectifiable, measurable phenomena. Readily observable and discrete events that covary or are causally related for groups of people are more likely to be investigated, whereas those aspects of experience that are harder to classify because they are more molar, idiosyncratic, or affective/cognitive (rather than narrowly behavioral) are less likely to be studied. In his approach to the integration issue, Kazdin does not emphasize the role of psychoanalysis in promoting insight or in modifying important but subjective aspects of self-experience. Rather, he considers the behavior therapies and psychodynamically oriented treatments principally as they affect presenting problems and produce behavior change. Psychoanalysis, insofar as it is a therapy having the goal of symptomatic and adaptational improvements, can be studied using controlled experimental designs. However, in order to study psychoanalysis as a method for illuminating subjective experience, for uncovering private and idiosyncratic references, and for developing multiple and complex meanings, descriptive and clinical methods must be utilized along with controlled experimentation.

CONCEPTUAL INTEGRATION

Kazdin's position is that empirical study best proceeds when phenomena are viewed atheoretically. In developing useful integrations, he is reluctant to retain constructs derived from one school of therapy or another because he considers them to be laden with theoretical baggage; that is, their referents are predetermined, they are often difficult to operationalize and measure, and they tend to carry considerable connotative as well as denotative meaning. This in turn is seen as hampering research efforts. Kazdin concludes that, in order to study the common ground between the behavior therapies and psychodynamic approaches, new atheoretical constructs (such as "response covariation") must be developed and that existing ones must be utilized more fully. In our view, existing theoretical constructs do not *necessarily* pose the problems that Kazdin cites, and, in light of this, abandoning them for purposes of research represents an overreaction.

Kazdin employs the arguments just cited in his critique of integration on the conceptual (theoretical) level. In particular, he questions the usefulness of "extend[ing] the meaning or application of general concepts beyond the phenomena they were proposed to explain." Although we share Kazdin's view that integration on the level of theory may be hampered by certain inherent limitations, we disagree on the reasons for this. We maintain that integration that involves reconciling the "basic assumptions" of the two schools is limited by important philosophical differences (cf. Messer & Winokur, 1980). However, we are more optimistic about theoretical integrations that involve applying constructs derived from one school to phenomena described by clinicians of a different school. That is what we present in our chapter when we discuss the inadvertent activation of unconscious fantasies in the behavior therapies.* Another example of the profitable use of one approach in considering data generated by another is Wachtel's (1977) application of the behavioral concepts of "exposure" and "desensitization" to a consideration of the anxiety-reducing properties of the dynamic psychotherapies. We would maintain that, as long as the constructs involved can be operationally defined and empirically tested, integrations of this type can enhance research efforts by suggesting sources of variance that might otherwise be overlooked by workers who conceptualize therapeutic change solely from one vantage point.

EXPERIMENTAL STRATEGIES

We are of the opinion that more is known about psychoanalytic constructs and psychodynamic relationships and that more is potentially knowable by use of methods that currently exist than Kazdin indicates. Thus, in discussing the construct "symptom substitution," Kazdin argues both that the construct is untestable and that, more generally, causal relations between symptoms and underlying psychological factors cannot be demonstrated. Both these positions, we think, warrant reconsideration. In regard to the second, more general point, we agree that methods for dem-

* To the extent that *unconscious fantasy* is considered a superordinate construct that subsumes phenomena observed by behaviorists and psychoanalysts, its use coincides with the approach referred to as "integration on the level of strategy." However, because the term unconscious fantasy derives from psychoanalytic theory and has connotative meanings associated with that theory we recognize that it differs from the atheoretical prototypes proposed by Kazdin.

onstrating the *independent* existence of causal factors analogous to those used in physical medicine are not available to researchers studying the psychological determinants of behavior. However, we would call attention to two experimental methods that have provided substantial amounts of data that, in a more limited sense, do, indeed, demonstrate causal relationships between psychodynamic factors and behavior that are in keeping with particular psychoanalytic formulations. These are the subliminal psychodynamic activation method (described in our chapter and summarized in Silverman, 1982) and the use of hypnotic induction of paramnesias as developed by Reyher and his co-workers (summarized in Silverman, 1976). The results from these studies show that the activation of unconscious psychodynamically relevant motives (motives involving the kinds of unconscious wishes, anxieties, and fantasies that are an essential part of psychoanalytic thinking) can produce ("cause") symptomatic changes predicted by clinical psychoanalytic theory.* Moreover, the results from some of these studies demonstrate *specific* relationships between particular unconscious motives and symptoms. With regard to the subliminal psychodynamic activation method, in one study (Silverman, Bronstein, & Mendelsohn, 1976) different clinical groups were each exposed to two experimental conditions as well as to a control condition. In one experimental condition, subjects from a given clinical group received subliminal exposures of a stimulus that, on the basis of theory and prior experimentation, was expected to intensify the symptoms characteristic of that group. In the second condition, the subjects were exposed to a stimulus that met neither of these criteria but that met both criteria for a different clinical group. The results were that the "relevant" stimulus in each case temporarily exacerbated symptomatology in the targeted group whereas the "irrelevant" experimental stimulus did not. Thus, for example, a stimulus suggesting the theme of incest intensified homosexual feelings in a group of male homosexuals, whereas a stimulus suggesting oral aggression directed against mother did not. Conversely, a group of schizophrenics showed increased thought disorder after the oral-aggressive stimulus but not after the incest stimulus.

The idea that specific psychodynamically relevant unconscious motives affect specific forms of behavior was further demonstrated in two

* In considering psychological causality from a more restrictive perspective, we are distinguishing between what may be termed *psychodynamic causality* and *etiological causality*. In the present context, the former refers to changes in symptoms or adaptation that follow from a psychodynamically relevant intervention (e.g., the activation of a salient unconscious wish), whereas the latter refers to the full range of factors (constitutional, structural, situational, etc.) that may lead to the development of any symptom or mode of adaptation. The experimental methods we are discussing demonstrate *psychodynamic* rather than *etiological* causality.

more recent studies (Dauber, 1980; Schmidt, 1981). Samples of depressed college students were divided into two subgroups on the basis of their scores on a depression inventory developed by Blatt *et al.* (Blatt, D'Afflitti, & Quinlan, 1976). The first type was termed "introjective depression" and was found where guilt was presumed to underlie the depression and the second was termed "anaclitic depression" and was found where the depression was understood to be associated with experiences of loss. In each experiment, the effects of two subliminal psychodynamically relevant stimuli (as well as a control stimulus) were studied; one of these stimuli was designed to intensify feelings of guilt and the other, feelings of loss. In both studies, it was found that the introjective depressives were affected by the guilt-related stimulus but not by the loss-related stimulus, whereas the converse was the case for the anaclitic depressives.

Finally, mention should be made of one investigation using the hypnosis paramnesia paradigm in which the specificity of a particular psychodynamic activation was demonstrated. Karnilow (1973) found that, when two groups of male college students were hypnotized and a paramnesia suggesting sexual seduction by a woman was introduced, significantly more symptoms were generated when the woman was described (for one group) as older and married than occurred when she was described (for the other group) as younger and unmarried. This was viewed as supporting the notion that unconscious sexual wishes are more likely to be pathogenic when they are specifically linked to Oedipal themes than when they are not.

The preceding data, we submit, offer strong support for the psychoanalytic proposition that psychodynamically relevant factors have a causal relationship to the emergence of symptoms.* What about the more specific problem Kazdin raises, namely, experimentally studying symptom substitution? Although we do not subscribe to the view that a symptom "removed" as a result of nonanalytic (including behavioral) interventions will necessarily or even probably lead to the emergence of a "substitute" symptom, we do believe there is a method available that permits one to study the circumstances under which true "symptom substitution" (as opposed to "response covariation") occurs. This method was developed by Seitz (1951, 1953). Using a hypnotic procedure, he suggested to patients that a specific symptom would disappear and be replaced by other symptoms. Sometimes, he found, the suggestion worked, whereas at other times

* For purposes of validating clinical psychoanalytic propositions, such experimental data provide a necessary complement to the clinical data (projective test responses, dreams, free associations, parapraxes, etc.) that are traditionally used by psychoanalysts to infer the presence of underlying motives. Together these types of data provide a stronger basis for concluding that causal rather than merely correlational effects are present.

it did not, with his crucial finding being that the former situation prevailed when the suggested substitute symptom was thought to be "psychodynamically equivalent" to the symptom that was removed by suggestion. Unfortunately, the number of studies in which this method has been used has been meager, and crucial controls have not been employed, so that the data reported by Seitz can be seen as no more than suggestive. However, our point, for purposes of the present discussion, is that a method exists whereby the psychoanalytic construct "symptom substitution" can be experimentally studied and its applicability and limits more clearly defined. We believe that, utilizing proper controls, *predictions* about which symptoms can substitute for each other could be tested, and subject and situational variables that determine whether or not symptom substitution will occur could be identified.

INTEGRATION ON THE LEVEL OF TECHNIQUE

In closing, we would like to comment briefly on the problems associated with integration on the level of procedure or technique. Kazdin maintains that integration on this level is not likely to be productive because (a) procedures vary considerably *within* the psychodynamic and behavior therapies and because (b) it is unlikely that there can be agreement about the choice of outcome measures in evaluating the effectiveness of procedural combinations. Although we agree that procedural heterogeneity characterizes both schools of therapy, we believe that it is worthwhile to develop and to test promising combinations of techniques empirically (e.g., Feather & Rhoads, 1972a, 1972b; Wachtel, 1977). With regard to outcome research, given that theoretical differences among researchers have led to divergent outcome criteria, we would favor studies in which measures compatible with both theoretical orientations were used. In fact, utilizing a broad range of outcome measures may be recommended as a strategy for enhancing the informational yield of all outcome studies. Doing this as a matter of course should have the effect of sensitizing researchers to measures derived from different theoretical models and might lead to more meaningful dialogue between proponents of different schools of thought.

REFERENCES

Blatt, S. J., D'Afflitti, J., & Quinlan, D. Experiences of depression in normal young adults. *Journal of Abnormal Psychology*, 1976, *85*, 383–389.

Dauber, N. *An investigation of guilt, loss and the separation-individuation process in depression.* Unpublished doctoral dissertation, Loyola University of Chicago, 1980.

Feather, B. W., & Rhoads, J. M. Psychodynamic behavior therapy: I. Theory and rationale. *Archives of General Psychiatry,* 1972, *26,* 496–502. (a)

Feather, B. W., & Rhoads, J. M. Psychodynamic behavior therapy: II. Clinical aspects. *Archives of General Psychiatry,* 1972, *26,* 503–511. (b)

Karnilow, A. *A comparison of oedipal and peer sex through the use of hypnotically implanted paramnesias.* Unpublished doctoral dissertation, Michigan State University, 1973.

Messer, S. B., & Winokur, M. Some limits to the integration of psychoanalytic and behavior therapy. *American Psychologist,* 1980, *35*(9), 818–827.

Schmidt, J. M. *The effects of subliminally presented anaclitic and introjective stimuli on normal young adults.* Unpublished doctoral dissertation, University of Southern Mississippi, 1981.

Seitz, P. D. Symbolism and organ choice in conversion reaction. *Psychosomatic Medicine,* 1951, *13,* 254–259.

Seitz, P. D. Experiments in the substitution of symptoms by hypnosis: II. *Psychosomatic Medicine,* 153, *15,* 405–424.

Silverman, L. H. Psychoanalytic theory: "The reports of my death are greatly exaggerated." *American Psychologist,* 1976, *31,* 621–637.

Silverman, L. H. The subliminal psychodynamic activation method: Overview and comprehensive listing of studies. In J. Masling (Ed.), *Empirical studies in psychoanalysis* (Vol. 1). Hillsdale, N.J.: Erlbaum, 1982.

Silverman, L. H., Bronstein, A., & Mendelsohn, E. The further use of the subliminal psychodynamic activation method for the experimental study of the clinical theory of psychoanalysis: On the specificity of relationships between manifest psychopathology and unconscious conflict. *Psychotherapy: Theory, Research and Practice,* 1976, *13,* 2–16.

Wachtel, P. L. *Psychoanalysis and behavior therapy.* New York: Basic Books, 1977.

6

Psychoanalytic, Psychodynamic, Cognitive Behavior, and Behavior Therapies Compared

MERTON M. GILL

Psychoanalysis and behaviorism can be compared in many different ways. In these remarks, I will confine myself to their relationship as methods of therapy.

Because I believe there is a much greater incompatibility between psychoanalysis and behavior therapy than between psychodynamic therapies other than psychoanalysis and behavior therapy, I must distinguish between psychoanalysis and other psychodynamic therapies. Whereas all psychodynamic therapies explore the patient's mental content, only psychoanalysis makes the analysis of the transference, or, to use a formulation closer to the data, the analysis of the patient's experience of the relationship as its central task. It is in connection with the analysis of the transference that I will point to incompatibility between psychoanalysis and behavior therapy.

But first I shall deal with psychodynamic therapy other than psychoanalysis and behavior therapy. Any such comparison must postulate a common and defining feature for the various psychodynamic therapies, on the one hand and behavioral therapies, on the other hand. I propose

---

MERTON M. GILL • Department of Psychiatry, University of Illinois, Chicago, Illinois 60680. This chapter has been revised from a presentation at a meeting of the Association for the Advancement of Behavior Therapy, November 17, 1978.

that these common and defining features lie in a distinction between examining the meaning of behavior and attempting to alter behavior directly. The former is psychodynamic or cognitive therapy because it explores the patient's mental content, whereas the latter is behavior therapy because it attempts to influence behavior directly rather than by way of exploring its meaning. Psychodynamic therapies can differ widely from one another, depending on the theory of psychodynamics that the therapist uses, whereas behavior therapies can differ widely from one another, depending on the behavioral techniques that the therapist uses. Nevertheless, the common and defining feature of the psychodynamic therapies is the exploration of the patient's mental content, whether or not the therapist also attempts to influence the patient's behavior directly, whereas the common and defining feature of the behavior therapies is the attempt to influence the patient's behavior directly, whether or not the therapist also explores the patient's mental content. As a concrete instance, if the patient has a phobia, the behavior therapist works directly on the phobia, whether by desensitization or some other technique; the psychodynamic therapist explores the patient's mental content relating to the phobia, whereas the psychoanalyst does not focus on the phobia as such but assumes that the phobia will find some representation in the patient–analyst relationship and will be relieved if this relationship is established, examined, and altered.

Cognitive behavior therapy is a hybrid that attempts to integrate exploration of mental content and direct alteration of behavior. To the extent, then, to which the psychodynamic therapist adds techniques of the direct manipulation of behavior or the cognitive behavior therapist adds the exploration of mental content will psychodynamic and cognitive behavior therapy converge. The major shift on the current scene seems to be a movement of behavior therapists toward incorporating cognitive considerations into their work. Psychodynamic and psychoanalytic therapies are continuing as they were, though a few psychodynamic therapists are beginning to use systematic behavioral techniques also.

That psychodynamic techniques and techniques of direct behavioral intervention can be combined is no longer in question. They can be and are being combined. The combination differs from how psychodynamic therapists ordinarily work, in the abandonment of the stricture against direct behavioral intervention that was adopted from psychoanalysis.

When psychodynamic and behavioral techniques are combined, the examination of the repercussions on the mental content of the behavioral intervention may or may not be examined. When Freud (1910/1957) for example, recommended that, at a certain stage in the analysis of a phobia, it was necessary to urge the patient to put himself or herself in the phobic situation, he was combining psychodynamic (in this case, psychoanalytic) and behavioral techniques. He does not explicitly say whether one should then examine the repercussions on the transference of the therapist's urging the patient to dare the phobia. We may assume that he would have done so. The point here is that the repercussion on the mental content of the behavioral technique may or may not be examined. Insofar as it is, the therapy is closer to a strictly psychodynamic one than if it is not. Wachtel's (1977) proposal for combining psychoanalytic and behavioral techniques explicitly recommends examining the repercussions on the transference of the behavioral techniques employed.

Although I have suggested that psychodynamic psychotherapy and cognitive behavior therapy are not incompatible, I believe that psychoanalysis and even cognitive behavior therapy are incompatible. The ordinary psychoanalytic argument against direct behavioral intervention is that it interferes with the spontaneous and "uncontaminated" development of the patient's attitudes toward the analyst. The analyst is ideally considered to be engaging in only interpretive communication with the patient; that is, he or she is not in any other way behaving in relation to the patient. The counterargument is that the blank screen model of the analyst is a myth, that the very existence of the analytic situation means that even the silent analyst is engaged in a behavioral interaction with the patient. The examination of the transference, therefore, the counterargument continues, has to take the analyst's actual behavior into account. I agree that the blank screen analyst is a myth and that the analyst's behaviors, including his or her verbal interventions, have important nonverbal behavioral meanings that serve the patient as more or less plausible explanations of his or her experience of the relationship. Therefore, they must be taken into account in analyzing the transference. It is the failure to recognize these principles in much current psychoanalytic therapy that justifies the criticism that it is authoritarian. It is false to consider the patient's experience of the interpersonal analytic situation to be a distortion of reality rather than a view of that situation with its own plausibility and validity (Gill, 1982a; Hoffman, 1983)

Nevertheless, it is in connection with the analysis of the transference that techniques of direct behavioral intervention are incompatible. There are two main reasons. First, the relatively ambiguous and restrained stance of the analyst is designed to bring into prominence the prior expectations the patient brings to the therapy so that his or her contribution to his or her experience of the relationship is more likely to stand out. Direct behavioral intervention makes this more difficult because the meaning the patient attributes to the therapist's behavior becomes more completely accountable for by that behavior. It is more difficult for patients to see that their feelings that the therapist is belittling them are drawn from a prior expectation of their own, for example, if it arises in response to instructions to bring in a detailed report of their day's activities than if they feel "put down" simply because the therapist has made an interpretation. I concede that the distinction is not absolute, but it is hard for me to see how a therapy centrally concerned with a hierarchy of imagined situations to promote desensitization, for example, can be combined with a central concern with the patient's experience of the relationship that is designed to show how that experience is influenced by the patient's prior expectation. The more prominent, vigorous, and varied the therapist's direct interventions are, the more difficult will it become to clarify these prior expectations.

Second, there is an important difference between the inadvertent influence on the transference that the analytic setup and the analyst's behavior exert and the influence on the transference of deliberate behavioral interventions. In the first situation, the therapist can plausibly maintain the position of refraining from influencing the patient insofar as he can, but in the second situation he cannot. The crucial analytic atmosphere of neutrality is compatible with *inadvertent* but not with *advertent* influence.

The role of free association in the therapeutic process provides a ready illustration. Free association is also often misunderstood to be ideally uninfluenced by the therapist. But just as the therapist's behavior inevitably influences the patient's experience of the relationship, so too will his or her associations be influenced by the setup in general and by interventions in particular. Free association means only that time and again the patient is given the opportunity to speak his or her mind as freely as he or she can. Nevertheless, the employment of free association in an analysis involves an atmosphere in which initiative is handed over to the patient in a way that is vastly different from one in which directive interventions are used.

I have so far discussed the relationships among the several therapies in a way that I suspect will seem odd to my psychoanalytic colleagues. I mean, that to them, the difference between psychoanalysis and psychoanalytically oriented psychotherapy is already great, even if, as the literature attests, it is not too easy to specify, whereas the difference between psychoanalysis and behavior therapy and even psychoanalysis and cognitive behavior therapy is so vast that it is a mistake even to take seriously the idea of comparing them. In any event, I have attempted to state the differences in terms of the analysis of the transference because, in my view, the most crucially identifying feature of psychoanalysis is the attempt to carry out the analysis of the transference as far as possible. There are, however, other major differences between psychoanalysis and any other form of psychological therapy. I will state two of them in an effort to make more plausible why so many psychoanalysts would regard the very effort to compare the therapies as misguided.

First, the goal of psychoanalysis is more ambitious than that of any other form of psychological therapy. The goal of psychodynamic therapy other than psychoanalysis is usually to overcome a symptom that has brought the patient to therapy, whereas the goal of psychoanalysis is no less than the reconstruction of character, not only to overcome symptoms but to attain as effective a level of functioning as is possible.

Second, and related to the foregoing point, psychoanalysis aims to bring about a regression, that, one hopes, is confined to the analytic sessions. The purpose of the regression is to provide access to the infantile neurosis; that is, the original and early disturbance of development, which is putatively the basis of the present character structure and which must be resolved if that character structure is to be altered in any essential fashion. The ambitious goal and the regression I have described as characteristic of the analytic process mean that much more primitive and developmentally earlier mental content will be dealt with in analysis than in any other psychological therapy. Primitive mental content is much less likely to be evident in the more reality-oriented situation that is characteristic of other psychological therapies.

I consider it possible that, as psychoanalysis is conducted, a regression that is, to some extent, iatrogenic and unnecessary is induced, while at the same time, this regression is erroneously considered to be spontaneous rather than in any way induced. But this is not the appropriate place for the discussion of this point. What I am attempting to make clear is only the vast difference in conception between psychoanalysis and the other psychological therapies.

I return to the issue of the analysis of the transference that, as I have said, I consider to be the central identifying feature of psychoanalysis as a technique.

Two arguments have been advanced against what is considered by some analysts to be an overemphasis on the analysis of the transference, or at least on its alleged exclusivity, in the work of some analysts. One is that an overemphasis on the transference neglects the other two important areas in which work must be done, namely, developmental history and the patient's contemporary relationships outside of the analytic situation. The other is that there are limits to the range of interpersonal behaviors that can be expressed in the transference.

As to the first argument, the reconstruction and, if possible, recovery in memory of the developmental history are considered to play important roles in the resolution of the transference. It is part of the ambitious goal of psychoanalysis, and it plays a correspondingly lesser role in other psychological therapies.

I do not deny the importance of the exploration of the patient's history, but I do believe that a defensive flight to the past from the transference in the present is common and that significant work in the resolution of the transference can be accomplished in the transference as expressed in the present as well as in its explication by the past (Gill, 1982a).

The second argument against an overemphasis on the transference relates to work with contemporary relationships outside the therapy situation. It maintains that because there are limits to the range of interpersonal behavior that can be expressed in the transference, it is mandatory to deal with contemporary relationships outside the transference. This argument relates to the one offered by Wachtel for combining behavioral techniques with the exploration of mental content. To take a gross example, How can a young man's diffidence about approaching a girl to ask for a date be expressed in the transference to a bearded, elderly analyst? And, in Wachtel's view, is it not necessary or at least useful to encourage and even instruct the patient how to approach a girl in addition to exploring the meaning of the diffidence?

As a proponent of the centrality of the analysis of the transference, I would make two points about this second argument. The first is that although clarification of the nature and meaning of the patient's behavior outside the analytic situation is often a necessary prelude to understanding and interpreting the transference, *clarification* is to be distinguished from *interpretation.* Although I grant that clarification and interpretation can shade into one another, the distinction, in principle, is that clarification seeks only to make the patient's mental content more explicit, whereas interpretation proposes connections that were, at most, only preconscious to the patient. If the patient is discussing an exchange with his wife, questions that are designed to get a fuller and more explicit account of this exchange could be classified as *clarification.* However, a suggestion that the report of this exchange was also an allusion to what was thus far only an implicit reference to a similar situation in the transference would be classified as an *interpretation.* It is because the therapist is a participant in the transference, whereas in the exchange with the wife he is not, that makes it more reasonable to expect that he is in a better position to make a valid interpretation about the transference than he is about the exchange with the wife. This is not to overlook the argument that, as a participant, he may be more prejudiced than as an onlooker and that, therefore he may be less likely to make a valid interpretation from the position of participant. A reply to this counterargument is that, in the analytic situation, the dialogue between the two participants can lead to a progressively clear exposition of even contrasting assessments of the situation than when the patient and therapist are discussing what happened between the patient and a third party.

As a second counterargument to the argument that the range of situations expressible in the transference is inevitably limited by the realities of patient and therapist, I suggest that if the many disguises in which the transference is expressed can be deciphered it may well be that the range within which the patient's problems are expressible, and indeed are expressed, in the transference is considerably greater than is often considered to be the case.

For clarification, I must repeat that although there are analysts who are concerned with an overemphasis on the transference and therapists who propose combining behavioral techniques with analysis, both take their point of departure from the alleged limits on the types of situations that are expressible in the transference. They, therefore, propose differing remedies for this problem. The analysts suggest only exploration and interpretation of contemporary relations outside the transference, whereas those who would add behavioral techniques suggest direct behavioral interventions as well.

Another argument offered by Wachtel for adding behavioral to psychodynamic techniques is that work in the transference is not as genuine as it is in the patient's real life. I would counter that the combined interpersonal experience and cognitive integration of an examination of the experience of the relationship is unique and uniquely effective (Gill & Hoffman, 1980). Even those analysts who argue against the exclusivity of work in the transference agree on the unique effectiveness of what is accomplished in the transference. It is the interpersonal situation that is most fully and accurately known and the one in which immediate affective involvement is likely to be the greatest. It is rare that symptomatic behavior, a change in that behavior, and insight into the symptom and the new behavior take place in relation to the very person involved as the other participant in that behavior, except in the analysis of transference.

The related argument, that changes in the patient–therapist relationship are not carried over into life outside the therapy without additional specific techniques for that purpose, is contrary to analytic experience.

I am not offering a simple yes-or-no answer to the question of the compatibility of psychoanalysis and behavior therapy. I am, however, pointing to the difficulties of combining the central technique of psychoanalysis, namely, a primary concern with exploring the patient's experience of the relationship, with systematic techniques of direct behavioral intervention. Of course, if the kind of behavior therapy under consideration is one that excludes examination of the patient's mental content in principle, even cognitive behavior therapy, let alone psychoanalysis, is incompatible with behavior therapy by definition.

So that I may not be misunderstood as suggesting that psychoanalysis is the only desirable and useful therapy, I will conclude with three additional points. First, I am not addressing myself to the question of what therapy can produce the quickest change in a symptom but to whether behavior therapy and psychodynamic therapy and behavior therapy and psychoanalysis are compatible. Second, I believe the techniques of free association and the analysis of the transference can and should be used to whatever extent the particular circumstances permit, even with a lesser frequency of sessions and a shorter overall duration than is usually considered necessary for an analysis (Gill, 1982a). In other words, I distinguish between the use of analytic techniques and the carrying out of a full-scale psychoanalysis. What I have really addressed, therefore, is not the compatibility of psychoanalysis and behavior *therapy* but of psychoanalytic—which I distinguished from psychodynamic—and behavioral *techniques.* And third, insofar as therapy manipulates behavior covertly, although recognizing that it is doing so, it would seem to violate the principle of truthfulness between patient and therapist. Open suggestions for behavioral change are, in that sense, preferable to hidden suggestions. What I mean is that I believe the combination of behavioral and psychodynamic techniques as advocated by Wachtel is surely preferable to *advertent* manipulation of behavior that the therapist does not acknowledge and is probably preferable to the inadvertent but unexamined manipulation of behavior that I believe is inevitable in any psychological therapy that does not make the analysis of the transference its central technique. Psychoanalytic technique is the only one that, in principle, makes the analysis of transference central.

AUTOBIOGRAPHICAL STATEMENT

I have long been concerned with what seems to me to be the incorrect minimization of the role of new interpersonal experience as a mutative factor in psychoanalysis, in contrast to the alleged exclusivity of the role of insight. I have also long been cognizant of the argument that the interpersonal relationship is the common factor that brings about change in the various psychotherapies, even if one attempts to analyze it, as in psychoanalysis. In other words, although all those who claim they have a specific agent of change are likely to see the interpersonal relationship as the placebo in other methods, there are those who claim the interpersonal relationship is the specific agent in all methods (Frank, 1973). It was not until I was asked to be a participant in a symposium by the Association for Advancement of

Behavior Therapy in 1978 that I gave any particular thought to behavior therapy, beyond assuming that changes brought about in behavior therapy, allegedly due to its specific techniques, in fact resulted from the interpersonal relationship between patient and therapist. Furthermore, I had considered behavior therapy to be so different from psychoanalysis that it was idle to even think of comparing them. It was because the convention met in Chicago, my own city, and because the symposium to which I was invited to participate included persons whom I respected that I agreed to write the paper.

MERTON M. GILL, M.D.

REFERENCES

Frank, Jerome. *Persuasion and healing.* Baltimore: John Hopkins University Press, 1973.

Freud, S. The future prospects of psychoanalytic therapy. *Standard Edition* (Vol 11). London: Hogarth Press, 1957. (Originally published, 1910.)

Gill, M. *Analysis of transference, Vol. I, Theory and technique.* Psychological Issues 53. New York: International Universities Press, 1982. (a)

Gill, M. Merton Gill: An interview by J. Reppen. *Psychoanalytic Review,* 1982, *69,* 167–190. (b)

Gill, M., & Hoffman, I. Z. Some views on effective principles of psychotherapy. In M. R. Goldsmith (Ed.), *Psychotherapy Process,* special issue of *Cognitive Therapy and Research,* 1980, *4,* 271–306.

Hoffman, I. Z. The patient as interpreter of the therapist's experience. *Contemporary Psychoanalysis,* 1983, *19,* 389–422.

Wachtel, P. *Psychoanalysis and behavior therapy: Toward integration.* New York: Basic Books, 1977.

6

Psychoanalysis Contrasted with Psychodynamic and Behavior Therapies

Commentary on Merton M. Gill

JOHN M. RHOADS

Gill's chapter comparing psychoanalytic, psychodynamic, cognitive-behavioral, and behavior therapies was a joy to read because of his clear definitions of each of them. He states that the central task of psychoanalysis is the analysis of the patient's experience of the relationship with the analyst, in contrast to behavior therapy in which the goal is the direct alteration of the patient's symptom or behavior. Psychodynamic therapy is defined as the exploration of the patient's mental content that involves the analysis of contemporary relationships outside the therapy as well as analysis of the transference. The degree of the therapist's activity also constitutes a crucial difference among the three. Whereas the psychodynamic therapies share the goal of examining the meaning of behavior, behavior therapy attempts to alter that behavior directly. Gill sees cognitive behavior therapy as "a hybrid" that attempts to integrate exploration of mental content and direct alteration of behavior.

Psychoanalysis itself, as distinguished from psychodynamic therapy, is seen as incompatible with behavior therapy, a view with which I whole-

JOHN M. RHOADS • Department of Psychiatry, Duke University Medical Center, Durham, North Carolina 27710.

heartedly agree. Although the concept of the analyst as a blank screen is certainly a myth (if he was, it is unlikely that very much would happen), all actions by the analyst are seen as meaningful to the patient. Such matters as the way the analytic hour commences or ends, when the analyst chooses to interpret as well as what his or her tone of voice and mannerisms are, provide a mix of transference and reality. The article by Guntrip (1975) that contrasts his two analyses is a graphic illustration of how much the technique of two respected analysts may vary. Nevertheless, on a relative scale, the analyst is at one pole, and the behaviorist is at the other insofar as intrusion of the therapist's own personality through his or her actions is concerned. Gill's statement regarding development of transference that "the more prominent, vigorous, and varied the therapist's direct interventions, the more difficult will it become to clarify these prior expectations [of the patient]" exemplifies this differentiation.

Gill states that the goal of psychoanalysis is more ambitious than that of any other form of psychological therapy. The goal of psychoanalysis is stated to be "the reconstruction of character, not only to overcome symptoms, but to attain as effective a level of functioning as possible." He states that the goal of psychodynamic therapy is usually to overcome a symptom. I think many psychodynamic therapists would disagree with this statement. The various forms of psychodynamic therapy that vary in frequency of sessions and duration may aim not only for symptom relief but equally for character change. Such character change may have as its goal marked alterations of the patient's ability to accept his or her impulses, lessened strictness of his or her conscience, or the reverse—modification of masochistic character traits or the improvement of relationships fixated at or regressed to primitive levels.

For that matter, behavior therapy itself may aim at major characterological changes as is exemplified by Birk *et al.*'s (Birk, Huddleston, Miller, & Cohler, 1971) report of treatment of homosexuality by a combined method. Additionally, primitive mental content not only occurs as a result of regression in psychoanalysis, but it may be the basis for the symptom to be treated by behavior therapy. A crucial difference between all these therapies and psychoanalysis is that regression within the psychoanalytic sessions serves a vital therapeutic purpose, but it is not viewed as desirable in psychodynamic or behavior theories.

Despite the denials of early behaviorists, the phenomena of transference and resistance do occur in the course of behavior therapy (Rhoads & Feather, 1972) and should be, in fact in some instances must be, interpreted if the behavior therapy is to succeed.

Aside from psychoanalysis, contemporary relationships are discussed in all forms of therapy. Gill is quite correct in stating that transference interpretations are apt to be more accurate because the affect is fresher and more immediate and because the patient's responses are firsthand, assuming that the analyst's countertransference is not an issue. It is apt to involve less distortion than a response by the therapist to a secondhand relation of an outside interaction. One need only note the surfacing of different and sometimes corrective data when the spouse of a patient is interviewed.

To conclude, I agree that the basic techniques and goals of psychoanalysis and those of behavior therapy are different and that the two techniques are incompatible. It is in the intermediate therapies, psychodynamic and cognitive behavioral, that there can be a productive overlapping of psychoanalytic theory and behavioral methods.

Psychoanalysis is both a technique of therapy that has a limited application and a theory of personality that has a wide range of usefulness. It is in this latter category that it may serve as a basis for psychodynamic therapy and as an aid in behavior therapy. Psychodynamic psychotherapy has as its goal the understanding of the conscious or unconscious meanings and motivations of behavior. It is based on analytic principles and utilizes interpretation of content, resistances, defenses, and transference. Behavioral methods may be utilized in a number of ways to supplement it—as ego-strengthening techniques, to overcome specific resistances, or as an introduction. Behavior therapy has as its goal the alteration of symptomatic behaviors. Analytic insight into psychopathology may be used as a guide in the design of behavioral programs and as a basis for the interpretation of resistances or transferences that interfere with the progression of the behavior therapy. Interpretation of content may be a useful follow-up to behavior therapy. As Gill notes, many therapists are currently combining these in a variety of productive ways.

REFERENCES

Birk, L., Huddleston, W., Miller, E., & Cohler, B. Avoidance conditioning for homosexuality. *Archives of General Psychiatry*, 1971, *25*, 314–323.

Guntrip, H. My experience of analysis with Fairbairn and Winnicott. *International Review of Psychoanalysis*, 1975, *2*, 145–156.

Rhoads, J. M., & Feather, B. W. Transference and resistance observed in behavior therapy. *British Journal of Medical Psychology*, 1972, *45*, 99–103.

6

A Rejoinder to John M. Rhoads

MERTON M. GILL

Rhoads is correct in stating that the goal of psychodynamic therapy can vary widely from symptom relief to character change. Indeed, it can have a goal as ambitious as that of psychoanalysis, although it is more usually less so. Rhoads suggests that behavior therapy can also have an ambitious goal, but he includes the interpretation of transference and resistance in "behavior" therapy with an ambitious goal. I believe that a therapy that includes the interpretation of transference and resistance is not correctly designated a "behavior" therapy.

It is true that the generally accepted view in psychoanalysis is that a regression is a necessary part of an analysis. My somewhat idiosyncratic position is that a regression beyond that with which the patient enters the therapy is undesirable, true though it is that the analytic setting, especially if its inadvertent infantilizing suggestive effect is not interpreted, may lead to an iatrogenic regression. To make my view plausible, a distinction between a deepening regression and the making manifest of disguised but already existing regressive mental content must be made. The progressive clarification of such mental content may, and I hope it does, take place in a context of progression rather than regression.

I applaud Rhoads's insistence on a sharp distinction between analytic *technique* and analytic *theory*. He considers the technique to have limited application and the theory to have a wide range of usefulness. I agree that that is the generally accepted view. Again, somewhat idiosyncratically, I

MERTON M. GILL • Department of Psychiatry, University of Illinois, Chicago, Illinois 60680.

have argued (1982) that with a dyadic and perspectival view of the analytic situation, analytic technique becomes altered in such a way that it has a much wider range of applicability than is ordinarily considered optimal for psychoanalysis. That view requires a distinction between an analytic technique, employed with an indeterminate goal, and psychoanalysis proper, which is employed with a predefined ambitious goal (Gill, in press).

REFERENCES

Gill, M. Merton Gill: An interview by J. Reppen. *Psychoanalytic Review*, 1982, *69*, 167–190.
Gill, M. Comment on: "What is psychotherapy by J. Lifschutz." *International Journal of Psychoanalytic Psychotherapy*, in press.

7

Relationships between Psychodynamic and Behavior Therapies

JOHN M. RHOADS

Recent years have seen some constructive efforts at the reconciliation of behavior therapy and psychodynamic therapies (Marmor & Woods, 1980; Wachtel, 1977; Wachtel, 1982). These are in happy contrast to the antagonistic polemics that have taken place in the past. For the most part, adherents of each have had little comprehension of the goals and methods of the other and have simply reiterated their own idealistic stances rather than look for common ground or seek to understand the real differences. In view of recent cutbacks in insurance funding for mental health care, the erosive effects of inflation on income available for care, and the push to document the effectiveness of treatments, it seems imperative that we try to determine which therapy or which combination of therapies works best for what conditions and which are most cost-effective.

The antagonism is curious in a way, because both forms of practice have been in existence for millennia. The interpretation of dynamics is exemplified by Freud (1900/1958) in his reference to Aristander's interpretation of Alexander the Great's Dancing Satyr dream during the frustratingly long siege of Tyre. Aristander broke the word *satyr* into its two Greek component words and then interpreted the dream as meaning that "Tyre will be yours." Learning theory has been with us as long as animals

JOHN M. RHOADS • Department of Psychiatry, Duke University Medical Center, Durham, North Carolina 27710.

have been domesticated and trained, soldiers have been drilled, and students have been schooled. The unfriendliness seems understandable only in terms of mutual lack of understanding of each other's goals, methods, vocabularies, and the narcissism inherent in what is perceived as a threat to one's own belief system.

Some notable efforts have been made to reconcile the two methods of operation. French (1933) and Alexander (1963) made extensive efforts to compare analysis and behavior therapy. Marmor and Woods (1980) have collected a number of articles by various authors dealing with the interfaces between the two. Wachtel (1977) has made extensive clinical efforts to combine psychodynamic therapy with behavior therapy. He views his approach as a fusion of analytic and behavioral methods.

My impression is that many behaviorists are very good psychotherapists, and, whether they acknowledge it or not, they utilize such dynamic concepts as the doctor–patient relationsip, the patient's obstruction of the therapist's efforts to help him or her, motivation, and self-protective measures. The doctor–patient relationship may involve both the reality relationship and the transference. The former indicates the patient's perception of the therapist as he or she actually is—as the therapist relates to the patient, deals with business details, and appears knowledgeable. The transference refers to the patient's fantasies about the therapist that are based on past important relationships. Therapists of all types have to deal with the patient's unconscious obstruction of the therapist's best efforts to help. These resistances may include withholding information, distortion of information, unexplained or rationalized absences and latenesses, failure to take medication, and so forth. Motivation concerns the goals of the patient and the extent of his or her drive to achieve them. Everyone utilizes self-protection against hurt, including the familiar defenses of denial, projection, displacement, and rationalization.

In a similar manner, many analytical therapists, knowingly or unknowingly, utilize aspects of learning theory by approving or disapproving a patient's actions, changes, or thinking. Frequently, the analytical therapist, despite his or her efforts, serves as a model for his or her patient's thoughts and actions. By going over and over the same traumatic material, many patients, in effect, undergo a desensitization process.

Curiously, many refer to the other system as if it were a closed philosophy with uniformity of theoretical and clinical viewpoints among its adherents. This is hardly the case. One need recall only the volcanic emotions engendered by splits within psychoanalytic institutes! Similarly, some behaviorists attack others in a manner that is reminiscent of their psychoanalytic brethren.

How may behavior therapy and psychodynamic therapies coexist or complement one another? There are a number of ways.

1. Behavior therapy may serve as a reasonable introduction to therapy. Its focus on the patient's symptoms builds faith that the complaint is being taken seriously, it frequently gives a measure of relief promptly, and these factors cement a working relationship between the patient and therapist.

2. Behavior therapy may be an adjunct to psychodynamic therapy by dealing with certain specific aspects of the patient's difficulties.

3. Psychodynamic therapy may be an adjunct to behavior therapy by facilitating progress of the process through interpretation of resistances, by helping the patient to understand the nature and origin of his or her problems, and by providing the therapist with an understanding of which targets to choose for behavioral methods.

4. Behavior therapy may be a means of learning new behaviors and ways of thinking after some cognitive understanding of the problem has been gained. Conversely, psychodynamic therapy may be a useful follow-through after a dominating symptom has been removed and a characterological problem has thereby been exposed.

The therapies have in common the aspects of cognitive learning, corrective experiences, modeling and identification with the therapist, working through, reinforcement, the use of fantasy, and the analysis of antecedents and consequences. Thus, both therapies utilize education, and both aim at providing corrective experiences for the patient in the course of therapy. The behaviorist does this by prescribed behavioral programs aimed at altering behaviors of the patient, whereas the analytic therapist provides this by analysis of the resistances and transferences in the therapeutic situation as well as analysis of the cognitive aspects of events in the patient's past and present life. It is a common experience to find analysands imitating their analysts' characteristic mannerisms, clichés, and even tones of voice in the course of treatment. When I was a candidate in an analytic institute, it was easy for me and my fellow candidates to identify the training analyst of any of our colleagues by looking for the preceding identifying features. Fortunately, in most instances these disappeared, though a few were certain to linger on and to be incorporated into the candidates' individual styles. The behaviorist may utilize modeling as a specific technique in the treatment of certain phobias—as, for instance, requiring a germ-phobic patient to touch a phobic object after the therapist has done so. Both types of therapists utilize fantasy extensively. The analysis of dreams and fantasies constitutes a major portion of what goes on in psychodynamic therapies, whereas the use of fantasy in the behavioral techniques of implosion and desensitization is the essence of the treatment. Analysis of antecedents and consequences is utilized in behavior therapy to plan behavioral programs that may interfere with events leading to the undesired behaviors or providing pleasant or unpleasant consequences for actions of the client.

The major difference between dynamic and behavior therapies hinges on the relationship of the patient and therapist. In psychoanalysis the relationship, the fantasies about it, and the attitude that the patient attributes to the therapist are the core of treatment. This is somewhat less important in analytically oriented psychotherapy, but in it also the therapist must be constantly on the alert for transferences that are hidden in incidents the patient reports about his or her daily life. In behavior therapy, the focus is less on the patient's fantasy life, and very little, if at all, on his or her relationship with the therapist—unless something in the relationship interferes with the therapy. Some behaviorists (Bandura 1969) discount the importance of transference, viewing it as friendship or as a substitute gratification for those lacking in the client's real life. In general, the behaviorist strives for a positive working relationship with the patient, does not delve into it, and focuses on the patient's symptoms and behaviors rather than on his or her relationship to the therapist.

In the following pages, I will provide clinical examples of how the two approaches may be utilized in conjunction with one another.

BEHAVIOR THERAPY AS AN INTRODUCTION

Many patients, once an initial evaluation is completed, expect that they and the therapist will focus on the immediate alleviation of their presenting or crippling complaints. For some, an explanation to the effect that the symptoms seem to come from some inner difficulties that are best approached by a method akin to free association suffices; for others, it does not. Many patients either lack psychological mindedness, or they are so distressed by their symptoms that they find it difficult to focus on other issues in their lives, which they have not considered to be problems and therefore regard them as irrelevant. Although some of these may ultimately grasp the principles behind a psychodynamic approach, others never do, and so they seek help elsewhere or turn to a pharmacy for aid. A focus on the immediate cause for the visit to the therapist gratifies the patient by providing him or her with tangible evidence that the therapist is taking his or her complaint seriously and is making a sincere effort to relieve the patient's immediate discomfort.

CASE 1

A young man afflicted with a germ phobia washed his hands somewhere between 30 and 40 times daily after a morning shower lasting as long as 4 hours! A previous physician who had treated him for 1 year had focused on certain disordered aspects of the patient's life, but the patient had never been able to grasp the connection between them and his symptoms. These disordered aspects continued to such a degree that he was unable to work and had virtually abandoned all social life. He reported his family history as negative and insisted that everything was fine, though one could readily guess that there was a problem for this single 30-year-old heterosexual male's living in his parents' home and having social and sexual relationships with prostitutes only. The patient was hospitalized for treatment of his social and occupational disabilities. Baseline counts were taken of the number of hand washings, when they occurred during the day, and the length of the showers. A program of paradoxical intention with respect to the hand washing was instituted. Arbitrary times for a number of hand washings that were equal to the daily baseline count were rigidly presented. Gloves were taped onto the patient's wrists to be worn between required washings. He was encouraged to reduce the amount of time spent in the shower gradually. He was required to keep large charts (graphs) posted on his door with daily hand-wash counts on one and the time spent in the shower on the other. Gradually, the showers decreased in length. The patient began to cheat on the hand-washing regimen's requirements by removing the gloves or by not putting them on, but he did refrain from washing his hands at unauthorized times. He asked that the required number be reduced, and this was gradually done. This was seen as an effort by the patient to resist the control inherent in the program. The therapist objected only mildly and allowed the patient to discontinue the wearing of gloves because the goal of reduced hand washing was being achieved. Also, by objecting to the gloves, the patient was "saving face" by being more assertive, which was a desired objective. A good working relationship had been established by now, and the patient began to speak spontaneously of his fears of dating "virtuous" women. The behavior therapy was continued, but the patient himself now led the way into a discussion of some of the dynamics of his Madonna–prostitute split, his antagonism to his family, and his guilt about it. Not all patients will make this spontaneous transition, but many do if they sense that the therapist is interested in them, in their life, and its style.

Case 2*

An elderly woman belched up to 400 times daily for 3 years and refused all efforts by her internist to explain her symptom on the basis of family problems as well as by refusing referral for any psychiatric help. After 3 years of many tests, medications, and failures, she relented and allowed herself to be hospitalized in a psychiatric ward.

*This case was treated in conjunction with Carole S. Orleans.

The patient was required to keep hourly belch counts each day, which established the number of approximately 400 per day noted before. The daily counts were required to be continued throughout the hospitalization.

A program involving the use of massed practice and aversive conditioning was was instituted. The massed practice involved having this patient retire to the bathroom within her single room after closing both doors. A small x had been placed on the wall at nose level. The patient was required to stand a foot away from the x and belch continuously at the spot for 5 minutes four times daily. Each day the number of belches outside the required 5-minute solitary periods had to be recorded on a graph that was posted on the patient's door. It became apparent that other patients on the ward responded to the patient's belching with amusement at first but with irritation after a few days. Every effort was made by the nursing staff to avoid any response at all to the patient's belching, and similar instructions were given to the other patients at a community meeting. It was believed that a nonresponse would not duplicate the inferred negative response she received at home. Within a week's time the number of belches decreased dramatically to approximately 25 per day. At this point the program was changed such that when she had the feeling that she had to burp at a time other than that required, she would try to hold back as long as possible and then go to the bathroom and burp at the wall when it was no longer possible to hold it back. Initially, the forced burping occasionally caused nausea or even vomiting. Later this stopped. By the time the belching, other than that at required times, had subsided to approximately a dozen a day, the patient was deemed ready for discharge.

Within a week after the program had been instituted, she began to talk about some of her family difficulties. These involved much hostility in her relationships with the family members who had been taking advantage of the "nice lady" for years. Once the patient learned that she could control her symptom, she spontaneously spoke to the therapist of her feelings about her life situation—problems her internist had correctly guessed in his initial evaluation. To aid her in learning to cope with her angry feelings, she was placed in a course of assertive training. Meetings were held with the patient and her family after she had had some time to learn appropriate assertive techniques. The belching had served as a somatized method of expressing anger arising from various life situations with which she could not cope.

The preceding cases represent severe and disabling illnesses. In each, the patient either denied or was unable to see any connection between life circumstances and the disabling illness. All attention was focused on the symptoms. Each felt that life was out of control, but this was too overwhelming a recognition to face. Thus, in each instance the struggle was displaced to a disabling symptom. In many people's minds, a disabling symptom is reason enough for not dealing with one's living problems. From a psychodynamic standpoint, this resistance to dealing with life problems that were seen as unsolvable constituted a block to treatment. Neither patient was able to consider the illness as the consequences of their life situation. Both were quite willing to consider dealing with the symptom and were very cooperative. Once it was clear to them that they were able to control their symptoms, they gained faith that their therapists might be able to help them with the life-style problems and were willing to take a more involved look at the latter.

BEHAVIOR THERAPY AS AN ADJUNCT

Behavior therapy may serve as an adjunct during the course of psychodynamic therapy by dealing with certain targeted aspects of the patient's behavior. These may include the following: (a) a focus on specific symptoms or inhibitions, for example, utilizing biofeedback to help control symptoms such as muscle-tension headaches, or anxiety; (b) the use of desensitization techniques to deal with certain phobic aspects of a patient's behaviors; (c) providing ego techniques that were previously lacking, such as assertive training to enable the patient to take appropriate aggressive actions in instances in which inhibitions had hampered them previously; (d) the control of undesirable behaviors such as heavy smoking by referral to an antismoking program; (e) dealing with certain resistances (see Case 6); and (f) coping with the special patient's dynamic problems by means of forced fantasies, which involved asking the patient to fantasize certain situations. Thus, in a case reported by Rhoads and Feather (1974), a masochistic transvestite was required to fantasize dealing with a woman in a sadistic manner. Having to imagine sadistic behavior led the patient to a greater appreciation of the extent and nature of his masochism and of the underlying hostility turned upon himself. This enabled him to recall the origins of his sexual masochism and to begin a corrective approach to it.

CASE 3

A patient in intensive analytic psychotherapy was disabled by overwhelming anxiety. He was referred to a behavior therapist for training in relaxation because the endless recounting of his anxiety symptoms wasted many hours during his therapy and because the symptoms themselves were disabling in his everyday life. When some assistance had been gained through his learning of relaxation techniques, the analytic therapy was able to proceed more efficaciously.

The referral to another therapist for relaxation training was made because it was feared that the analytic therapist's shifting from a passive interpretive role to an active educator–instructor role would interfere significantly with the development of transferences. It is probably easier to go the other route; that is, from behaviorist to analytically oriented therapist. In the latter instance, the therapist initially becomes an authority figure but one in whom the patient reposes trust and faith—that is, if the behavior therapy works well! For the therapist in this case, to turn to a more passive interpretive role was apparently easier for a patient to adjust to than was the reverse; that is, to go from a passive interpretive role to an authoritarian one and then back to a passive interpretive one.

In this particular instance, the patient, who had spent almost his entire hours relating the infinite dreary details of his anxiety, was able to complain to the analytic therapist about the authoritarian manner of the behaviorist, even though he appreciated the fact that behavior therapy had enabled him to feel more comfortable. This paradox proved an opening wedge for analytic therapy when the patient brought out his ambivalence to the analytic therapist because he was "ineffectual and had to refer me elsewhere for relief." The patient also told the therapist that "you were wise to make a referral to someone for a specific technique which helped the therapy get under way."

Case 4

A 38-year-old woman trapped in a unhappy sexless marriage recognized her hostility to her passive-aggressive husband but was unable to do anything about it in spite of encouragement in both individual and group therapies. A period of assertive training enabled her to begin to voice her specific complaints to her husband. This promoted a partial resolution of her agoraphobia by enabling her to give vent to some of the pent-up hostility that had been projected onto the environment, leading to her fear to leave her house. After the expression of anger at her husband, she was able to spend more time in the dayroom and from there to enlarge her world to the rest of the hospital and ultimately to outdoors.

Case 5

A 55-year-old woman who had had a prior psychotic episode was in supportive–directive psychotherapy following resolution of the psychotic state. Understanding was gained about her pathologic relationship to her sister, her resentment of the sister, and the guilt feelings that made her unable to cope with the sister's exploitation of her. The psychotherapy proceeded relatively well for several years, but it was noted that she suffered from recurrent severe episodes of bronchitis and that whenever tensions arose in her relationships with other people her smoking increased to the point of three to four packs of cigarettes a day.

The smoking evidently served as a tension-release mechanism, but it was clearly an unhealthy displacement. She was referred to an antismoking clinic where behavioral methods were utilized, which enabled her to decrease her smoking behavior. For a brief time her anxiety increased, but this provided more focus for psychodynamic work. And, in fact, much of this might not have been brought out had the displacement not been blocked by the successful work done in the smoking clinic. However, my belief is that had this been done earlier, soon after the resolution of the psychosis, the process might not have worked as well and might have blocked what was, for a time, a necessary outlet.

CASE 6

A couple were seen in conjoint marital therapy. As is usually the case in such instances, they were on the verge of divorce and could barely stand the sight of one another. Each professed a desire for the marriage to continue, but during the first several hours of therapy it was apparent that their marital life was comparable to that of the fabled two cats from Kilkenny. I politely suggested that they seemed to prefer fighting to any other behaviors, a proposition with which they disagreed—though its correctness was manifested clearly. They were assigned the task of holding hands for 5 minutes in the morning and in the evening. Both objected, which presented the opportunity to reiterate the previous interpretation and to point out the resistance. They reluctantly agreed but carried out the instructions. Each separately reported that while holding hands there were many temptations to resume fighting, but somehow they found it more difficult during those brief periods. They were then instructed to pay each other two compliments during the 5 minute hand-holding periods. No other instructions were given. Subsequently, each reported that it was difficult to find anything to compliment the other about, but they did manage to find a few items.

These behavioral methods enabled the couple to recognize and discuss how serious was the disruption of their marriage. Yet each was about to recognize that they wished the marriage to continue and that if this was to take place each would have to make a greater contribution. Initially, the wife brought out the mismanagement of finances by the husband. He apologized repeatedly but always in an aggrieved, angry tone. The words were right, but the affect was not, and the wife continued her assault over the misuse of her money and his "freeloading" along with unfavorable comparisons of her husband to her father. This latter comparison infuriated him each time it came up. She came from a very wealthy but cold family. The wife had inherited a considerable amount of money and had no training at all about what to do with it. The husband came from a family of rather modest means, felt inferior and inadequate, and had mistakenly used his wife's money in an ill-fated venture that he had undertaken in an effort to prove himself worthy of her. When the venture failed, his feelings of inadequacy increased. Her attacks on him had unerringly focused on his weakest point; therefore, to avoid being "subjugated" and overwhelmed, he would counterattack. When these dynamics were able to be interpreted, the husband was able to apologize in a more meaningful way, and the wife was able to reduce her attacks on him after recognizing his vulnerability. In this case, the behavior therapy was utilized to get treatment underway by utilizing a degree of physical intimacy as a counter to the verbal fighting. The intervention of compliments conteracted the almost totally negative atmosphere that was of such intensity that it preempted those positive aspects of the marriage that continued to exist. Because calm had been inserted into the interchange, the couple were able to voice some of their fears and hostilities rather than merely to swap insults.

PSYCHODYNAMIC THERAPY AS AN ADJUNCT

During the course of behavior therapy, one encounters resistances like those one finds in the course of analytic therapy. As is well known, patients can find innumerable excuses for not making counts, not keeping charts, for miscounting, for constructing graphs in an unintelligible manner, and for not carrying out recommended actions. It is frequently helpful to mention to the patient the fact that he or she is resisting and, if possible, to note some of the reasons for it. Often, pointing this out to the patient brings an amused nod of recognition followed by a compliant response but with no follow-through in action. Open rebellion may be missing, but the passive resistance is all too obvious. It is useful to have the patients discuss their feelings about assignments, to relate this, if possible, to what is known about their similar behaviors in other life circumstances and possibly even to the origins of this resistive behavior in their earlier life settings.

In the first case previously discussed, the patient "forgot" to time the starting of his shower ritual for a number of sessions. He "lost count" of the number of hand washings; therefore, it was impossible to get accurate daily counts. He reported that he had great difficulty working with the primary nurse assigned to him, whose duty it was to assist him in record keeping, to oversee the hand washing and other such tasks. He reported that he could work much better with another nurse. The first nurse herself asked to be transferred to another case. It was noted that the first nurse was young, exceptionally pretty, religious, and clearly a "nice" girl. The other nurse was somewhat older and had a more motherly approach. The first nurse's request was refused, and the transference situation was explained to her. This gave us the opportunity to bring the matter to the patient's attention and to point out that the Madonna–prostitute split in the patient's mind carried over not only from his family to his social relationships but also to the hospital setting as well. We were able then to discuss his attraction to the nurse, his fears and guilt about it, and his efforts to solve the problem by avoidance and by turning to the older, more motherly nurse.

With the interpretation of his resistance and his transference to the two nurses, the patient's compliance with the behavior therapy protocol improved remarkably. I believe that being able to interpret his transference resistance led to better compliance with the behavior therapy and ultimately to an improvement of the symptom to the point where he was able to return home to work, to recognize the nature of his life problem, and to be willing to be referred to a dynamic therapist close to his home. The referral was necessitated by the fact that the patient lived so far from the hospital that it made follow-up impractical.

In the second case, the burping lady had been given a counter to count and record the number of belches per day. She reported difficulty working the counter; therefore, another one was obtained for her. Next she equivocated over whether a tiny squeak counted or whether it had to be a resounding roar in order to be enumerated. In addition she would "lose count" or say, "There were too many to count at once." It was pointed out to her that this represented an effort on her part to avoid dealing with other problems in her life. To this she made no response, but it was noticeable that counts were more prompt and accurate thereafter.

Targets for behavioral approaches may be selected on the basis of an understanding of the patient's psychodynamic pathology. In the following case, treated by systematic desensitization, the hierarchies were evolved on the basis of a psychodynamic understanding of the patient's problem, which involved a symbolic displacement. Ignoring the displacement, the focus was on the original feared object and situation, which was treated behaviorally.

Case 7

Feather and Rhoads (1972) reported the treatment of a woman with a cockroach phobia who had not seen a roach for many years. Her illness had begun 4 years previously with a severe washing compulsion that was related to a fear of contamination by cockroaches. Her disability reached the point at which she was spending 12 to 18 hours a day in compulsive rituals and had a bleeding dermatitis in her hands and arms. The illness had begun coincident with the death of her mother and the discovery of an unwanted pregnancy at age 37. Because she had not seen a roach for over a year, it seemed logical that roaches were a symbolic substitute for some more basic real fear. The pregnancy had occurred after years of presumed sterility. Following it, she developed a strong feeling of revulsion for her husband. Sex was out of the question, and even being touched casually by him led to feelings of revulsion and disgust. She rationalized that she was too preoccupied with cockroaches and cleanliness to bother with sex. It was inferred that cockroaches must therefore symbolize sexual contact with her husband, and for this reason we decided to desensitize her to her husband and to sex rather than to cockroaches. A program that reduced cleaning and scrubbing to 6 hours a day was instituted, and all compulsive cleaning had to be restricted to those times. She was taught muscle relaxation, and a desensitization hierarchy around the theme of physical contact with her husband was developed. Because even looking at a photograph of her husband elicited disgust, the initial scene in the desensitization hierarchy had to be a neutral one of a snow-covered mountain. The rest of the hierarchy consisted of imaginary scenes—first, looking at photographs of her husband and then directly at him, then touching him, and, finally, imagining intercourse and orgasm. The hierarchy had to be revised downward frequently because of feelings of revulsion and disgust. When she was able to imagine all the scenes in the hierarchy comfortably, she was instructed to begin carrying them out in reality, starting with the ones that were the lowest and moving to subsequent ones only when she felt free of discomfort. By the 25th session she was able to have intercourse with orgasms. She wished to retain 1 hour 3 days a week when she could scrub things as she felt like it. This was agreed to. She no longer thought about cockroaches or contamination except during the ritualized scrubbing time. She was able to leave her home, regain her weight, dress more attractively, and regain functioning. The case was seen as illustrating the application of systematic desensitization to a conflict underlying an obsessive-compulsive neurosis. The preoccupation with avoiding cockroaches and scrubbing represented a symbolic displacement of her fears of sex.

AN INTEGRATED APPROACH

As mentioned previously, there is usually some difficulty in shifting back and forth between the two approaches. In general, it appears easier to move from a behavioral approach to an analytic one, but this is not always the case. The case to be discussed next illustrates that it is sometimes possible to move from one to another and back, utilizing whichever method is most useful at a given time for special problems.

CASE 8

Rhoads and Feather (1972) reported the case of a young divorced woman who was treated for an anxiety state. Not until she had been in analytically oriented therapy for a year was she able to allow herself to be seen by a gynecologist, who determined that, although she had been married for several years, she was still a virgin. She herself had not known whether or not her marriage had been consummated, and for years she had not been able to touch or look at her own genitals. A desensitization procedure was then devised to be carried out by her at home that involved first looking at pictures of women's genitals in an anatomy text across the room and then gradually looking at the book at closer range. Next, she examined herself in a mirror, at first across the room and then gradually closer. She finally looked directly at her genitals and touched them. This enhanced familiarity and acceptance of herself enabled her to begin to talk about her unresolved Oedipal relationship with her father, his seductive behavior toward her even as an adult, and its interference with her ability to relate to men. The treatment had now shifted to a psychodynamic approach. Ultimately, she was able to remarry, and this time she was able to have a satisfactory sexual relationship.

DISCUSSION

No psychotherapeutic treatment is without its difficulties and complications. In some of the examples cited in this chapter, I have alluded to or described some of the specific difficulties encountered and how either mode of therapy may be utilized to deal with resistances arising in the course of the other. A major problem in the course of any approach is in dealing with the transference relationship. Such a relationship inevitably evolves between patient and therapist. In a short-term counseling or behavioral treatment, a relatively simple positive working relationship is all that is necessary, and no interpretations are called for. However, in some instances, a transference develops quickly, and its nature and ramifications must be kept in mind. The transference to the nurse noted in the first case gives a rather clear illustration of how an understanding of transference can be useful in the course of a behaviorally oriented therapy. In the second case, the therapists assumed an authoritative role in order to enforce compliance with what they believed were necessary tasks. Interpretation was also utilized, but no interpretation of the relationship between patient and therapist was necessary. In general, it is fairly easy to move from being directive, as in a behavioral approach, to being interpretative, as in a more analytic approach. It is more difficult to move in the former direction, especially if the analytic method is proceeding more or less successfully. I believe that moving in this direction results in such a mixed and confused transference that the patient and therapist find it difficult to continue working with one another. My experience, as exemplified in the third case, leads me to believe that if I am treating a patient with analytically oriented therapy, it is better to refer the patient to another therapist for the behavioral intervention. Although the referral in itself may be taken as evidence of more active intervention in the patient's life by the therapist, it is usually not an insurmountable one as long as the reason for it is clearly understood by both and as long as the analytically oriented therapist's own behavior does not change. Going the other direction seems to pose fewer difficulties. Patients, having begun to deal with the symptom, find it relatively easy to discuss more personal details of their life with the therapist, and the switch from more active to less active by the therapist seems less confusing for them. Case 8 represents an exception to the preceding and is included for that reason.

Which therapy or which combination is best for what problems? This is a perplexing question that must await more extensive and more carefully planned research. Sloane, Staples, Cristol, Yorkston, and Whipple (1975) have done a careful study of outpatient treatment of certain neuroses showing that either therapy was more effective than no therapy (waiting list) and that, in terms of results, there was little difference between behavior therapy and brief analytically oriented psychotherapy. One can reach some relatively self-evident propositions. Behavior therapy would seem to be indicated for the eradication of "ghost symptoms" (for example, phobias no longer serving a dynamic purpose but that have become habits), certain dangerous or disabling symptoms (such as a case cited by Rhoads in 1981 of a woman with the compulsion to put in and take out her contact lenses many times daily), for simple phobias that prevent an individual from carrying out essential daily tasks, and the use of operant methods to deal with certain types of disabling psychotic behavior (such as the token economy use of rewards for such desired behaviors as personal cleanliness, eating meals, etc.). Psychonalytically oriented therapy or psychoanalysis would appear to be indicated for neuroses involving inner conflicts, narcissistic disorders, and particularly for those instances where successful treatment is deemed to depend on the understanding and interpretation of transference and its various ramifications. I find it difficult to conceive of a behavioral method being other than partially successful at best in dealing with an individual's suffering from multiple sexual deviations, a man with an inability to relate to women to whom he feels close, a narcissistic problem of self-esteem maintenance (grandiosity vs. inferiority), or an unresolved Oedipus complex. Such cases depend on uncovering the unconscious roots of the problem, interpretation of the transference neurosis, and transfer of the knowledge gained by patients to their everyday life. On the other hand, it is possible to use an integrated approach in certain of these complex neurotic disorders. To illustrate this, a man in therapy for a chronic anxiety neurosis found it difficult to relate to his wife. He was angry with her, afraid of her, and dealt with her in a passive-aggressive manner. He confused her in his mind with his autocratic mother, though she was not at all like her. He found it difficult to cope with his mother, primarily because he could not deal with her manipulations, which left him feeling angry, guilty, and impotent. He was referred to a colleague, who, by means of role playing, desensitized him to his mother's behavior. Once he was able to cope better with his mother in reality, he no long needed to displace his angry feelings to his wife. This was something that could then be interpreted to him effectively and with the desired carry-over to an improved relationship with her.

SUMMARY

Much work has been done by a number of investigators on the relationship and the integration of psychoanalytic psychotherapy and behavior therapy. It is abundantly clear that both are effective methods of treatment for a number of psychiatric disorders and that, in some instances, a combination of the two methods can be utilized to shorten treatment or to facilitate it. It is to be hoped that further work will be done to clarify these relationships, to demonstrate scientifically for which conditions they are most effective, and to make possible greater efficiency in the therapy of mental disorders.

AUTOBIOGRAPHICAL STATEMENT

Nothing is so firmly believed as that which we least know.

MONTAIGNE

Reared in the psychoanalytic thinking that dominated residency training from the end of World War II until the advent of effective medications and behavior therapies, I was fortunate to have had O. Spurgeon English as a chief. He advised me when I began my residency to listen to and consider views that differed from those advocated by my immediate preceptors. This advice has stood me in good stead throughout my professional life. When tempted toward insularity, I have remembered his words and listened a little more carefully to those whom I did not understand or with whom I intuitively disagreed. It should be obvious to anyone who practices any form of therapy that no one form of psychiatric or psychologic therapy is 100% successful. It is unreasonable to blame this on the patient/client and equally so to attribute it to some hidden flaw in the technique of the therapist. With this background, I was prepared by the mid-1960s to look for effective, briefer, and less costly psychological forms of treatment as an addition to psychoanalytically oriented therapy.

Ben W. Feather and I had been collaborating in the treatment of some cases, not all of them successful, and we had wondered about the behavior therapies that were new at that time. He had just completed his Ph.D. in experimental psychology and was quite familiar with the rather limited literature on the subject at that time. At first, we were discouraged by the polemics indulged in by some of the early behaviorists, but we finally agreed that we should try them because, looked at from a theoretical standpoint, they did make sense. We agreed that whichever of us saw a likely case first, we would refer the patient to the other for behavior therapy, while continuing to observe the patient. I happened to see the first such case, referred the patient to Feather, and it was this patient who was written up in our initial publication in 1972. Feather used a creative and imaginative approach, basing his behavioral methods on our understanding of the patient's psychodynamics. The outcome of what seemed to be an impressively difficult case was surprisingly good! We followed it with a series of cases, alternating which one of us was the behaviorist and which was the observer. In this series of cases, we noted that, contrary to what some behaviorists said, one saw phenomena such as resistance and transference in behavior therapy as well as in psychodynamic therapies. At the same time, we gained an appreciation for the creativity and skill of many of the behavior therapists. Initially, we followed the methods of Joseph Wolpe and found that his writings gave clear, concise, and useful descriptions of his methods. We also came to admire his skill in preparing patients for behavior therapy, something we overlooked with some later cases.

Subsequently, Feather left Duke Medical Center to become chairman of the Department of Psychiatry at Brown University, and after a few years our collaboration regretfully ceased. My own work in the area has continued as appropriate cases present themselves. I would say that in addition to Wolpe, I have been most influenced by the writings of Isaac Marks, Paul Wachtel, Lee Birk, Victor Meyer, and S. Rachman.

Let us hope that in the future psychiatrists and psychologists will be able to provide their patient/clients with whichever form of therapy provides the most efficacious, least expensive, and most rapid relief for their illnesses.

JOHN M. RHOADS, M.D.

REFERENCES

Alexander, F. The dynamics of psychotherapy in the light of learning theory. *American Journal of Psychiatry*, 1963, *120*, 440–448.

Bandura, A. *Principles of behavior modification.* New York: Holt, Rinehart & Winston, 1969.

Feather, B. W., & Rhoads, J. M. Psychodynamic behavior therapy II. Clinical aspects. *Archives of General Psychiatry*, 1972, *26*, 503–511.

French, T. M. Interrelations between psychoanalysis and the experimental work of Pavlov. *American Journal of Psychiatry*, 1933, *89*, 1165–1203.

Freud, S. The interpretation of dreams. In *Standard Edition* (Vol. 4). London: Hogarth Press, 1958. (Originally Published, 1900.)

Marmor J., & Woods, S. M. *The interface between the psychodynamic and behavioral therapies.* New York: Plenum Press, 1980.

Rhoads, J. M. The integration of behavior therapy and psychoanalytic theory. *Journal of Psychiatric Treatment and Evaluation*, 1981, *3*, 1–6.

Rhoads, J. M., & Feather, B. W. Transference and resistance observed in behavior therapy. *British Journal of Medical Psycholology*, 1972, *45*, 99–103.

Rhoads, J. M., & Feather, B. W. The application of psychodynamics to behavior therapy. *American Journal of Psychiatry*, 1974, *131*, 17–20.

Sloane, R. B., Staples, F. R., Cristol, A. H., Yorkston, M. A., & Whipple, R. Short-term analytically oriented psychotherapy versus behavior therapy. *American Journal of Psychiatry*, 1975, *132*, 373—377.

Wachtel, P. L. *Psychoanalysis and behavior therapy: Toward an integration.* New York: Basic Books, 1977.

Wachtel, P. L. *Resistance: Psychodynamic and behavioral approaches.* New York : Plenum Press, 1982.

7

Differing Views of Transference

Commentary on John M. Rhoads

MERTON M. GILL

WIDE DISPARITY

The gap between Rhoads's perspective and mine seems to me so wide that I despair of making any genuine contact. I come to that conclusion in large measure because of the many indications of the gulf between us in our understanding of transference. I say this despite the fact that he does agree that a transference relationship develops in every therapy, whatever the approach, that even a referral has meaning in the transference, and that he cites problems in which behavioral methods cannot be more than partially successful at best.

Let me give an example. Rhoads says that if one begins with behavior therapy—and is successful—the therapist becomes a trusted authority figure. One is led to suspect that he regards such a transference as appropriate for an interpretive therapy and not something that may conceal transference trends that themselves require interpretation. He distinguishes between the psychodynamic therapist as passive and the behavior therapist as active. I consider this seriously misleading because it fails to recognize how interpretation is also an activity that always has repercussions on the transference.

Another indication of Rhoads's essential disregard of transference in my terms may be seen in his failure to say much about the transference

MERTON M. GILL • Department of Psychiatry, University of Illinois, Chicago, Illinois 60608.

meanings of the gross manipulations he describes. He does mention that the man with the obsessional washing shows evidence of disliking what he perceived as the coercion of the instructions as well as his preference for a young, pretty nurse rather than an older, motherly one, but these are only the grossest kinds of transferences. He says nothing about how the belching woman may have experienced the task she was assigned. I find it hard to believe that that experience did not include a significant element of feeling ridiculed. Some people may indeed find a particular cure worse than the disease and give up at least the overt manifestations of the disease. But should we not be especially curious about the fate of such cures after the patient is released from the immediate influence of the therapist? I realize that a psychoanalyst is hardly in a position to decry the absence of follow-up data, but I believe such data would be especially important in the kind of situation Rhoads describes.

A third example relating to our different views of transference is this: Rhoads makes the usual citation offered in discussions such as these of a patient who failed at an extended psychodynamic therapy (e.g., Cases 1 and 3) and who then responds well to behavioral therapy. How can I evaluate a psychodynamic therapy about which I am told only that the therapist "had focused on certain disordered aspects of the patient's life, but the patient had never been able to grasp the connection between them and his symptoms?" It is especially difficult for me to credit the dynamic therapy as well done when I can interpret such a statement to mean a dogged persistence on the therapist's part, even when what he was doing made no sense to the patient. In other words, the meaning of the therapist's activity was not being dealt with in the transference.

ADJUNCTION VERSUS INTEGRATION

Rhoads argues that psychodynamic and behavioral methods can be used in adjunctive and integrative ways. I fail to see that he has shown any difference between adjunctive and integrative uses. What he calls *integrative* turns out to be simply a triple sequence of the two treatments—interpretive, behavioral, interpretive—rather than the double sequence—interpretive behavioral or behavioral interpretive—that he calls *adjunctive.*

A genuine integration would be the intermingled use with interpretation of the transference meaning of behavioral intervention and behavioral intervention dictated by the transference patterns unearthed, as in Wachtel's (1977) proposal for integration. One is led to suspect, however, that Rhoads may consider a genuinely integrated approach to risk such a mixed and confused transference that the patient and therapist find it difficult to continue working with one another. He does approach this issue when he refers to the difficulty of changing from behavioral to interpretive therapy and the reverse. He believes the former is easier, so much so that an interpretive therapist who wants to add behavior therapy should refer the patient concurrently to another therapist. The basic theme of my own exposition is that there is a fundamental difficulty in principle in both manipulating and interpreting the transference in a treatment that attempts to integrate behavioral and interpretive techniques.

DOES EACH USE THE OTHER'S TECHNIQUES WITHOUT REALIZING IT?

Rhoads makes the usual suggestion that the behaviorist employs psychodynamic techniques, whether he or she admits it or not, and that the interpreter uses learning techniques—he instances desensitization—whether he or she admits it or not. But that failure to admit may be the key to whether we can ever understand each other, much less persuade each other. The genuinely formidable obstacles standing in the way of an understanding between behaviorists and analysts may be glimpsed if I ask how can one possibly learn what may be the transference meaning of a manipulation if one does not inquire into the mental content relating to it? And how could Rhoads go about showing that a reiterated interpretation exerted its effect by way of desensitization? How would he counter my suggestion that the effect may be a transference one, with the patient finally surrendering to get the therapist to stop harping on the same point? And how could I persuade him that an initial symptom amelioration by behavioral techniques that he says leads the patient to feel he is being taken seriously and will be helped may be explained on the basis of a transference effect? In fact, the early subsidence of symptoms is also a common phenomenon in an analysis and is there also ascribed to such factors as being taken seriously. Rhoads's invoking of such a factor at the same time that he ascribes the effect to a behavioral technique illustrates the way common-sense psychodynamic explorations are casually employed, only to be overlaid by the allegedly true explanation drawn from learning theory.

CONCEPTUAL CONFUSION

Rhoads is not careful enough about the concepts he uses in our two different systems of thought. Early in his chapter he refers to the use of both interpretive and behavioral practices for millennia, but he slips too easily from learning to learning theory. Of course any therapy includes learning. But the principles accounting for that learning are not necessarily those expressed as schedules of reinforcement and extinction. Another example of the blurring of what may well be major distinctions as to types of learning may be seen in Rhoads's lumping together the domestication and training of animals, the drilling of soldiers, and the schooling of students. Should he so readily assume that learning principles for animals and man and for different activities are necessarily the same? Rhoads says approving or disapproving patients' actions, changes, or thinking is utilizing an aspect of learning theory. What learning theory? Are not *approval* and *disapproval* terms in the language of interpersonal interaction? Is modeling, whether witting or unwitting, to be explained in learning or interpersonal theory? To speak of the analysis of fantasy in psychodynamic therapy and the use of fantasy in implosion and desensitization as if they are comparable is a travesty. If one goes to such a high level of abstraction as "both therapies utilize education, and both aim at providing corrective experiences for the patient," a specious convergence is obtained that may produce professional harmony but can only obstruct genuine understanding. I believe the same objection holds even for the more specific, differentiated elements that Rhoads suggests the two therapies have in common—cognitive learning, modeling and identification, working through, reinforcement, the use of fantasy, and the analysis of antecedents and consequences. This list ranges from specific mechanisms in two very disparate theoretical systems—identification and reinforcement—to the highly abstract affirmation of a scientific outlook: There are antecedents and consequences. Far more cogent as a statement of the differences a would-be integrator must confront is this statement by Rhoads:

> The behaviorist does this by prescribed behavioral programs aimed at altering behaviors of the patient, whereas the analytic therapist provides this by analysis of the resistances and transferences in the therapeutic situation as well as the cognitive aspects of events in the patient's past and present life.

Yet, even here, a major disparity in formulation may be seen: The behavioral reference is descriptive of the therapist's manifest activity, whereas the analytic reference already employs terms of a theoretical system like resistances and transferences. My own formulation (Gill, 1973) that the one manipulates the transference whereas the other analyzes the transference likewise uses terms from a system of explanation, but at least it is a single system.

BRIDGING THE GAP

Have I any suggestions for bridging the gap? I offer three. First, we need a more differentiated view of the systems we are comparing. Rhoads distinguishes only between analytic and behavioral methods, whereas I distinguish psychoanalytic, psychodynamic, cognitive, and behavioral methods.

Second, we will never understand each other if we communicate in summaries of case vignettes alone. We need detailed, even verbatim, studies of therapies, and what is even more important and difficult, we must figure out some way in which the mental content of a patient's being treated by behavioral methods can be elicited without interfering with the behavior therapy. I do not know whether it would be possible in purely behavioral therapy, although some retrospective method or some apparently uninvolved observer might help. Perhaps it can be done only in a therapy that genuinely integrates the two methods.

My third suggestion is, in a sense, the antithesis of attempts at theoretical integration of the two therapies, but it may nevertheless turn out to be the more fruitful activity. It is already being done to a greater or lesser extent. Let each system attempt to explain all the findings of the other in its own terms, that is, in its own language (Schafer, 1976) or from its own point of view (Gill, 1983). I am not suggesting that any language is as good as any other and that the ultimate goal is consistency. I believe, rather, that the attempt at mutual translation will show which is the more inclusive language that is more suited to the facts—and I am not overlooking the fact [*sic*] that the facts are to some degree defined by the language employed. I need not say which language in my opinion will turn out to be the better one.

Of course behavioral and dynamic *techniques* can be combined, but knowing that tells us little or nothing about the explanation of what is going on when they are.

REFERENCES

Gill, M. Analyzed and unanalyzed transference. *International Journal of Psychiatry*, 1973, *11*, 328–335.

Gill M. The point of view of psychoanalysis: Energy discharge or person. *Psychoanalysis and Contemporary Thought*, 1983, *6*, 523–551.

Schafer, R. *A new language for psychoanalysis*. New Haven: Yale University Press, 1976.

Wachtel, P. *Psychoanalysis and behavior therapy*. New York: Basic Books, 1977.

7

A Rejoinder to Merton M. Gill

JOHN M. RHOADS

I find it rather difficult to respond to Gill's commentary inasmuch as we seem to be speaking different languages and to have different goals regarding the subject under discussion. This is illustrated in his comment about the belching woman in which he wonders whether her response to the behavior therapy included an element of feeling ridiculed and whether she gave up the overt manifestation of the illness to avoid such a feeling. Such questions are irrelevant. They would be relevant had she objected, but she did not. His questions indicate an intellectual view of the treatment and leave out the practical aspects of need for rapid results in the case of third-party payers for relatively indigent patients.

To comment further on the case, it seemed apparent from the start that there was a family problem, and one could readily postulate that this woman's belching behavior was a means of protesting something about it. Inquiry met with steadfast denials, and because she already had resisted referral to a psychiatrist for several years, it seemed apparent that some other approach had to be tried. The behavioral approach, utilizing massed practice, made it possible for her to gain control over her symptoms in a short period of time. In the course of gaining this control, her anger at her family became apparent and could then be addressed as such. A point in dealing with this case was that it is likely that if her hostility toward her

---

JOHN M. RHOADS • Department of Psychiatry, Duke University Medical Center, Durham, North Carolina 27710.

family had not been dealt with, that symptom or some other one would probably have recurred. But because the psychodynamics had been "smoked out," as it were, by the behavioral method, they could be dealt with in a short time span. I might mention that we have a 2-year follow-up with no recurrence. The case followed the intervention sequence of behavioral, interpretive, and behavioral (the latter *behavioral* was assertiveness training to help this woman deal with her family). Perhaps this is sequential and not integrative, as Gill points out, but the use of assertiveness training *is* based on the psychodynamic understanding of the patient's failure during her lifetime to develop a means of dealing with her family's aggression against her and could be seen as constituting the remedy of an ego defect.

I have the impression that Gill looks at all phenomena through a psychoanalytic microscope. His comment that an initial symptom amelioration by behavioral techniques may be explained on the basis of a transference effect seems to me to be perfectly obvious. The problem is that some patients regard an analytic approach as not taking them seriously, and my point is not to deny that transference is present in each instance. My point is simply to fit the method to the patient rather than the patient to the method. Some patients clearly prefer an exploratory approach and respond to it, whereas others prefer a behavioral approach. In addition, Gill's comment on my statement about the psychodynamic therapist being passive and the behavior therapist active is misleading and simply misses the point. Of course an interpretation is an activity; I thought it was fairly clear that my reference was to the difference in quantity of interventions and the directiveness furnished by the behavior therapist as compared to the psychodynamic therapist.

I do not agree with Gill's formulation that the behaviorist manipulates the transference whereas the analyst analyzes it. This uses terms from one particular system of explanation and, in the process, attributes to the other a pejorative act. Finally, Gill's suggestion that in order to aid communication between behavioral and psychoanalytic therapists the mental content of a patient who is being treated by behavioral methods be elicited and reported without interfering with the behavior therapy has already been carried out (Rhoads & Feather, 1972).

To conclude, Gill seems to have the impression that I am comparing the value of psychoanalysis and behavior therapy as techniques. Such was never my intention. Each has its place in the treatment of psychiatric disorders. The questions that confront us are: Which therapy or combination of therapies is best for a particular disorder, which is most economical while at the same time effective, and how can we offer patients the best therapy for them rather than the therapy at which we happen to be best?

REFERENCES

Rhoads, J. M., & Feather, B. W. Transference and resistance observed in behavior therapy. *British Journal of Medical Psychology*, 1972, *45*, 99–103.

8

On Conceptual and Technical Integrity in Psychoanalysis and Behavior Therapy

Two Fundamentally Incompatible Systems

CYRIL M. FRANKS

American psychology has long been polarized with respect to the nature and role of unconscious mental processes. If early metaphysical behaviorists steadfastly rejected both unconsciousness and consciousness, psychoanalysts resolutely continued to espouse a complex structure of unconscious mental processes (Shevrin & Dickman, 1980). At the intellectual level, it is reasonable to conclude that the mutual antagonism between behavior therapy and psychoanalysis that characterized the early development of behavior therapy stemmed in part from this dichotomy. At a more pragmatic level, there were other driving forces.

In the early days, circa 1958–1968, many words but few data were dedicated to the edict that behavior therapy was "superior." Circumscribed studies were eagerly paraded to bolster the proclaimed advantages of behavior therapy. Later, the naive question of which form of therapy *per se* was more effective was abandoned in favor of comparisons of specific treatments under specific circumstances for specific purposes. For reasons that were not entirely scientific, the argument that each type of intervention

---

CYRIL M. FRANKS • Graduate School of Applied and Professional Psychology, Rutgers University, Busch Campus, Piscataway, New Jersey 08854.

had merit under certain circumstances became increasingly fashionable (e.g., Luborsky, Singer, & Luborsky, 1975). This, it may be speculated, led to retrenchment and a superficial easing of tensions between the two warring factions. Questions about behavior therapists—primarily psychologists—receiving third-party payments and demands that all clinicians be held accountable for and demonstrate the efficacy of their interventions could well have created a vexing predicament. On the one hand, it became increasingly apparent that generally applicable yardsticks of comparative effectiveness were not to be readily established by simple experiment. On the other hand, external agencies were accelerating their demands for scientific evidence that therapy was effective and the general public was becoming lawsuit conscious. Neither faction could comfortably endure those pressures. Implicit agreement on the expediency of shared concepts, the effectiveness of selected interventions, and the value of certain common professional tactics might well have favored the movement toward some form of integration and the joining of forces against a common external threat. The changing climate, with its increasing emphasis upon information exchange and innovation, which was encouraged by the media, also contributed to an acceptance of hybrid intervention systems and a breakdown of rigid patterns of therapy.

It is, of course, most unlikely that members of either camp will admit to the possibility of such motivations as contributing factors, and the argument for détente is usually couched in some professionally more acceptable form (see Franks & Barbrack, 1983). The debate usually revolves around the feasibility of integration at various levels, ranging from the highly conceptual to day-to-day practice.

Regardless of the possibility of harmony at more esoteric levels, the notion of some form of technical alliance is clinically enticing. It is hard to justify the rejection of any procedure that seems to offer hope to a human being in distress. But this should not blind us with respect to the basic issues. Is conceptual or philosophical integration possible? Is integration at the more utilitarian level of techniques possible and, if so, under what circumstances? Even if technical eclecticism, the application of procedures that seem effective regardless of theoretical origins, is shown to be helpful in the treatment of specific patients, under what circumstances—if any—is this likely to lead to long-term advancement in our understanding of the principles of therapeutic intervention? The position adopted here is that, in the long run, the call for rapprochement is likely to herald neither an era of scientific progress nor patient benefit (see Franks, 1982). A spirit of tolerance, if not acceptance, of two vigorously promulgated, vehemently but not rigidly defended, fundamentally different positions is advocated as a possible alternative either to destructive antagonism or futile integration. That position is the basis of the argument that follows. It is to be regarded primarily as the perspective of one behavior therapist and as a starting point for further refinement and development rather than a fully articulated thesis.

THE QUEST FOR INTEGRATION

In its least thought-through version, integration consists simply of the concurrent deployment of techniques regardless of theoretical origins or conceptual implications (e.g., Cohen & Pope, 1980). Sometimes the call for eclecticism is defended on pragmatic rather than philosophic grounds (e.g., Karasu, 1979). For others, cognition is the royal road to integration (e.g., Sollard & Wachtel, 1980). But whereas psychodynamicists stress inner psychic structures and unconscious processes of a highly speculative nature, cognitivists generally avoid this way of thinking. It is assumed that behavior therapy is guided by potentially conscious determinants that are amenable, at least in principle, to experimental investigation and therefore to change through systematic manipulation. Although acknowledging certain common elements, the subjective inferences of psychodynamic theoreticians and the total disregard of the role of cognition by applied behavior analysts are unacceptable to the cognitive-behavioral therapist. Unfortunately, as Mahoney (1980) and R. Lazarus (1980) quite independently have pointed out, rapprochement is more easily said than done. Many assumptions about diverse perceptions of reality and the nature of health and pathology are left unexplored. It is questionable whether either theory or procedure in cognitive therapy is as yet adequate to contribute significant advances to our understanding of human behavior and maladaption.

Goldfried's (1980) approach to integration is somewhat more sophisticated. Based upon a recognition of the growing discontent among therapists of both orientations, his starting point is the assumption that some form of integration is feasible and desirable. The psychotherapeutic process is conceptualized in terms of a three-tier hierarchy, ranging from what is directly observable to the highest level of abstraction. The latter is envisaged as primarily conceptual and theoretical, with an emphasis upon how and why change occurs and the philosophical context surrounding these formulations. As Goldfried correctly notes, the search for commonality between the two orientations is not likely to reach common ground here.

At the lowest level of abstraction lie the actual procedures used during the intervention process. Although commonalities across approaches may readily occur with respect to specific techniques, it is unlikely that such comparisons would reveal more than trivial points of similarity. It is in between these two—at the so-called level of clinical strategy—that Goldfried sees the possibility of meaningful consensus. Were these strategies to have a clear empirical foundation, Goldfried would refer to them as principles of change. In the absence of such a precise basis, Goldfried has to settle for a more vague and less satisfactory characterization. He refers to these strategies as the "clinical heuristics that implicitly guide our efforts during the course of therapy" (1980, p. 996).

Examples of such clinical strategies include the provision of corrective experiences and direct feedback. According to Goldfried, proponents of each camp advocate the use of such strategies, and many others wait to be uncovered. To this end, Goldfried proposes large cooperative efforts that are designed to search for, discuss, and reach consensus on commonalities in the therapeutic enterprise. Correctly anticipating the many problems that could arise from possible paradigm clashes involved in such a collaborative endeavor, Goldfried makes the questionable assumption that those concerned would be willing and able to relinquish their habitual world views for the common good.

Now, psychology is still an emerging science, which is somewhat akin in its developmental history to physics and chemistry in the 16th century. New *paradigms,* in the way we use this term here, are rare—Copernicus, Newton, or Einstein come to mind as trailblazers in this respect—and it seems probable that psychology is still in a preparadigmatic stage (see Franks, 1980, for a more extended discussion of this thesis). It is therefore with trepidation that we should invoke the Kuhnian notion of paradigm shift as it might apply in clinical psychology.

According to Kuhn (1970), whose schema was developed for the natural rather than the behavioral or social sciences, paradigm shifts occur only in times of crises when traditional problem-solving approaches no longer work and, even then, only under certain conditions. For a defunct paradigm to precipitate a crisis, it is essential that the effects of the incorrect paradigm be of major practical significance. Even if the assumption is made that there are conflicting paradigms within clinical psychology, as yet, there is no great sense of crisis, perhaps because these conflicts have not created pressing practical problems such as loss of livelihood or threat of a devasting lawsuit. Were this to occur, the ensuing crisis could conceivably set the stage for the kind of paradigm shift that might facilitate either an entirely new system or a move toward integration. In the meantime, the prospects for integration would seem to be negligible, even at Goldfried's level of clinical strategy.

A call for therapists to work together to achieve a consensus of clinical strategies is certainly appealing. What is more questionable is the meeting place. On what common ground can therapists of different theoretical persuasions meet? Messer and Winokur (1981) make the compelling point that Goldfried's examples of shared principles actually illustrate fundamental incompatibilities rather than commonality. For instance, Goldfried detects consensus around the clinical strategy of offering direct feedback for change, whereby "patients/clients are helped to become more aware of what they are doing and not doing, thinking and not thinking, and feeling and not feeling in various situations." (Goldfried, 1980, p. 995). To make his point, Goldfried compares and contrasts the position of the psychoanalyst Wilhelm Reich with the behavior therapist's use of self-monitoring (in the instance cited, of the number of cigarettes smoked) and its consequences. First, Goldfried quotes Reich:

> What is added in character-analysis is merely that we isolate the character trait and confront the patient with it repeatedly until he begins to look at it objectively and to experience it like a painful symptom; thus, the character trait begins to be experienced as a foreign body which the patient wants to get rid of. (Reich, 1933/1949, p. 50)

This form of feedback is then juxtaposed with McFall's (1970, p. 60) serendipitous observation that "when an individual begins paying unusually close attention to one aspect of his behavior, that behavior is likely to change even though no change may be intended or desired."

For Goldfried, the similarity between these two positions is "striking." For Messer and Winokur (1981), what is more striking is the difference, in both content and process, between these two clinical situations. I concur. In the former, the precursors and antecedents to these maladaptive behaviors are typically unconscious, covert, and extremely difficult to measure. More importantly, the analyst insists that there are powerful forces opposing their recognition. In the latter situation, no such assumptions are made nor have they been shown to be necessary. The proposed change principles take on a very different quality depending upon the philosophical/conceptual perspectives of the observer. These crucial distinctions are overlooked by Goldfried and others who seek to integrate behavior therapy and psychoanalysis.

For psychodynamicists Messer and Winokur (1980), the incompatibility of behavior therapy and psychoanalysis stems from their essentially irreconcilable visions of reality. Behavior therapy is characterized as embodying the comic vision in the theatrical sense of following the structure of dramatic comedy. It emphasizes the possibility of non-ambigous happy endings leading to security and gratification through direct action and removal of situational obstacles. By contrast, psychoanalysis is characterized by an emphasis upon the "tragic, the inevitability and ubiquity of human conflict, and the limits placed by the individual's early history on the extent of possible change." Thus, for Messer and Winokur (1981), Goldfried's vision is essentially "comic" in that the main difficulties in reaching consensus about the principles of change are social, economic, and political. The quite different vision of reality embodied in the psychoanalytic model and the problems engendered by any attempt at synthesis are not considered by Goldfried.

Despite their convincing arguments with respect to the incompatibility of the respective visions of reality held by the two systems, ultimately it is what Messer and Winokur (1980) term the "romantic element" that prevails in their thesis (see Franks & Barbrack, 1983). Refusing to close tight the door against integration, Messer and Winokur (Chapter 2, this volume) suggest that therapists strive to maintain a "dual focus" between subjectivity governed by the ground rules of hermeneutics (the art and "science" of interpretation as typically applied to literary and historical texts) and the objectivity of the traditional methods of science. As Franks and Barbrack observe, this is more akin to semantics than solution because it requires conditions that cannot coexist. It is possible to begin with the hermeneutic approach and then to incorporate these impressions into an objective, quantifiable framework. At this stage, the hermeneutic way of thinking is necessarily abandoned. The two cannot coexist, it is not possible to think in terms of the *hic et nunc* objectivism of the behavioral scientist and the hermeneutic pastoriented framework of the psychoanalyst at the same time. Thus, in describing how behavior therapy and psychoanalysis might benefit from integration and cross-fertilization, Messer and Winokur unwittingly strengthen the position held here that such an integration is not feasible at this time.

Of the many attempts to establish consistent theoretical and practical foundations for integration, Wachtel's (1977) is the most comprehensive and sophisticated in that it attempts to offer a conceptual framework for his mode of integration rather than an ill-fitting patchwork. As a group, behavior therapists are taken to task by Wachtel for failing to pay adequate attention in either theory or practice to thinking, feeling, values, wishes, impulses, interpretation, and inference. Traditional psychoanalysts are faulted for their failure to respond to neo-Freudian developments and to advances in neurophysiology. There is a reluctance among these die-hard psychoanalysts either to make the necessary theoretical changes to bring concept and practice into agreement or to question traditional hermeneutic ways of thinking about data and methodology in the light of new developments as they arise.

Recognizing, on the one hand, the deficits of Freud's 19th-century hydraulic model of mental functioning, which was rooted in a medical model and a now partially outmoded neurophysiology, and the limitations and insensitivities of certain behavior therapists, on the other hand, Wachtel proposes an innovative synthesis of his own, which is calculated to capitalize upon the strengths of both systems and obviate their weaknesses. Attempts to integrate these highly disparate models raise two far-reaching questions. First, at the conceptual level, is such an integration possible without profound distortion of both models to such an extent that neither camp would find the synthesis acceptable? Second, at the more practical level and regardless of the acceptability of this synthesis to traditional psychoanalysis and behavior therapists, would such an integration pay off in terms of demonstrable clinical dividends over the long haul as well as in short-term benefits? It is to a consideration of these concerns that we now turn.

SOME ISSUES TO BE NEGOTIATED EN ROUTE

"Technical eclecticism," a term coined by Lazarus (1967), pertains to the strategy of seizing upon whatever seems to work in the immediate clinical situation, regardless of theoretical origins or potential for conformity to some dominant conceptual framework. Technical eclecticism and integration are conceptually different, despite certain areas of tactical overlap. Technical eclectics maintain that integration of behavior therapy and psychoanalysis at the conceptual level is logically impossible but that this impasse need not and should not prevent the clinician from seizing upon whatever seems to work at the level of practical implementation, regardless of theoretical origins or even lack thereof. Thus, although the thoughtful technical eclectic is conceptually far from integration, many an integrationist would probably favor the practice of technical eclecticism if not the rationale upon which it is predicated. These distinctions will be developed further at a later stage in this chapter.

Technical eclecticism is a clinically seductive notion that could lead to opportunism rather than eclecticism. Witness, for example, the plethora of popular prescriptive texts now on the market (e.g., Blanco, 1972; Schaefer, Millman, & Levine, 1979). The parameters of technical eclecticism, particularly with respect to an amalgam of behavior therapy and psychoanalysis, and the circumstances, if any, under which such an integration could lead to a clearly articulated therapeutic system of *demonstrable* benefit, remain unknown. In the absence of such information, it may be preferable to confine both research and clinical activities to one system or the other but not to both.

To transform mere opinion into an informed position, a more rigorous analysis than that presented here is required. It is with this caveat in mind that the following tentative conclusions are offered as starting points for discourse. First, integration is impossible at the conceptual level without doing injustice to quite different but equally cherished notions about methology that are held by behavior therapists and psychoanalysts. Second, even at the clinical level, although some form of technical eclecticism might benefit an individual patient, the speculative argument could be put forward (evidence is lacking) that, in the long run, advancement in clinical practice is more likely to emerge out of programmatically and rationally derived techniques spawned within a clearly articulated system than out of an indiscriminate deployment of whatever seems to work, regardless of its origin.

To develop this thesis, it would first be necessary to examine the focal characteristics of both contemporary psychoanalysis and behavior therapy. In so doing, it would be important to differentiate between psychoanalysis and psychodynamic therapy and between theory and practice in behavior therapy. Psychoanalysis as a theoretical system and psychodynamic therapy or applied psychoanalysis, which employs somewhat different ground rules, are not necessarily totally congruent. It is possible to explore a patient's mental world in terms of a psychodynamic framework without making the analysis of the relationship (the transference situation) the core task. Similarly, it is necessary to distinguish between behavior therapy as a set of theoretical and methodological assumptions shared by most behavior therapists and the behavioral techniques that virtually any clinician, regardless of orientation, or even a lay person can use (Erwin, 1978).

Psychoanalysis, stated in an overly simplified form that fails to reflect the many nuances involved, refers to a conceptual system with a more or less clearly defined set of generally applicable postulates for the understanding of the human psyche, its structure, development, and therapeutic implications. Mental illness derives from otherwise insoluble intrapsychic, largely unconscious, early childhood experiences and thus represents inadequately resolved infantile conflicts. Prior to illness, these conflicts may have been successfully handled by way of a complex, idiosyncratic patterning of defense mechanisms and configurations that, in combination with certain constitutional endowments, make up the enduring personality structure of that individual.

Previously effective methods of maintaining a homeostatic equilibrium fail due to a variety of stresses from within and without. Inner conflicts arise, the defense mechanisms no longer function effectively, and disruptive symptoms emerge. Together with certain other characterological structures, the nature and organization of these symptoms reflect these inner conflicts, how the ego tries to cope with them and the more enduring psychic structure of the person concerned. Psychoanalysts attempt to remedy this situation by way of a small number of nondirective strategies that arise out of this conceptual framework and that are couched in the nomenclature of the medical, or disease, model. Thus, psychoanalysis is both an approach and a formulation with a more or less circumscribed set of procedures. Regardless of school (classical Freudian, Horney, ego analytic, etc.) or some prevailing pop variant (primal scream therapy, transactional analysis, etc.), in essence this model applies even though its proponents might think otherwise. All share a belief in subconscious symbolically represented mental processes and an acceptance of a methodology and definition of science and its acceptable yardsticks that are quite alien to the behavior therapist. This can lead upon occasion to quite striking differences in approach. For example, psychoanalysts make the claim that, in the final analysis (no pun intended), the only fit commentators upon psychoanalysis are those who themselves have undergone satisfactory analysis. "Satisfactory," of course, is determined by the analysts concerned. It need hardly be underscored how at odds this is with the behavioral tradition.

"Objectivity," the proudly proclaimed hallmark of behavior therapy, is at best of secondary significance in either psychoanalytic theory or method. The data of psychoanalysis are primarily derived from the personal, unique, and private relationship between analyst and analysand. As such, they neither permit nor require the checking and external validation operations mandated by the behavioral scientist. Thus, in the way behavioral scientists use the term, there is no "fact" in psychoanalysis. Psychoanalysts do not observe for its own sake; they interpret. The analytic situation is not reducible to a direct description of a set of observables that are meaningful primarily, if not exclusively, in themselves or with respect to some closely related referents. Psychoanalytic methods of validation and the rules governing the nature, validity, and determination of data are not those of the natural and behavioral sciences. Psychoanalysis is an exegetical or interpretative science (Ricoeur, 1970).

The essence of any science is not so much the existence of a body of facts as the method and manner in which these facts are systematically sifted and appraised (Sherwood, 1969). The advance of science depends upon this process. For there to be communication and orderly process or argument within a particular science or between sciences, there must be rules. If we cannot agree about these ground rules, communication and dialogue become impossible.

Nagel (1959) expects the science of psychoanalysis to conform to the canons of behavioral science ("a credible theory must be confirmed by observational evidence, and also be capable of being negated by such evidence"). But it is inappropriate to impose these rules upon a system that makes no claim to accept, follow, or be judged by these standards. For psychoanalysts, validation becomes a matter of historical interpretation rather than empirical observation.

Behavioral scientists insist upon precise rules to anchor concepts to operationally defined, quantifiable observables. If a theory is to be capable of refutation and therefore to qualify as a science, this is essential. This should not be taken to imply even tacit endorsement of a return to the more primitive operationalism of the 1930s. There is no objection to the study of processes that are not directly observable, as in physics or cognitive behavior therapy, for that matter. In both of these areas, investigators are at pains to trace out the inferential paths leading from putative processes to directly observable changes. In psychoanalysis, this is not only unnecessary, but it could even be undesirable in that it could interfere with the subtleties of the analyst–analysand relationship, thereby distorting the hermeneutic process.

The appeals to parsimony and precisely articulated testable predictions, the *sine qua non* of respectability for the behavioral scientist, offer further examples of methodological and, by extrapolation, conceptual alienation between the two systems. One person's economy of postulates is another's poverty of explanation. The typical lean-line, narrowing focused prediction generated by the behavior therapist "assumes less, [it] postulates less, and by golly [it] explains less" (Cheshire, 1979, p. 321). Those of us who have encountered both the behavior therapist's painstaking attention to precise but sometimes trivial detail and the psychoanalyst's willingness to have a ready explanation for virtually everything will readily appreciate the vast gulf between the two systems.

In psychoanalysis, subjective data derived entirely from the clinical situation are regarded as valid.* For the reasons stated, direct behavioral intervention is never acceptable. Psychoanalysts rarely distinguish facts from their interpretation. Observations are usually valued not for their own sakes but as springboards for second and higher order conjectures. Even investigators such as Shevrin and Dickman (1980), who are seemingly committed to the utilization of empirical-observational data, function in this fashion. These are the declared ground rules of psychoanalysis, and it is within this setting that psychoanalysis is appropriately appraised. The rules of one system cannot legitimately be applied to another system that rejects them. For example, as a vehicle within which to conduct therapy, it is difficult to see how the behavioral goal of direct intervention can be

* An implicit distinction is drawn here between subjective and self-report data as utilized by the psychoanalyst and behavior therapist, respectively. Subjective data acceptable to the psychoanalyst are, by their very nature, not amenable to objective verification. By contrast, self-report data, at least in principle, are amenable to empirical scrutiny.

combined with a primary concern for therapeutic experience of the relationship in terms of prior subjective and often symbolic patterns.

It might be thought that some of these rules are not conflicting and that certain goals are compatible. For example, at first examination, it might seem that the goals of psychodynamic insight and behavioral change are in accord and even complementary. But psychoanalytic *insight* is a concept with a meaning that is inextricably interwoven into the psychodynamic fold. For the behavior therapist, this specialized meaning does not exist. In terms of the goal of behavioral, cognitive, and affective change, insight is primarily a matter of awareness of contingencies and their impact. For the psychoanalyst, the direct pursuit of behavior change impedes the attainment of insight. In classical psychoanalysis, insight is usually an end (not the only one) in itself, and behavior change for its own sake is irrelevant or, at best, ambiguous. (I say "ambiguous" because the behavior in question, for example, smoking, might be modified for a variety of reasons, some of which the analyst would regard as trivial and others as closely related to the acquisition of therapeutic insight.) Insight is given fundamentally different meanings in the two systems, a fact that integrationists tend to overlook. Perhaps *outsight* might be a better term for the insight that occurs during the process of behavior therapy.

In behavior therapy, the ground rules are quite different. The enduring postulates are fewer, less structured, and more open to within-house debate by behavior therapists who are operating within different frameworks (e.g., social learning theory, applied behavioral analysis, classical conditioning). Although certain leading figures stand out, there is no single founder, and there is much less of an abiding core to which all behavior therapists subscribe. There is no carefully worked out personality structure with unfolding stages of human development. Even though couched within some broad-based S–R (stimulus-response) learning theory framework, there are fewer fixed clinical strategies or invariant therapeutic goals. There is no clear-cut set of procedures or techniques for evaluation and intervention. To use Yates' (1970) term, behavior therapy is more of a learning theory-oriented "methodological prescription" for therapeutic intervention based upon precise notions about what constitutes acceptable data and scientific methodology that it is a distinctive theory. If the framework is usually classical conditioning, operant conditioning, or some type of formal learning theory, this is by no means essential.

In behavior therapy, far fewer global statements are made about personality as an enduring structure. The preference is for predictions confined, in the main, to specific situations. Formulations in terms of probability statements about more general categories or possible options are in order but are not preferred by most behavior therapists. For data to be acceptable, they must conform to the hypothetico-deductive or some related methodology of the behavioral scientist. It is easy to declare that behavior therapists must accept data from any source, examine these data, subject them to the canons of science, and then rise to the challenge of incorporating these data into a behavior therapy framework (e.g., Phillips, 1977, p. 266). But what constitutes acceptable data is another matter. To assert that scientific methodology and a data-based orientation are the forté of behavior therapy without first making it clear that we are playing by certain rules about the nature of data and methodology is not good enough. Acceptable as these rules are to behavior therapists at this juncture, it has to be recognized that they are not the only possible rules for all sciences, for all scientists, and for all time. Conceivably, one could develop a third set of rules that conform in part to those of behavior therapy and psychoanalysis and add unique innovative elements that may or may not be acceptable to advocates of either or both systems. To deny this possibility is to be unnecessarily rigid. However, to embrace this possibility at this time might be at the cost of a premature rejection of psychoanalysis and/or behavior therapy and the distinctive contributions that each has to offer within its own frame of reference.

Despite the considerable latitude that prevails within the broad complex of behavior therapy, it is conformity to a generally accepted set of rules that constitutes one essential unity of contemporary behavior therapy. For example, it is these rules that distinguish cognitive researchers in behavior therapy—whether they are called cognitive behavior therapists, social learning theorists, or what have you—from those who make use of cognition, introspection, and the like in various nonbehavioral frameworks. It is this that is what behavior therapy in large part is all about. What is at issue here is not only whether cognitions or other postulated internal states can legitimately be included within some sort of behavioral framework but also the methods whereby they are to be incorporated. Those who affirm that much of contemporary behavior therapy is not behavioristic and that the current "cognitive connection" implies some sort of integration of behavior therapy with nonbehavioral models may be missing the point. It is possible to adopt a cognitive position and still remain committed to the methodology of the behavioral scientists. Similarly, the failure of conditioning theory to account for many phenomena in behavior therapy is not necessarily indicative of a falling apart of behavior therapy. There may be no convincing evidence of operant and classical conditioning as either viable concepts in their own right or as useful explanations of complex adult human behavior (see Franks & Wilson, 1980). Despite its focal position, conditioning is not a cornerstone of behavior therapy in the same way that, for example, the unconscious is of psychoanalytic theory.

Even radical changes in our notions about the nature and process of "conditioning" would only temporarily affect the viability of contemporary behavior therapy as a conceptual approach. The fact that behavior therapy is not totally dependent on any such foundation may be one of its strengths—just as the lack of an integrative model of personality and of human beings may be one of its weaknesses at this time.

If modern behavior therapists, with their acceptance of certain intervening variables and their rejection of metaphysical behaviorism, are behavioral rather than behavioristic, they share with behaviorists a common methodology and view of data that is alien to that of most psychoanalysts. If contemporary behavior therapy has its inferences (e.g., W. Mischel's 1977 "person variables"), these concepts are viewed quite differently by behavior therapists and psychoanalysts. When behavior therapists such as Eysenck search for person variables, they are at pains to ground them in empirical observations and testable predictions relating to specific situations that have direct meaning within themselves. By contrast, psychoanalysts tend to regard these variables as avenues to still more complex and logically distant inferences.

EXPANDING HORIZONS WHILE REMAINING ON COURSE

Intellectual autobiography is rarely as interesting to the general public as the central figure would have us believe. Nevertheless, with the reader's forebearance, it seems appropriate at this stage to help place the present discussion in context by engaging in some personal reminiscence. Some 20 years ago it was all very clear. There was proof positive, at least to my mind, of the ineffable superiority of the methodology of behavioral science and hence of its findings. Today, although this remains without question my strategy of choice, I no longer believe that objectivity and quantification are the only avenues to understanding. My behaviorally distinct bias remains strong; it is the evangelical intolerance that has weakened. As Cheshire (1975) forcefully comments, numerocracy is not always an effective substitute for creative thinking: It could be that the prestige that the more established physical sciences rightly derived, and still do, from their spectacular achievements served as a model for a psychology that was anxious to acquire an intellectually respectable pedigree. In the name of objectivity and rigor, objectivist psychologists—and these included myself in the early days of behavior therapy—hammered their data into quantifiable form and into the only true shape upon the altar of *scientism* rather than science. Thus, in our own fashion, argues Cheshire, we revived that sectarian exclusiveness that has fortified theologians from the Dark Ages to the present.

In the words of Saint Augustine: "There is no salvation outside the Church."

With Popper (1935), we accused those who suggested that data gathered in accord with criteria other than those set forth by behavioral scientists could be meaningful of being unscientific and illogical. We were inclined to dismiss facilely the possibility that contributions to "knowledge" (itself a debatable concept) have been made throughout the ages by a variety of learned individuals in such diverse fields as history, literary commentary, archaeology, and linguistics who knew nothing about, and cared even less for, the methodology of the behavioral scientist. To view such nonscientific enterprises as imprecise and capricious could be a myopic and self-centered way of looking at knowledge and its acquisition. There is many a mystic who flatly rejects the data base of both behavior therapy and psychoanalysis as inadequate and irrelevant to the acquisition of knowledge. Who can with certainty say, in any absolute sense, that they are wrong? As Alexander Pope put it in his *Essay on Man,* "trace science then, with modesty thy guide" (Cheshire, 1975). Ultimately, our committment to science, however this term is defined, is part of our belief system.

It is certainly true that extremists in the psychodynamic camp have shown a culpable disregard for even minimal standards of evidence, objective observation and scientific acumen in their speculations about people. But it is equally true that some behavior therapists overreach themselves and assume that only their notions about methodology, observation, fact, evidence, accuracy, and sound reasoning could possibly lead to advances in knowledge. For such individuals, the rationale of scientific discovery as spelled out by Popper in the 1930s remains the alpha and omega of empirical truth, even though contemporary physics is itself departing from such a stance. For example, Heisenberg's uncertainty principle led to the shattering discovery that, at the subatomic level, there is no such thing as the "exact sciences." There are limits beyond which, neither in principle nor in practice and no matter how hard we try, the processes of nature cannot be measured accurately. In other words, there exists an ambiguity barrier beyond which we can never pass without venturing into what Zukar (1979) termed the "realm of uncertainty." In Zukar's graphic words,

> As we penetrate deeper and deeper into the subatomic realm, we reach a certain point at which one part or another of our picture of nature becomes blurred, and there is no way to reclarify that part without blurring another part of the picture. (p. 111)

As the physicist Heisenberg (1958, p. 55) wryly commented, what we observe is not nature itself but nature exposed to our method of questioning. There may be no "objective" reality for the exact sciences to study, and alternative methods may have to be developed. If, under certain circumstances, the distinction between objective and subjective becomes blurred, then the new physics, if it leads us anywhere, leads us back to ourselves.

Thus, it could be that the physical sciences and their methods are not the sole repositories of rationality or fact. There may be more to the study of human beings than slogans about objectivity, measurement, prediction, and controlling variations, and there may be a place, after all, for those who wish to engage in the interpretative approach of psychoanalysis and even for those who are beyond science at any level—behavioral or hermeneutic. In making this point, it needs to be reaffirmed that the fact that such alternative intellectual styles cannot be ruled out is no reason for behavior therapists to abandon their conviction that, for behavior therapy to progress, it is an objectivist methodology that is most likely to yield fruitful results rather than an alternative system or some form of integration of the behavioral and psychoanalytic approaches. There would seem to be no compelling evidence that integration, either in terms of the early dictionary construction of Dollard and Miller (1950) or in the more sophisticated endeavors of Wachtel (1977), yields scientifically valuable dividends.

A CURRENT POSITION

With this point established, let us return to psychoanalysis and behavior therapy. As has been stressed repeatedly, these are two models that differ fundamentally. They employ different language systems and different data bases. They differ drastically with respect to such matters as what constitutes acceptable methodology, data, and outcome evaluation. What the behavior therapist regards as essential scientific requirements could be regarded as naive and unnecessarily restrictive by the psychoanalyst. The two frameworks differ with respect to what constitutes research, clinical evidence, and the goals of therapeutic change. Behavior therapists prefer to evaluate more discrete behaviors, but they are quite prepared to work with any type of behavior as long as it can be specified in objective, quantifiable terms—and this is where one major problem lies. Psychoanalysts prefer to work with more global criteria, perhaps in part on the grounds that the complex variables of personality structure are difficult to measure. Further, and many modern physicists would sympathize with this position, psychoanalysts would argue that, quite apart from distorting the subtleties of the patient–therapist relationship, any attempt at precise measurement would influence the very variables they are trying to measure.

When psychoanalysts do take note of specific behaviors, their purposes and terms of reference are quite different.

Arguments are rarely about facts as such; they are more usually about how the facts are to be conceptualized and understood. The controversy between proponents of behavior therapy and psychoanalysis is often pictured as a controversy about the "depth" or "permanence" of the changes produced (T. Mischel, 1977). This makes it seem as if what is at issue could be resolved empirically, but this is not so. The still-ongoing debate about symptom substitution is very much a case in point. Empirical studies that purport to show that specific behavioral procedures, as contrasted with psychoanalysis, do or do not lead to symptom substitution raise similar conceptual issues to those that they are supposed to resolve. "Symptom substitution" is a construct that has precise and quite different meanings within each camp. The term can be meaningfully employed within a psychoanalytic context because the notion of "symptom" has meaning within this context. It is quite appropriate to discuss and evaluate the data of so-called "symptom substitution" within a behavior therapy context but not the notion. It is appropriate to appraise such data *and* the notion of symptom substitution within a psychoanalytic context. For the behavior therapist, "response substitution" has a clear and precisely defined meaning within a behavioral content. Because the concept of a symptom is quite alien to behavior therapy (even though some behavior therapists quite incorrectly include this notion within their so-called behavioral repertoires), it is meaningless and therefore fruitless to engage in debate over whether symptom substitution does or does not occur within any behavioral context. Nevertheless, something does happen within the intervention process that can be observed and recorded—sooner or later the patient does certain things that are clinically unacceptable and that were not evident prior to the intervention. These events exist and can be observed, discussed, and incorporated into either a behavioral or a psychoanalytic formulation. Within a behavioral context, it is meaningful to discuss these events in terms of the data themselves and some appropriate behavioral conceptualization but not in terms of the alien notion of symptom substitution. Within a psychoanalytic context, it is appropriate to discuss both the data and the inferred notion of symptom substitution because this is a term within this setting.

For the behavior therapist, response substitution can occur and should even be expected to occur under certain circumstances (see Bandura, 1969). The difference between symptom substitution and response substitution is far more than semantic. Each has a specific contextual meaning and intimately interwoven series of conceptual linkages that make the two notions incompatible. Each becomes logically meaningful only within its own context. For example, in the treatment of enuresis, simplistic behavioral intervention with respect to the presenting complaint without a thorough behavioral analysis of the full range of potentially reinforcing contingencies could well result in the emergence of new, unwittingly reinforced, maladaptive behaviors as responses to certain environmental contingencies. This is response substitution. By contrast, symptom substitution implies the emergence of new symptoms, not in response to environmental contingencies alone, but as part of the complex psychic superstructure that constitutes the psychoanalytic model. What is not meaningful and therefore not constructive is the discussion of behaviorally formulated issues and concepts within a psychoanalytic setting and vice versa. On this basis, how can there be any conceptual integration?

Similarly, it may be argued that judgments about the superiority of behavior therapy, even specific behavioral programs, as contrasted with psychoanalysis either as competing systems or therapeutic devices, are futile, unproductive expenditures of time and energy. Such judgments detract from the obligation of each system to go about its business, and they might even lead to misleading or otherwise nonproductive comparisons. There is no specific clinical entity called "behavior therapy" that can be meaningfully compared with psychoanalytic psychotherapy.

In a somewhat related vein, just as psychoanalysis as a theoretical system has to be differentiated from psychoanalytic psychotherapy, so behaviorism as a theoretical system (actually there are at least two kinds of behaviorism and possibly more—methodological behaviorism and metaphysical behaviorism) has to be distinguished from the practice of behavior therapy. It is perhaps meaningful to compare two conceptual approaches called *behavior therapy* and *psychoanalysis*, respectively. It nevertheless is relatively meaningless to attempt a general, clinical comparison of something called "the practice of behavior therapy" with psychoanalytic psychotherapy. All we can compare are specific treatment strategies and procedures that are derived from the conceptual approach called "behavior therapy," that are geared towards specific patients with specific problems, and that utilize specific therapists with specific agreements about mutually acceptable goals, with similarly specified procedures derived from the psychoanalytic tradition. Whether the therapies concerned could ever agree about the many issues at stake is another matter!

Arguments about the utility of behavioral, as opposed to psychodynamic, taxonomies cannot be resolved empirically because the empirical findings are subject to interpretation in terms of radically different types of theories. Both approaches are interested in understanding the determinants of human functioning—normal as well as abnormal. These approaches differ, as the late T. Mischel (1977) pointed out, because they disagree about what the determinants are. They also differ in that they have radically different conceptions about what a theory to explain human functioning would have to look like. The argument is thus conceptual; it is an argument about the type of explanatory theory psychology should use to understand human behavior. The argument would seem to be sterile and likely to produce little of a constructive nature.

Thus, at the conceptual level, it would seem that, if the integrity of either system is to be preserved and if each is to develop within its own domain to its maximum potential, there can be no convergence. Integrity is an important aspect of integration conceptually as well as semantically. Such a synthesis could lead to the bowdlerization, distortion, and dilution of both systems—to a patchwork integration of a modified form of psychoanalysis that is unacceptable to most psychoanalysts and to a modified form of behavior therapy that is unacceptable to most behavior therapists. Theories are not meant to be regarded as eternal dogma. A good theory, like a good therapy, is the best approximation we have until a better one comes along. To keep the integrity of a theory intact for no other reason than to retain its integrity will not do. But in the present instance, as we have tried to indicate, there are good reasons why we should do so for now.

Certainly, Wachtel's synthesis goes beyond the dictionary construction integration of Dollard and Miller (1950). Dictionary construction or translation is a hazardous game to play. As the Italian phrase *traduttore traditore* succinctly puts it—to translate is to betray. For example, a translation of psychoanalytic concepts into conditioning terms is to distort, even lose, the focal core of the psychoanalytic belief that man is dominated by potent unconscious strivings. Wachtel transcends this dictionary construction activity in his attempt to reformulate the notions and practices of behavior therapists and psychoanalysts alike. His criticisms of both camps are well taken, as is his conclusion that integration at the conceptual level is not a viable proposition. Wachtel's position with respect to the merits of collaboration at the level of clinical practice might seem at first blush to be quite defensible: Techniques drawn from different systems can be usefully deployed without necessarily accepting the conceptual frameworks of the theories that spawn them. Unfortunately, those who espouse "technical eclecticism," to use Lazarus's (1967, 1981) term, all too often are tempted to use questionable techniques without questioning their validity in terms of *any* system.

There is a vast difference between clinical practice and programmed research. Practitioners are primarily interested in helping their clients. They are not overly concerned with *what* models are more likely to explain *what* data. In systematic research, it is not possible to be eclectic: If bigotry is an anathema, bias is mandatory. If past experience is any guide, good science is more likely to emerge by working consistently within one framework than through an eclectic dip into whatever happens to be around or from a transplant that is probably doomed not to take.

For the clinician, the position is more debatable, and two somewhat contrasting points of view can be distinguished. It could be argued that, in the long run, more useful information and thus more help for the patient might accrue by a consistent approach within one theoretical framework. After all, there are a vast number of techniques to be dreamed or dredged up. Therefore, it would seem more efficient to focus on the investigation and development of those that emerge logically as part of a consistent, stepwise program of thinking, research, and accumulation of data within a particular framework.

It is useful to conceptualize the scientific method at three levels or stages in a continuum. At the top—the *rational* level—the emphasis is upon logical theory construction, the formulation of hypotheses, and the generation of testable predictions. Early behavior therapists liked to think of themselves as scientists, working primarily at this rarified level. Next comes the level of *empirical* validation with an emphasis upon well-designed studies to amass empirical evidence about the utility of a specific procedure used under specific circumstances. Much of medicine functions and continues to function at this level and so does much of contemporary behavior therapy. At the lowest level, the *notional,* the appeal is to whim and fancy, with no regard for evidence of any sort. Saying makes it so, and many of the fad therapies of the day operate exclusively at this level. This, of course, is not to gainsay the hunch or appeal to the notional as a starting point for eventual elevation to the other two levels. And by the same token, there is usually an intuitive element present in seemingly rational strategies. The interactive ideal embraces all three levels.

If it is not always possible to work effectively and exclusively at the rational or theory-derived level, this does not mean that it is necessary to descend to the level of the notional and the whim, grabbing at any technique regardless of validating data. There is always the intervening, more methodological, level of empirical validation. It is possible that facile integration at the technique level may tempt clinicians to use procedures whose validation has been overlooked within both the behavioral and the psychoanalytic systems. Thus, it may be that, even as far as clinical practice is concerned, integration may be less than desirable.

It might also be difficult in actual practice for behavior therapists to abandon their customary objective approach to all patients and proceed largely in terms of the more subjective, intuitive feeling and interpretative style of the psychodynamic clinician.* Similarly, it might be hard for psychoanalysts to abandon their basic commitment to regarding all patients as free and responsible individuals who must be left to themselves to work through and be in touch with their feelings, forming their own decisions, and deciding upon their own courses of action without the imposition of even implicit directions from the therapist or even from themselves. One might also wonder how the technically eclectic therapist is going to adopt one intellectual stance for one patient and then switch to the other during the next therapy hour—let alone switching positions during the same session to match whatever technique is being used at that particular moment.

The alternative possibility—the case for technical eclecticism—is best exemplified by Lazarus (1967, 1981) who takes the position that, if a scientist cannot afford to be eclectic and if theoretical integration is unrealistic, the clinician cannot afford *not* to be eclectic. It would be nice, so the argument goes, if we had enough knowledge for clinical commitment to one theoretical system and to procedures closely derived therefrom. But unfortunately, at this time we do not. For reasons that are currently unknown, certain patients occasionally behave in an idiosyncratic fashion. Seemingly unpredictably, they respond to techniques or strategies that have no empirical foundation whatsoever other than clinical experience. In the interests of the hapless patient, Lazarus argues persuasively, we have to use clinical trial and error and to latch onto almost anything that we have reason or intuition to think or feel might possibly be helpful. For most patients, at most times, it may be possible to proceed systematically and planfully within a consistent framework and to rely upon validated procedures—but not for all.

Lazarus's only stipulation is that such techniques have a modicum of empirical support and that empirical methods be used to monitor clinical effectiveness. In so doing, Lazarus stresses the necessity to maintain theoretical integrity in the formulation of conceptual models and overall clinical strategy if not in the specifics of the procedures used. It is regrettable that he fails to explain the logistics whereby the practice of technical eclecticism and the holding of an internally consistent philosophical framework can coexist. No technique is ever formulated or applied in a conceptual vacuum devoid of an explicit or even implicit underlying framework. There is no such thing as a concept-or theory-free clinical procedure

* This, of course, is not to deny the value of the hunch or notion in the practice of behavior therapy. But, for the behavior therapist, such subjective intuition is of value not for its own sake but only as an avenue to empirical validation in terms of the *methodology of science* as he or she uses this term.

that is related exclusively or even primarily to the technique itself rather than to any implicit underpinnings. The argument that such considerations are of secondary significance is a weak one in practice in terms of both data and strategy.

Empirical evidence bearing upon the value of technical eclecticism is meager. Self-styled eclectic behavior therapists claim to use a broader and more varied range of therapeutic techniques than do those who endorse a particular behavioral orientation (Swan & MacDonald, 1978). The question of whether and under what circumstances the use of a broader range of techniques results in more effective, efficient, or durable changes has not as yet been seriously addressed. Conceivably, technical eclecticism could facilitate the development of an enriched therapeutic armamentarium. Conversely, it could foster an overemphasis upon technique, to the detriment of theoretical and conceptual appreciation of the issues at stake. Even more important, with a myriad of techniques or potential techniques awaiting investigation, what guiding principles would be utilized in selecting priorities? Few practitioners read the literature, even uncritically, and even fewer gather data for themselves. The temptation would be strong for the busy eclectic clinician to assume a validity for the technique in question that did not exist, not even in the mind of the inventor who dreamed it up.

A PROVISIONAL SUMMING UP BUT NOT THE JOURNEY'S END

It is suggested that, at the present stage of knowledge, behavior therapy and psychoanalysis are fundamentally incompatible at the conceptual level. Arguments can be presented for and against the advantages of integration at the clinical level. The position taken here is that, even at this level, integration is highly impractical and is likely, certainly in the long run and probably in the short run, to be disadvantageous both to patient welfare and the advancement of clinical practice within either a behavioral or a psychoanalytic context.

Behavior therapy is now entering its third decade. The first, the 1960s, was the pioneering era, characterized by naiveté, ideology, and militant evangelism. The second was characterized by consolidation and a search for new horizons within its own domain. Concepts, methodologies, and ways of viewing data beyond those of traditional conditioning and learning theory were introduced. More sophisticated methods of treatment and outcome evaluation were developed. The third decade is characterized by constructive within-house, behaviorally committed but open-minded discourse. There is a shift from a climate of implacable and mutual antagonism between behavior therapy and psychoanalysis to an atmosphere of limited tolerance that coincides with an acceptance of the fundamental and pervasive incompatibility of the two systems. The call, then, is to both behavior therapists and psychoanalysts for commitment to a vigorously supported and vehemently advanced bias that is coupled with caution, humility, and a recognition of the possible limitations of scientific methodology as behavior therapists and psychoanalysts know this term. This, at least from the behavioral perspective of the present writer, should not be taken to imply a laissez-faire tolerance of demonstrably invalid or nonvalidated clinical procedures. There is an ethical obligation to members of the mental health profession and the unsuspecting public to define and pursue effective approaches and to limit clinical access to those that could be detrimental or that have no clear utility. Acceptance of the rights of psychoanalytic clinicians and thinkers to pursue and work within their own conceptual and clinical framework should not detract from the behavior therapist's obligation to avoid condoning that which, in his or her view, is demonstrably not in the public interest.

AUTOBIOGRAPHICAL STATEMENT

Past behavior is a useful guide to present and future activities. In 1947, I completed a degree in physics and mathematics in the University of Wales, acquired a graduate diploma in education plus a few additional frills, and became an instructor in the London Nautical School, a training facility for cadets seeking to enter the British Merchant Service. I found that I knew much about physics, mathematics, and electronics but little about "Johnny." To remedy this deficit, I enrolled in intensive evening and weekend classes in the University of London and acquired a solid background in psychology. In 1951, I had the good fortune to be accepted into the clinical training program at the University of London Institute of Psychiatry (Maudsley Hospital) where I came under the influence of Hans Eysenck and a group of psychologists who were seeking objective methods for understanding and modifying human behavior.

The postwar society was one of mild privation, change, and emerging problems with which most of us were ill-equipped to cope. In the main, mental health intervention was confined to the good intents of caring people or to sedatives and one or two tranquilizers when caring proved insufficient. Psychotherapy, to the extent that it was available at all, was primarily in the hands of psychodynamic psychiatrists who were specializing in the elitism of intensive one-to-one treatment for the few who had the time, money, and education for such capers.

The painstaking search for alternatives stemming out of our training as psychologists (defining psychology as "the scientific study of behavior") led us to S-R learning theory as the only area of psychology that was sufficiently established to generate testable predictions. And for us, this marked the start of behavior therapy—a far cry from its present form. (It should be noted that contemporary behavior therapy has many roots, and this is but one.)

We were aided by two developments, among others. First, Wolpe's desensitization yielded a promising conditioning-based alternative to either psychotherapy or medication for use with the sophisticated individual who was generally to be found on the psychoanalyst's couch. Second, Dollard and Miller's (1950) influential treatise dealing with the ancillary role of learning theory in the enrichment of the psychodynamic model provided a model of what to avoid. By implication, Dollard and Miller viewed psychodynamic principles as ultimate truths to be made more understandable and possibly more amenable to experimental investigation by translation into a language acceptable to behavioral scientists. It was this dictionary-construction allegiance to something unrelated to the tradition of psychology that we sought to avoid.

In those simplistic and intolerant years, our main aim was to prove our superiority. Fortunately (as it turned out), as the years sped by it became increasingly evident that our techniques were rarely as superior as we had proclaimed and that our strengths lay elsewhere—in the uniqueness of our methodology; in our concerns with accountability, outcome evaluation, experimental rigor, and the like; and in foundations rooted in the science of psychology, as we viewed this term. It was at about this stage that I moved to the United States in late 1957.

The other transition point in my conceptual development was the founding of the Graduate School of Applied and Professional Psychology (GSAPP) at Rutgers University in 1970, with its stress upon eclecticism, professionalism, learning by doing, and the clinician as the consumer of research rather than its creator. Two quite different and distinct kinds of professional clinical psychologists lived, and still live, in the same house: one committed to behavioral science and the other to psychodynamic theory and practice (the systems and community tracks came much later). Over the years, I was forced, willy-nilly, into intellectual relationships with students and adjunct faculty whose views were alien to my own. At first, I was convinced that my behavioral approach was the only one that would ever advance the cause of professional psychology. I had nothing but a thinly veiled contempt for those who subscribed to a psychodynamic model. Gradually, two developments occurred. Increasing interaction led to the realization that we were arguing about two totally different, irreconcilable, and incompatible viewpoints. It was as capricious to place these two camps in the same training program as it would be to expect chemistry and art history to cohabit. Although one could, and possibly should, study chemistry *and* art history, to view them as different facets of one program was clearly absurd. The problem was, and still is, that chemistry and art history are obviously different in content and application. Their relationships are not fraught with antipathy and misunderstanding. Regrettably, this did not—and still does not—always apply to our two tracks in GSAPP. It took years to recognize this painful fact.

The second development that led to tolerance, if not acceptance, was the many interchanges that I had with the only nonbehavioral member of our core faculty—Stanley Messer. Despite all inclinations, I was forced to recognize the disquieting fact that here was a committed psychodynamicist of integrity and knowledge with whom I could engage in open-minded dialogue and enjoy the process.

This sums up the convoluted path from those early days in the Maudsley Hospital over a quarter-century ago to my present position. I remain convinced that my route is the best for me at this time, and I still find psychoanalysis scientifically incomprehensible, not to mention unrelated to the needs of contemporary society—but who knows for certain. The journey continues, and it is volumes such as this that may point the way toward directions as yet uncharted.

CYRIL M. FRANKS, PH.D.

REFERENCES

Bandura, A. *Principles of behavior modification.* New York: Holt, Rinehart & Winston, 1969.

Blanco, R. F. *Prescriptions for children with learning and adjustment problems.* Springfield, Ill.: Charles C Thomas, 1972.

Cheshire, N. M. *The nature of psychodynamic interpretation.* London: Wiley, 1975.

Cheshire, N. M. A big hand for Little Hans. *Bulletin of the British Psychological Society,* 1979, *32,* 320–323.

Cohen, J. H., & Pope, B. Concurrent use of insight and desensitization therapy. *Psychiatry,* 1980, *43,* 146–154.

Dollard, J., & Miller, N. E. *Personality and psychotherapy.* New York: McGraw-Hill, 1950.

Erwin, E. *Behavior therapy: Scientific, philosophical and moral foundations.* New York: Cambridge University Press, 1978.

Franks, C. M. On behaviourism and behaviour therapy—not necessarily synonymous and becoming less so. *Australian Behaviour Therapist,* 1980, *7,* 14–23.

Franks, C. M. Behavior therapy: An overview. In C. M. Franks, G. T. Wilson, P. Kendall, & K. Brownell, *Annual review of behavior therapy: Theory and practice* (Vol. 8). New York: Guilford Press, 1982.

Franks, C. M., & Barbrack, C. R. Behavior therapy with adults: An integrative approach. In M. Hersen, A. E. Kazdin, & A. J. Bellack (Eds.), *The clinical psychology handbook.* New York: Pergamon, 1983.

Franks, C. M., & Wilson, S. T. Behavior therapy: An overview. In C. M. Franks & S. T. Wilson (Eds.), *Annual review of behavior therapy: Theory and Practice* (Vol. 7). New York: Brunner/Mazel, 1980.

Goldfried, M. R. Toward the delineation of therapeutic change. *American Psychologist,* 1980, *35,* 991–999.

Heisenberg, W. *Physics and philosophy.* New York: Harper & Row, 1958.

Karasu, T. B. Toward unification of psychotherapies: A complementary model. *American Journal of Psychotherapy,* 1979, *33,* 555–563.

Kuhn, T. S. *The structure of scientific revolutions (2nd ed.).* Chicago: University of Chicago Press, 1970.

Lazarus, A. A. In support of technical eclecticism. *Psychological Reports,* 1967, *21,* 415–416.

Lazarus, A. A. *The practice of multimodal therapy.* New York: McGraw-Hill, 1981.

Lazarus, R. S. Cognitive behavior therapy as psychodynamics rendered. In M. J. Mahoney (Ed.), *Psychotherapy process: Current issues and future directions.* New York: Plenum Press, 1980.

Luborsky, L., Singer, & Luborsky, L. Comparative studies of psychotherapies: Is it true that everyone has won and all must have prizes? *Archives of General Psychiatry*, 1975, *32*, 995–1008.

Mahoney, M. J. Psychotherapy and the structure of personal revolutions. In M. J. Mahoney (Ed.), *Psychotherapy process: Current issues and future directions.* New York: Plenum Press, 1980.

McFall, P. M. Effects of self-monitoring on normal smoking behavior. *Journal of Consulting and Clinical Psychology*, 1970, *35*, 135–142.

Messer, S. B., & Winokur, M. Some limits to the integration of psychoanalytic and behavior therapy. *American Psychologist*, 1980, *35*, 818–827.

Messer, S. B., & Winokur, M. Therapeutic change principles: Are commonalities more apparent than real? *American Psychologist*, 1981, *36*, 1547–1548.

Mischel, T. The concept of mental health and disease: An analysis of the controversy between behavioral and psychodynamic approaches. *The Journal of Medicine and Philosophy*, 1977, *2*, 197–219.

Mischel, W. On the future of personality measurement. *American Psychologist*, 1977, *32*, 246–254.

Nagel, E. Methodological issues in psychoanalytic theory. In S. Hook (Ed.), *Psychoanalysis, scientific method and philosophy.* New York: New York University Press, 1959.

Phillips, E. C. *Counseling and psychotherapy: A behavioral approach.* New York: Wiley, 1977.

Popper, K. R. *The logic of scientific discovery.* London: Hutchinson, 1935.

Reich, W. [*Character analysis*] (T. P. Wolfe, Trans.). New York: Orgone Institute Press, 1949. (Originally published, 1933.)

Ricoeur, P. *Freud and philosophy.* New Haven: Yale University Press, 1970.

Schaefer, E. C., Millman, H. E., & Levine, G. L. *Therapies for psychosomatic disorders in children.* San Francisco: Jossey-Bass, 1979.

Sherwood, M. *The logic of explanation in psychoanalysis.* New York: Academic Press, 1969.

Shevrin, H., & Dickman, S. The psychological unconscious. A necessary assumption for all psychological theory? *American Psychologist*, 1980, *35*, 421–434.

Sollard, R. N., & Wachtel, P. L. A structural and transactional approach to cognition in clinical problems. In M. J. Mahoney (Ed.), *Psychotherapy process: Current issues and future directions.* New York: Plenum Press, 1980.

Swan, S. E., & MacDonald, M. L. Behavior therapy in practice: A national survey of behavior therapists. *Behavior Therapy*, 1978, *9*, 799–807.

Wachtel, P. L. *Psychoanalysis and behavior therapy: Toward an integration.* New York: Basic Books, 1977.

Yates, A. *Behavior therapy.* New York: Wiley, 1970.

Zukar, G. *The dancing Wu Li masters: An overview of the new physics.* New York: Bantam Books, 1979.

[illegible]
[illegible]
[illegible] Basic Books, 1967.
[illegible]
[illegible] Baltimore [illegible] Press, 1968.
[illegible]
[illegible]
Wolpe, J. [illegible] New York: Pergamon Press, 1960.

8

The Behavioral Scientist as Integrator

Commentary on Cyril M. Franks

LEON SALZMAN

Cyril Franks makes a cogent and powerful argument for avoiding a too early marriage between two immature partners whose philosophies, understanding, and emotional attitudes toward facts and phantasies are at great variance. Perhaps they should wait until each has matured and learned more about life and each other, especially in the areas of the organization of the brain as well as the mind. This will permit each of them the freedom to be expansive, curious, and inventive before succumbing to a joint enterprise that requires compromise in order to be collaborative.

Franks's thesis is well documented, provided we can agree (and here again is the dilemma) on his definitions and the boundaries of the disciplines he is talking about. He attempts to be specific, but there is still much confusion about which psychoanalysts and which behavior therapists he is talking about. If it is the rigid orthodox who pursue Freud's original formulations undeviatingly, then he is wasting his brilliant exposition. In my opinion, this segment of the psychodynamic view of human behavior is gradually disappearing for theoretical as well as practical reasons. They may have already made their contributions, which will forever be the shoulders on which further progress will be made.

If Franks is speaking about the more eclectic psychoanalysts, then he

LEON SALZMAN • School of Medicine, Georgetown University, Washington, D. C. 20057.

must define that group more clearly because they comprise a diverse group of psychotherapists, some of whom view psychoanalysis as a modifiable discipline but prefer to maintain the name. There is also another growing group of therapists who prefer to call themselves "psychotherapists" and who do not hold to a hierarchical notion of the discipline, with psychoanalysis at the top and psychotherapy at the bottom. The label of "psychotherapy" has been applied to every conceivable involvement of two individuals where the human psyche plays some role. At times, this group includes those who have made bizarre extensions of minimal psychodynamic insights and form cultist and mystical groupings. However, the more scientifically based eclectic psychotherapists have retained many of the psychological findings that are derived from a view of behavior that postulates out-of-awareness influence on behavior and a view of personality development that is ontological and is based on interpersonal interaction. They hold that early experiencing plays a determining role in the ultimate character structure of the individual. They accept the significance of biogenetic, constitutional factors and the role of character and conditioning but recognize that human existential needs such as love, avoidance of loneliness, and awareness of one's mortality strongly motivate a person's behavior. They may drop the "psychoanalytic" label because of its historical and scientific limitations and use the embracing term "psychotherapy." They will view the physiology and psychology of behavior as a unity and not as a series of subspecialties that need to be integrated.

This type of behavioral scientist will need to be developed out of training programs that recognize the validity of the tributaries from all branches of the behavioral sciences rather than be a contest of institutional converts of a particular conceptual hypothesis. These disciplines will then comprise informed developmental psychologists as well as aetiological specialists whose notion of behavior will automatically incorporate all these viewpoints. At that time, we will have an integrated science of human behavior that will not dichotomize psychoanalysis, behavior therapy, drug therapy, and the rest as separate approaches to the healing of mental dysfunctioning. In this group there would be a loosening of rigid doctrinaire orientation, and the members of this group will have goals that are shared by those who have a concern for observation and verification and a valid interest in the objective quantification of valid subjective experiencing wherever it is possible. They would avoid untestable hypotheses, and in the present state of enormous complexity of the mind and brain, they would permit alternative viewpoints when they add to the understanding and relief of psychic disorders as well as advancing theory.

Franks's review has too many remnants of the doctrinaire elitist behavioral scientist who is still caught up in institutional warfare, while advocating a commitment to a vigorous bias, coupled with caution, humility, and recognition of limitations. In my opinion, the call should be for a vigorous openness without bias, for a scientist who can accommodate without capitulating. Perhaps this must wait on the new professional behavioral scientist who has not been caught up in the medical-nonmedical institutional warfare and is trained in a new profession where all present-day theoretical systems are explored and judged on the basis of present understanding.

Franks suggests that premature rapprochement is not likely to produce scientific progress. Although this is true if there are no shared concepts or theories, it seems to me that it is not true with regard to behavior therapy and psychotherapy. In fact, these disciplines share many basic concepts, although they still have major differences. We should, if we maintain our individual integrity, utilize the acceptable insights of other disciplines to forestall much wasted time and energy in fruitless research. Clearly, the methodology that Franks suggests is widely discrepant in both disciplines, but an enlightened investigator can pursue an agreed-upon methodology, even while disagreeing on some essential issues. Both are studying human beings and their failures in adaptation and behavior. Both can agree on observable data while questioning the validity of interpretation as an objective reality. Both can agree that the source of many behaviors is unknowable by direct observation and must be extrapolated on the basis of agreement regarding motivation or goal-directed behavior. If there cannot be agreement on these essential issues, then I would agree with Franks that integration is premature and go further by saying that it is impossible.

The issue of technical eclecticism as a therapeutic gambit cannot be used to define or validate theory. In the realm of the psyche, too many unknown variables influence behavior. Our theories must be defined in ways other than the traditional model because it has subjectivity as its base. Franks's description of the psychoanalytic model as a universally shared subconscious that symbolically represents mental processes does not take into account the range of out-of-awareness phenomena that are equally available to all behavioral scientists. The controversial issue is how these processes influence behavior rather than their existence.

There is no argument about the tendency of dynamic theorists to put too much emphasis on interpretation that is based on disputable concepts and their failure to acknowledge the culture bias of some of their theories. However, the very essence of their methodology precludes the required control of variables and repeatability of their findings. On these matters, they should not be judged as defective scientists but rather viewed as attempting to develop a science where subjectivity and nonrepeatability are intrinsic to the science. The behavior therapist often presumes to be more scientific, yet he or she fails to take into account his or her tendency to accept clinical syndromes and disease categories that come out of the tainted science of psychodynamics and then to prove how more successful he or she is in treating these disorders.

Similarly, in presuming to treat symptoms rather than behavioral dysfunctions, the behavior therapist has unwittingly but in a mercantile fashion entered the world of healing without a thorough understanding of the physiology and anatomy of disease and malfunction. When the behavioral therapist attempts to alter or remove rituals, he or she claims to be curing the obsessive-compulsive disorders. This, behavioral therapists can only do because in their ignorance they assume that the obsessive-compulsive disorders consist of obsessions and compulsions and in their alteration they have cured that disease. To alleviate the cough does not necessarily cure the tuberculosis. Thus, what appears to be good statistical research often turns out to be a numbers game where the definitions are drawn to suit only the players without reference to the validity of the game in the first place.

Psychotherapy must be integrated with other treatment modalities that have some shared views on human functioning, particularly when they can accelerate or deal more effectively with pieces of the puzzle. Whether now is an appropriate time will depend on the maturity of the practitioners in their own specialized areas and the state of the science itself. We should make a start to see where the impediments are, in order to remove them, or agree to proceed with some agreement about the disputed issues.

8

A Rejoinder to Leon Salzman

CYRIL M. FRANKS

What Salzman fails to appreciate is that I am not writing about specific psychodynamic and specific behavior therapists. My primary concern is with two distinct approaches that characterize psychodynamic therapists, on the one hand, and behavior therapists, on the other, regardless of their individual positions on either the psychodynamic or behavioral spectrum. Salzman is certainly correct in his contention that contemporary psychoanalysts and psychodynamic therapists are less rigid, more eclectic, and more open to new ideas than were their predecessors. And, as I have often tried to make clear, a similar state of affairs exists within the domain of behavior therapy. But, and this is a very big *but*, whatever the position of a particular psychodynamically oriented clinician or researcher is with respect to any specific postulate, nearly all give allegiance to a conceptual model that embraces similar notions about such matters as the unconscious, the goals of therapy, motivating variables, outcome evaluation, the nature of data, and what constitutes acceptable clinical and research methodology. A similar, if contextually very different, commonality characterizes behavior therapists.

In his well-intentioned but, in my view, mistaken ecumenical plea, Salzman seems to gloss over the preceding facts of life and continues in the vain hope that so-called "enlightened investigators" can agree. It is when he attempts to make this point explicit that additional confusion occurs. What, for example, does "both can agree on observable data while

CYRIL M. FRANKS • Graduate School of Applied and Professional Psychology, Rutgers University, Busch Campus, Piscataway, New Jersey 08854.

questioning the validity of interpretation as an objective reality" mean? How can one reconcile the two parts of this statement? Salzman himself seems, at least implicitly, to recognize certain fundamental divergencies between the psychodynamic and behavioral models when he writes that

> the very essence of their [psychodynamic] methodology precludes the required control of variables and repeatability of their findings. On these matters, they should not be judged as defective scientists but rather viewed as attempting to develop a science where subjectivity and nonrepeatability are intrinsic to the science.

I find myself in accord with his statement: "If there cannot be agreement on these essential issues, then I would agree with Franks that integration is premature and go further by saying that it is impossible."

Salzman rejects my plea for bias, defined as a hypothesis to test that arises out of some investigative program that is generated within a preferred conceptual framework, coupled with humility defined as a recognition of limitations and a live-and-let-live encouragement of alternative models. In its place, he would substitute a call for "a vigorous openness without bias, for a scientist who can accommodate without capitulating." Salzman does not tell us, however, what accomodating without capitulating means and how one can do or not do either without a position from which to start. As Montaigne succinctly put it long ago: No wind blows in favor of a ship that has no direction.

To my mind, methodological commitment and bias and the importance of being theoretical need not imply a rigid orthodoxy. All theory is, of necessity, an oversimplification in the first instance—how else could one embark on the process of systematic investigation? But, by the same token, good theory, like good therapy, is merely a working approximation until better theory or therapy comes along. But this "coming along" is *not* a matter of chance. It is more likely to occur within the disciplined exploration of some theoretical framework than in either an eclectic pursuit of whatever happens to be around or a premature integration of two systems that, to my way of thinking, are clearly incompatible and best left, at least for the time being, to develop independently.

In sum, contemporary behavior therapy is a sophisticated approach to the whole person. It is by no means simplistic and in no way assumes, to use Salzman's example, that altering the obsessions and compulsions of an individual so afflicted is all that is required to bring about full mental health and adaptive functioning. Psychodynamic therapists might begin by thinking through the precise meaning of the word *symptom* in psychoanalytic theory, its total lack of meaning within the behavioral framework, and how behavior therapists contend conceptually and practically with the fact that working with the presenting complaint alone is rarely, if ever, adequate.

9

The Activation of Unconscious Fantasies in Behavioral Treatments

ERIC MENDELSOHN and LLOYD H. SILVERMAN

The learning of new responses and the deconditioning of maladaptive behaviors are identified as the principal mutative factors in behavioral treatments in most discussions found in the behavior therapy literature. In this chapter a different perspective will be offered; behavioral treatments will be discussed from the vantage point of a theoretical construct that is traditionally associated with psychoanalysis—the unconscious fantasy. The discussion will proceed as follows: A rationale for considering alternative or additional ways of accounting for behavior change in the behavior therapies will be presented. The thesis will be advanced that the construct *unconscious fantasy*, as it is used by psychoanalytic theorists, refers to many of the same phenomena that commonly employed constructs such as *nonspecific effects, cognitive mediation, expectancies,* and *relationship variables* do when they are discussed in the behavioral/experimental literature. It will be maintained that many of the phenomena referred to by such terms can be conceptualized as instances of activated unconscious fantasies. Hypotheses about the activation and mediating effects of specific unconscious fantasies in behavioral treatments will be presented. The findings from a series of controlled experiments demonstrating that the activation of certain

ERIC MENDELSOHN • The New York Hospital-Cornell Medical Center, Westchester Division, White Plains, New York 10605. LLOYD H. SILVERMAN • New York Veterans Administration Regional Office, New York, New York 10001 and Department of Psychology, New York University, New York, New York 10003.

unconscious fantasies produces behavior change will be reviewed. Results from several studies where specific unconscious fantasies have enhanced the effectiveness of behavioral treatments will be described, and some suggestions will be offered about how to investigate further the role of unconscious fantasies in mediating behavior change in the behavior therapies. The implications of this research for clinical practice and training will be considered, and the chapter will conclude with a brief discussion of the integration of psychoanalysis and behavior therapy.

KEY CONSTRUCTS

The *behavior therapies** are not a homogeneous entity; technical procedures and their theoretical foundations vary considerably. As a consequence, broad characterizations of the group of behavior therapies are likely to be, at best, somewhat imprecise. Nevertheless, certain general statements about how behavior change and therapy process are conceptualized in the behavior therapy literature can modestly be offered. Partly because of their origins in experimental psychology and academic learning theory, the behavior therapies emphasize the analysis and modification of observable behaviors rather than having as a method or a goal the understanding of mental processes. The primary therapeutic concern is with variables currently implicated in the maintenance of the patient's difficulties (Wachtel, 1977). To the extent that a historical perspective is employed, it tends to be focused; it is the learning history associated with the problem at hand that is emphasized. The result of these emphases is that behavior therapists conceptualize psychological difficulties more as discrete phenomena than as aspects of broad, general patterns of disturbed adaptation (Wachtel, 1973, 1977). Treatment philosophy follows from these conceptualizations.

A major goal of clinical research in the behavior therapies is to identify the factors that account for positive and negative outcomes and to utilize these findings to devise effective therapeutic techniques (e.g., Davison & Wilson, 1972; Stuart, 1980). As a consequence, increased attention has been paid to the role of heretofore "unspecified" factors (i.e., those that are not attributable to the direct effects of technical procedures). In this section, the terms used to designate such factors will be defined and the phenomena they refer to will be described. Certain factors that are thought

* Throughout this chapter the designation *behavior therapies* will be used when referring to the group of treatments derived from learning theory. This is done in recognition of the heterogeneity of this grouping. Specific treatment techniques will be referred to in the singular; that is *systematic desensitization* or *assertiveness training*, though a review of the literature suggests much variability *within* each of these types of treatments as well.

to be common to all therapies will then be described and previous attempts to consider the behavior therapies from a psychoanalytic vantage point will briefly be reviewed. The term *unconscious fantasy,* a construct derived from psychoanalytic theory, will then be defined and its phenomenology explicated. It will be proposed that a considerable amount, though not all, of the phenomena adumbrated by such constructs as *nonspecific effects, cognitive mediation, expectancies,* and *relationship variables* can be conceptualized as reflecting the activation of unconscious fantasies. A further theoretical advantage of applying the construct *unconscious fantasy* to the study of these therapy process variables will then be considered.

Definitions

It will become apparent in the following discussion that there is considerable overlap in the definitions and phenomenology of nonspecific effects, cognitive mediation, expectancies, and relationships variables. Nonspecific effects is a superordinate term; the others represent specific cases (though expectancies are products of cognitive mediation). In order to understand fully the relations between these terms and grasp their relevance to the present discussion, a brief review of each follows.

Nonspecific Effects *

As indicated earlier, discussions of therapy process in the behavior therapy literature tend to focus on the opportunities for new learning, the deconditioning of maladaptive behaviors, skills acquisition, and so forth that are afforded by standardized therapeutic techniques (e.g., Marks, 1978). Researchers seek to identify which aspects of therapeutic procedure are critical in accounting for therapeutic gains. As a next step, researchers ask what factors, beyond the procedures themselves, are mutative. Collectively, the set of factors other than the direct effects of procedures of presumed efficacy are referred to as *nonspecific* factors.† There is debate among behavior theorists as to whether or not such factors will eventually be understood in terms that are compatible with S-R learning theory or its variants (cf. Gomes-Schwartz, Hadley, & Strupp, 1978).

* Inclusion of this term for purposes of the present discussion should not be interpreted as an endorsement of its usefulness by the authors. *Nonspecific effects* are neither "nonspecific" nor "effects." More correctly, they may be termed "as yet unspecified factors." See Grunbaum (1981) for a discussion of definitional problems in this area.

† *Placebo effects* is a term often used synonymously with *nonspecific effects,* though their definitions differ somewhat. See Shapiro and Morris (1978) for an excellent, scholarly discussion of placebo effects in medical and psychological treatments.

Lists of nonspecific factors tend, by definition, to be lengthy and loosely formulated; however, those most commonly cited include the following: suggestion, the therapeutic relationship (Klein, Dittman, Parloff, & Gill, 1969), expectancies, facilitative therapist behaviors such as providing advice, encouragement, and focused attention (Marks & Gelder, 1966), and the patient's perception of the treatment and understanding of the procedures (Goldfried & Davison, 1976). There is increasing debate about how best to account for the effectiveness of behavioral treatments (Gomes-Schwartz *et al.,* 1978). Recent methodological reviews have indicated, for example, that the majority of studies of nonspecific treatment effects in systematic desensitization have not adequately controlled for subjects' expectancies (Kazdin & Wilcoxon, 1976). Other studies of systematic desensitization have indicated that many of the specific techniques used in Wolpe's original procedure such as deep-muscle relaxation, graded hierarchies, and the reciprocal inhibition of anxiety may well be unnecessary to obtain therapeutic outcomes (Kazdin & Wilcoxon, 1976). Findings such as these have spurred interest in the study of nonspecific effects.

Cognitive Mediation

Cognitive mediation refers to mentation occurring following the reception of stimuli and preceding the enactment of responses. It represents both the integration of the stimulus and the preparation for the response (Ryle, 1978). It is a term associated with social and cognitive behaviorism and refers to phenomena originally considered outside the domain of traditional behavioral analysis. Murray and Jacobson (1978) summarized the theoretical shifts embodied in the introduction of this term.

> The changes include an abandonment of the basic behaviorist model with its exclusion of consciousness, direct environmental causation, and the mechanistic conditioning process. What is taking its place is a cognitive model in which the human being is viewed as an information processing organism, capable of symbolization and thought, self-controlling and controlling the environment. Cognitive, personality and social variables are considered fundamental parameters of the learning process. (p. 663)

The authors observed that, even in classical conditioning experiments, subjects do not passively respond to stimuli but rather strengthen or inhibit certain response tendencies as a function of their *interpretations* of events. Ryle (1978) made similar points in describing the limitations of S-R models of learning and concluded that an adequate theory of learning must, of necessity, take into account the mental processing that is both a product of past experience and a reflection of the *meaning* assigned to experiences. Self-regulatory processes such as "self-efficacy" (Bandura, 1982) and experimentally manipulated "sets;" that is being told a given procedure is either "therapy" or "experiment" (e.g., Rosen, 1974, 1976), are examples of therapy process variables that fall within the domain of cognitive mediation. The consideration of cognitive mediation renders the behavior therapies more mentalistic and less strictly behavioristic.

Expectancy

Expectancy is the nonspecific factor most frequently studied in behavior therapy research (Gomes-Schwartz *et al.*, 1978). It refers to a person's predictions about treatment. Although some investigators contend that expectancy effects have not been adequately demonstrated (e.g., Wilkins, 1973), most writers maintain that expectancy effects account for a considerable degree of the improvement in certain behavioral treatments such as systematic desensitization (Franks & Wilson, 1976; Lick, 1975; Marcia, Rubin, & Efran, 1969). Expectancies may be deliberately manipulated by therapists, they may be activated or modified inadvertently, or they may be "brought" to the treatment by the patient as a result of earlier experiences (Shapiro & Morris, 1978). It has been demonstrated that induced expectancies can enhance the effectiveness of behavior therapies (Wilson & Evans, 1976) and that manipulated positive expectancies are associated with more positive outcomes (Ingram & Goldstein, 1978). The anticipation of cure is one frequently studied expectancy (Murray & Jacobson, 1978). Expectancies fall within the domain of cognitive mediation and are mentalistic phenomena.

Relationship Variables

Relationship variables refer to all aspects of the patient–therapist relationship that affect treatment process and outcome. These include observable behaviors, overt and covert responses to these, and more enduring attitudes and affects that are relatively difficult to recognize and even harder to measure. It is not known to what extent relationship variables affect outcome (Marks & Gelder, 1966), and the number of clinical reports far exceeds the number of controlled studies (Gomes-Schwartz *et al.*, 1978). Because of the complexities involved in undertaking controlled research in this area, most of the experimental studies have involved manipulations of a single variable (usually some aspect of the therapist's behavior) in the context of a standardized treatment protocol of somewhat questionable clinical relevance. The findings from a number of such studies (Davison & Wilson, 1972; Goldfried & Davison, 1976; Kahn & Baker, 1968; Morris & Magrath, 1979; Morris & Suckerman, 1974a, 1974b; Ryan & Moses, 1979) indicate that relationship variables, when evaluated in comparison to the influence of therapy technique, play a relatively small role when the technique is effective and the presenting problems are minor. Relationship variables play a relatively large role when the technique is less powerful and when the presenting problems are more serious. A number of writers have described a somewhat defensive attitude on the part of behaviorists—who wish to maintain that their therapies are solely "technique oriented"—when it comes to recognizing and identifying relationship variables (e.g., Rhoads & Feather, 1972; Wilson & Evans, 1976). It has been proposed that success in the behavior therapies is dependent upon recognizing and controlling for such factors, not only upon refining technical procedures (Braff, Raskin, & Geisinger, 1976; Goldfried & Davison, 1976; Strupp, 1979; Stuart, 1980; Wilson, Hannon, & Evans, 1968). Such contentions have been supported, though not proven, by the finding that patients who had completed a behavioral treatment (as well as patients who had completed expressive psychotherapy) rated the relationship with the therapist as the most important factor affecting outcome (Sloane, Staples, Cristol, Yorkston, & Whipple, 1975).

In keeping with the prevailing clinical and theoretical zeitgeist, discussions of relationship variables in the behavior therapy literature deal principally with observed behaviors and consciously experienced attitudes. Terms like *transference* and *resistance,* given their association to psychoanalytic theory and their connotation of unconscious processes, infantile origins, and so forth are not typically used, and their phenomenology is not usually considered to be within the purview of the behavior therapies. However, some writers have maintained that transferences and resistances are ubiquitous (e.g., Wolf, 1966) and are at least experienced, if not analyzed, in the behavior therapies. Wachtel (1977), in an extensive analysis of the behavior therapies and psychoanalysis, concluded that although certain characteristics of behavioral treatments (i.e., the brevity and focused quality of the therapies, the active stance of the therapist, etc.) typically prevent the development of full-blown regressive transferences, some aspects of "irrational influence" nonetheless remain.

Crisp (1966) attempted to measure and assess the impact of transferences in behavioral treatments. Using a standardized instrument to measure selected prevailing interpersonal attitudes, he plotted shifts in patients' feelings about their therapists alongside symptomatic changes. He concluded that major clinical changes during the treatment were accompanied by changes in the transference and found that, in some cases, a change in the transference preceded and predicted a symptomatic change.* Finally,

* In interpreting the results of this study, the following qualifications are in order: (a) As Crisp (1966) himself pointed out, the measure he employed only "indirectly assessed some of the possible 'transference' attitudes" (p. 182); and (b) the results represent correlational rather than causal data.

Shapiro and Morris (1978), in their discussion of the placebo effect, pointed out that the therapist–patient relationship is characterized by such disparate phenomena as: (a) discrete responses to the behaviors of the other; (b) responses on the part of therapist and patient to the attitude of the other toward treatment; (c) conscious perceptions of the other; and (d) unconscious attitudes carried over from early in life and activated in the treatment. Together, these phenomena are thought to constitute a considerable component of the effects not attributed to specific techniques.

Factors Common to All Psychological Therapies

The terms previously discussed refer to factors other than the direct effects of techniques affecting outcome in the behavior therapies. It has sometimes been pointed out that these factors are not unique to behavioral treatments and may be common to all psychological therapies. Differences in descriptions of such factors vary as a function of the theoretical orientation (language) of the observer. The purpose of this section is to briefly map out some of the terrain described by various writers who have studied mutative factors operating in all therapies.

Marks (1978) contended that outcome in any psychological treatment is influenced by the patient's motivation to seek out and complete therapy. This factor is, in turn, determined by four prior ubiquitous factors: previous motivation, social pressures, suggestion, and the credibility of the therapy and therapist. Friedman (1963) stated that certain expectancies, particularly those for symptomatic improvement, were common for all therapies. Appelbaum (1975) cited a number of mutative factors that are presumably operative in all therapies: presence of a concerned other, the activation of hope, the extinction of fears, corrective emotional experiences (typically involving benign responses by the therapist to behaviors that had previously evoked aversive responses), the provision of a rationale to account for psychological difficulties, opportunities for new learning, the provision of experiences of success, and the state of mind of the person seeking help (conceptualized as involving conditions of "special readiness"). Meyer and Chesser (1970) identified suggestion, expectancies, and the therapeutic relationship as mutative factors in all treatments, and Luborsky, Singer, and Luborsky (1975) in an extensive review of psychotherapy research concluded that motivational variables and the quality of the patient–therapist interaction were important contributors to outcome in all therapies. Finally, the writings of Wachtel (1977), Crisp (1966), Wolf (1966), and others who have discussed transferences, resistances, and other psychodynamic aspects of the behavior therapies can be interpreted in such a way as to suggest an additional ubiquitous therapy-process variable—namely, the *meaning* a particular procedure or interpersonal encounter has for a patient (cf. Gelder, Bancroft, Gath, Johnston, Mathews, & Shaw, 1973).

Previous Discussions of the Behavior Therapies from the Vantage Point of Psychoanalysis

Several thoughtful discussions of the behavior therapies utilizing constructs derived from psychoanalysis may be found in the literature. A very brief review of some central points follows. Wachtel (1977) stressed that patients always form impressions of psychological interventions and said, "Understanding the range of conscious and unconscious meanings that the intervention can have can be critical to whether or not the intervention succeeds" (p. 140). Crisp (1966), as described earlier, emphasized the influence of transference reactions in the behavioral treatments. He pointed out that powerful emotional reactions to the therapist may be activated and may affect outcome. Wolf (1966) argued that it was crucial in the behavior therapies, as well as in psychoanalytic treatments, to monitor and control countertransference reactions in order to prevent harmful responses to patients' disturbed interpersonal behaviors. Weitzman (1967), by analyzing the imagery produced in desensitization treatments, hypothesized that the mechanism of therapeutic improvement was the deconditioning of previously unacceptable unconscious wishes. Finally, Ryle (1978) argued for a translation of both psychoanalysis and the behavior therapies into the language of cognitive psychology. He pointed out that an adequate theory of behavior change has to account both for the formation and strengthening of associations and for the construction of organized mental representations.

Let us summarize the discussion up to this point. Traditionally, behavior therapists have been concerned with developing therapeutic techniques that will provide opportunities for new learning and for the deconditioning of maladaptive responses. The major focus in behavior therapy research has been on observable behaviors and their immediate environmental precipitants. In recent years, increasing attention has been paid to the role of cognitive and interpersonal factors in mediating behavior change. Thus, clinicians have begun to consider such "nonspecific" factors as cognitive mediation, relationship variables, and expectancies in treatment outcome. In addition, common factors between the behavior therapies and other psychological treatments have increasingly been studied. Writers who analyzed the behavior therapies from a psychoanalytic perspective have stressed the activation of unconscious processes and the effects of patients' impressions of the procedures and the therapeutic relationship in determining outcome. Thus, there is a tradition of conceptualizing the process of therapeutic change in the behavior therapies from a vantage point that (a) considers the effects of factors other than specific techniques, (b) is mentalistic, (c) is concerned with responses activated in the present but rooted in the prior history of the patient, and (d) is concerned with meaning and interpretation. This, then, provides a backdrop for utilizing the construct *unconscious fantasy.*

Unconscious Fantasy

Unconscious fantasy is a construct derived from psychoanalytic theory. Laplanche and Pontalis (1973) pointed out its early use in Freud's writings to designate a set of mental representations in which the depiction of everyday images is transformed by the influence of unconscious wishes and defenses. Unconscious fantasies were seen as components of dream and symptom formation, and in their central features, they were thought to be relatively stable and enduring, expressing important aspects of the infantile mental life. Rycroft (1968) also stressed the intermingling of contemporary elements with concerns carried over from early in life in the construction of unconscious fantasies. He stated that the unconscious components of fantasy were, in essence, expressive of loving and aggressive feelings toward infantile objects. In the course of being incorporated as fantasies, these were said to undergo symbolic elaborations. For purposes of the present discussion, *unconscious fantasy* will be defined as follows: It is an organized configuration of unconscious ideas and images, motivated (to varying degrees) by libidinal and aggressive wishes, anxieties, defensive operations, and adaptive strivings. When a behavior emerges, intensifies, diminishes, or disappears without any apparent conscious instigation (i.e., perception, memory, anticipation, or other cognition), the activation of some unconscious fantasy (or some element thereof) is likely to be causative (Silverman, 1979, 1982a). Unconscious fantasies are often activated by immediate environmental events, though in their enduring aspects they reflect the influence of usually long-standing unconscious motives. Their activation may lead to behavior change, and these may be adaptive or maladaptive (Silverman, 1982a).

Using the terms explicated in the present discussion, unconscious fantasies are (a) products of *cognitive mediation* (that is, their activation occurs "between" the stimuli encountered in the therapy and the responses by the patient to these); (b) they reflect the influence of *expectancies* (those that are situation specific as well as those that are enduring); and (c) they are frequently related to the patient's experience of the *therapeutic relationship* (that is, they are activated in the context of a meaningful, often emotionally laden involvement with a therapist). A major thesis of this chapter follows: *Unconscious fantasies activated in the behavioral therapies account for a portion of the therapeutic gains attributed to nonspecific effects.** Use of the construct *unconscious fantasy* thus allows for the organization of considerable clinical data.

In stating the thesis in this manner, it would appear that the role of unconscious fantasies in mediating behavior change was being considered apart from the effects of specific therapeutic techniques. To some extent this is correct because unconscious fantasies logically may be expected to be activated by the act of entering *any* therapy, by the person (sex, manner, age, etc.) of the therapist, by the perception of symptomatic changes, and so on. However, it is also possible to consider unconscious fantasies in conjunction with the effects of specific therapeutic techniques. In this regard, unconscious fantasies may be conceptualized as ideas or images that reflect the influence of unconscious wishes, anxieties, defenses, and adaptive strivings as these are activated by specific immediate events in the treatment—that is, specific treatment interventions or therapist behaviors. Fantasies activated in this way must be presumed to reflect, in part, the patient's *interpretation* of the events of the treatment. Thus, such fantasies become a principal way of organizing and representing the experience of treatment. A second thesis, one that will be discussed in more detail later, is the following: *Specific unconscious fantasies are likely to be activated in particular behavioral treatments, and these may play a role in mediating behavior change.* Thus, not only can the activation of unconscious fantasies be conceptualized as one nonspecific factor accounting for a portion of the therapeutic improvement in the behavior therapies, but it may be predicted that the predominant fantasies will vary as a function of the type of treatment (including technique, stance of the therapist, setting, etc.).

UNCONSCIOUS FANTASIES

This section will be organized as follows: Hypotheses will be offered concerning two unconscious fantasies that are likely to be activated in certain behavioral treatments. The key elements of these fantasies will be described, and their activation will be linked to specific aspects of commonly practiced behavioral treatments. Experimental data relevant to these hypotheses—and to the broader theses presented in the first section—will be reviewed in the third section.

* For a discussion of the role of unconscious fantasies in mediating therapeutic improvement in *psychoanalytic* treatments, see Silverman (1982a).

Hypotheses

1. *What may be termed symbiotic-like gratification fantasies are frequently activated by the treatment situation and/or the therapist's behavior in the behavior therapies and may often play a role in mediating therapeutic improvement.*

2. *What may be termed sanctioned impulse-gratification fantasies are frequently activated by the treatment situation and/or by the therapist's behavior in the behavior therapies and may often play a role in mediating therapeutic improvement.*

It is presumed that these fantasies are activated *inadvertently,* that is, without the conscious intent or knowledge of the therapist. Further, their effect is on an unconscious level; patients remain unaware of the fantasies activated in the treatment. These fantasies will now be described.

The Symbiotic-like Gratification Fantasy

This fantasy involves the unconscious idea that a state of oneness has been achieved with an important object (usually the mother or some substitute for the mother). Such a fantasy has been understood in psychoanalytic theory as having its origins in the symbiotic stage of development, as has been described by Mahler, Pine, and Bergman (1975). This phase can be defined as the period when the infant, who is enormously dependent upon the mother for his or her physical and psychological well-being, is as yet incapable of formulating a sense of self that is distinct from the mother. A fantasy of oneness with the mother—more precisely, a fantasy in which *some but not all* mental representations of self and mother are merged is understood as serving a number of defensive and adaptive needs. The oneness fantasy serves to reassure that mother's presence is "guaranteed" so that nurturance, affection, and protection always seem available. Further, in this fantasy, feelings of weakness, defectiveness, helplessness, and ineffectuality can be remedied by feeling at one with mother or by magically sharing her strength. Thus, in infancy, oneness fantasies can reduce anxiety and dysphoria and provide a sense of security and well-being. Symbiotic-like fantasies continue to be invoked later in childhood, though typically less frequently and less completely (i.e., with fewer self- and object representations merged).

Symbiotic-like gratification fantasies can be understood as a legacy of these early experiences. People are found to vary considerably in the degree to which wishes for such experiences continue to motivate their behavior. It is presumed, however, that for all people, wishes for nurturance, protection, power, reassurance, and the like will, to some extent, continue to be sought in the manner of infancy. A corollary to this is that many aspects of experience toward which many people are drawn owe a large part of their attraction to their ability to activate fantasies of symbiotic-like gratifications. It has been proposed that "silent" experiences of symbiotic-like gratification underlie everyday, seemingly incidental occurrences that suddenly result in improved adaptation and feelings of well-being (Rose, 1972). It is also assumed that for the activation of such fantasies to enhance adaptation, the experience of oneness must be delimited. Optimally, this means that experiences of oneness should be countered by some reinforcement of one's sense of differentiation and separateness (Silverman, Lachmann, & Milich, 1982).

The Sanctioned Impulse Gratification Fantasy

This fantasy involves the idea that some person or agency (usually one invested with moral authority) has sanctioned the expression of impulses that are otherwise taboo or highly conflictual. Examples of such fantasies include those involving the expression of derivative Oedipal wishes or those involving competitive strivings that are rooted in penis envy. For purposes of illustration, the derivation and phenomenology of one such fantasy—the "sanctioned Oedipal gratification" fantasy—will be discussed.

During the Oedipal phase—as compared to the symbiotic phase—the mother is experienced less as part of the self and more as an external object. Thus, she can become, for the boy, the primary object of his sexual desires and, for the girl, the rival for father's affections. For both boys and girls, in part because the sexual wishes for the opposite-sex parent are largely ungratified, these urges get to be experienced as taboo, and they become subject to defensive operations. Likewise, the competitive and aggressive wishes toward the same-sex parent are feared and defended against.

To varying degrees, people remain motivated by Oedipal wishes throughout their lives. Depending upon the degree to which the infantile Oedipus complex is not resolved, the wish for sexual closeness with the opposite-sex parent and wishes to be rid of, or at least defeat, the same-sex parent continue to be important motivators in adulthood. Thus, many aspects of adult behavior can be viewed (in part) as derivative expressions of Oedipal strivings. For example, sexual relations between men and women can contain as a component of their meaning the gratification of incestuous wishes. Participation in competitive sports can express competitive feelings toward the same-sex parent. And vocational achievements can represent surpassing or outdoing the Oedipal rival.

Thus, behaviors and activities, such as those that have been described, can be understood as owing part of their attraction to their ability to activate fantasies of sanctioned Oedipal gratification. That these gratifications must be experienced as sanctioned is of crucial importance because, in contrast to the symbiotic-like wishes discussed earlier, Oedipal wishes are understood as much more likely to remain taboo, and therefore they are highly conflictual. Thus, even for *derivative* gratifications (i.e., those that represent modulated or regulated departures from the original sexual and aggressive aims and/or those directed toward objects other than the parents) to be allowed, society or some external figure (identified with the superego) must be viewed as sanctioning the behavior.

Possible Activators of Symbiotic-like Gratification Fantasies in Behavioral Treatments

In general, it may be expected that symbiotic-like gratification fantasies are most likely to be activated in treatments where the therapist adopts a comforting, reassuring, empathic stance and, in other respects, displays characteristics that are associated in fantasy with the mother of the symbiotic era. When other aspects of the treatment situation are congruent with or reinforce this perception of the therapist, the chances of such a fantasy's being activated become greater.

Systematic desensitization, as it is commonly practiced,* may be considered an example of a behavioral treatment in which symbiotic-like gratification fantasies are likely to be activated. A brief review of the key elements of this treatment (as presented in Goldfried & Davison, 1976) indicates that many aspects of the technique, the setting, and the therapist's stance may combine to produce a sense of reassurance, well-being, and connection to the therapist that include symbiotic-like elements.

The relevant *therapist behaviors and attitudes* would seem to be the following. The therapist adopts a calm, reassuring manner that promises protection against excessive anxiety. There is consistent support and encouragement; there are invitations to "go deeper" and "relax further" during the relaxation procedure; assistance is offered in formulating imagery, and there is prompt intervention when anxiety intrudes. *Techniques* that likely facilitate the activation of such fantasies include the use of deep-muscle relaxation and/or deep-breathing exercises, the provision of sug-

* *Systematic desensitization* actually involves a wide range of procedures and techniques, with choice of interventions varying as a function of the practitioner and the presenting problem. Though research indicates that learning an anxiety-competing response, such as deep muscle relaxation, and constructing graded hierarchies of anxiety-provoking situations are not essential for positive outcomes (Kazdin & Wilcoxon, 1976), these procedures continue to be utilized frequently in clinical practice (Goldfried & Davison, 1976; Walen, Hauserman, & Lavin, 1977).

gestions to promote relaxation, recordings of the therapist's voice to take home for practice sessions, and cue words to reinvoke experiences associated with the treatment. Relevant aspects of the *setting* may be the prone position and the darkened, quiet room during the relaxation procedure.

It is hypothesized here that these elements, which are frequently included in systematic desensitization (especially when it includes deep-muscle relaxation), produce a pull toward a state of tranquility, pleasurable passivity, and safety. Such a state is thought to have as its prototype the experience of oneness with the mother that was originally enjoyed during the symbiotic phase of development.

As suggested earlier, considerable uncertainty exists about which, if any, of the most frequently employed techniques are necessary for positive outcomes in systematic desensitization. Marks (1978) postulated that exposure to anxiety-provoking stimuli, accomplished by *any* strategy that proves effective in helping patients remain "in the presence" of such stimuli, is the essential element in desensitization procedures. Murray and Jacobson (1978) characterized systematic desensitization as a complex interpersonal encounter in which the therapist transmits the expectation of therapeutic gain to the patient. What is clear, however, is that the mechanisms underlying the transmission of positive expectancies are not known, nor is it known what processes occurring within the patient enable him or her, with the help of the therapist, to remain "in the presence" of fear-arousing stimuli. It is suggested here that the activation of symbiotic-like gratification fantasies may be one factor mediating such processes.

It is further proposed that such fantasies may be activated—and may mediate therapeutic gains—in other behavioral treatments where such key elements of the "oneness" experience are suggested by the techniques and/or the therapist's stance. Whereas certain therapeutic procedures and therapist behaviors may be more likely than others to activate oneness fantasies, whether or not such activation occurs is most likely dependent upon a complex interaction between technique, the personality of the patient, and the personality of the therapist.

Possible Activators of Sanctioned Impulse Gratification Fantasies in Behavioral Treatments

In general, sanctioned impulse gratification fantasies will most likely be activated in treatments where the therapist adopts an active, directive stance and implicitly or explicitly encourages libidinal or aggressive behavior that has been taboo or deeply conflictual for a particular patient in the past. In such cases, the therapist may be experienced as a permissive superego representative who is sanctioning the fulfillment of previously forbidden wishes. When other aspects of the treatment procedures are congruent with this perception of the therapist, the chances of such a fantasy's being activated become greater.

One example of a behavioral treatment in which such fantasies are likely to be activated is *assertiveness training*. In particular, it is likely that "sanctioned Oedipal gratification" fantasies are activated in assertiveness training, and these may be one factor mediating therapeutic improvement. What aspects of this treatment are likely to activate such fantasies? The following features of assertiveness training (as described by Walen, Hauserman, & Lavin, 1977) would seem to be relevant. Patients often seek this form of treatment because they are inhibited in expressing affectionate or angry feelings. A major thrust of the treatment is to reassure the patient that such expressions are not only acceptable but are *sanctioned* by the therapist and/or the group.* Patients are encouraged to model the behavior of the therapist, to practice acting assertively, and to assert themselves with the therapist, all the while being told that such self-assertions are not harmful. The distinction between assertion and aggression is frequently reinforced. The modeling and rehearsal procedures often include exercises in which the patient is encouraged to give bodily expression to his or her emotions and practice sessions with the therapist that involve staring exercises, shouting, and tugs of war.

Walen *et al.* (1977) have presented several case vignettes illustrating the use of assertiveness-training procedures. In one of these, many of the presumed activators of sanctioned Oedipal gratification fantasies were present.

The patient was a divorced man who complained of nervousness and claustrophobia. In the initial interview, the patient said he "felt like a failure" and added that, to a considerable degree, he agreed with his father's derogatory views of him. The therapist told the young man that his anger was a key problem and that he was having trouble being assertive. The therapist distinguished between assertion and agression. He then went on to say that he thought that it was important for the patient to be able to confront his father about his insults and criticisms. In the course of modeling and rehearsing this confrontation, the patient revealed that he harbored murderous wishes against his father. The therapist attempted to get the patient to articulate and accept these while continually reassuring him that such feelings were normal and that fantasies differ from actions. Moreover, he *sanctioned* the young man's anger by saying that he too would feel that way in similar circumstances. The therapist role-played the pa-

* Assertiveness training is often conducted in a group setting.

tient's father and had the patient confront him. The patient went on to do this with his father, and he was reassured by his father's benign response. He was also gratified that the father said some positive things about him. By the fourth session the presenting symptoms had abated.*

In this case vignette (which, incidentally, indicates that the therapist conceptualized the case in psychodynamic terms), the material supports the hypothesis that the therapist sanctioned and prepared the patient for the expression of derivative Oedipal wishes.† It may be further hypothesized that any behavioral treatment where the technique or stance of the therapist is characterized by an implied sanctioning of forbidden wishes will likely activate sanctioned impulse gratification fantasies. We also propose that such fantasies may mediate therapeutic improvement. As was suggested earlier, the type of fantasy activated in any treatment situation will be a function of an interaction between technique and therapist and the patient's personality variables. Thus, although systematic desensitization procedures may be especially likely to activate symbiotic-like gratification fantasies and assertiveness-training sanctioned impulse gratification fantasies, in particular cases—given a therapist of a certain personality type and a patient with certain dynamics—a sanctioned Oedipal gratification fantasy could be activated in systematic desensitization, or a oneness fantasy could be activated in assertiveness training. The relative influence of technique, therapist, and the patient's personality variables in determining which fantasies are activated is an empirical question.**

The hypothesis that the implied sanction of taboo impulses is a mutative factor in certain behavioral treatments is consistent with views expressed by Weitzman (1967). Based on an analysis of the imagery produced by patients during a systematic desensitization procedure, Weitzman proposed that previously unacceptable unconscious wishes that were expressed in disguised form in the patients' visualizations were being deconditioned (through pairing them with relaxation and with nonaversive outcomes). Such "deconditioning" was said to occur because the disguised

* No data were presented concerning any other adaptational changes that occurred following these sessions.

† In this case, the patient's difficulties with self-assertion were experienced and later worked on *directly* with his father. Thus, the sanctioned Oedipal gratification was less derivative and closer to an original aim than is usually the case.

** The theses presented here concerning the activation of different unconscious fantasies in different behavioral therapies and their role in mediating therapeutic improvement can be applied to other treatments as well. See Silverman (1979, 1982a) for further discussions of this view.

expression of the taboo wishes was experienced in a benign, nonaversive context. Clinical support for this formulation may be found in the work of Feather and Rhoads (1972b) who demonstrated clinical improvement in several patients when they were desensitized to the unconscious wishes that were thought to underlie their phobic symptoms. We would posit that during such desensitization, sanctioned impulse gratification fantasies were activated.

Experimental data bearing on the effects of activated unconscious fantasies on behavior in clinical and nonclinical populations will be presented next.

LABORATORY STUDIES

In this section, a series of laboratory experiments that demonstrate that the activation of various psychodynamically relevant unconscious fantasies brings about behavior change will be reviewed. Results from studies where symbiotic-like gratification fantasies and sanctioned impulse gratification fantasies led to improvement in adaptive functioning will then be cited. The effectiveness of activating these fantasies as an adjunct in behavioral (and other) treatment programs will be documented. Finally, some suggestions for investigating the hypothesis that certain unconscious fantasies are activated in the behavior therapies and mediate therapeutic improvement will be offered.

During the past 20 years, an experimental method that is referred to as *subliminal psychodynamic activation* has been developed that allows for the controlled study of the effects of unconscious fantasies on behavior. Over 50 studies from various research laboratories have been extensively reviewed in a recent article (Silverman, 1983). Using the demonstrations of subliminal registration in Fisher's pioneering studies (e.g., 1954, 1956) and the later investigations stimulated by Fisher's work (summarized in Wolitzky & Wachtel, 1973) as a starting point, this method attempts to utilize the phenomenon of subliminal registration for stimulating unconscious fantasies in order to make a systematic, precise, and controlled appraisal of their influence on behavior. The implications of these findings for psychoanalytic theory have been discussed in several earlier reports (Mendelsohn & Silverman, 1982; Silverman, 1967, 1970, 1971, 1972, 1975, 1976, 1978).

The following is a description of the experimental design that has been used in many of these investigations (those designated as "laboratory" studies). Subjects are seen individually for an experimental session on one day and a control session on another with their order counterbalanced. In the first session, the experimenter explains the purpose of the study to the subject and seeks his or her cooperation. Then, the assessment procedures that will be used are described to the subject who is further informed that several times during these procedures he or she will be asked to look through the eyepiece of a tachistoscope and will see flickers of light that contain extremely brief exposures of verbal and pictorial stimuli. Subjects are told that they will be debriefed about the content and purpose of the stimuli at the conclusion of the experiment.

The session proper begins with an assessment of the subject's propensity for whatever behaviors are being investigated. Following this, the subject is asked to look into the tachistoscope and to describe the flickers of light. Four exposures follow of either a stimulus related to an unconscious fantasy (the experimental session) or a stimulus presumed to be of neutral content (the control session). Each exposure lasts for 4 msecs. Then the behavior in question is reassessed to determine the effect of whatever stimulus was exposed. The procedure for the second session is identical, except that a different stimulus is exposed between the baseline and reassessment task series. Subjects who were exposed to the fantasy-related stimulus in the first session are shown a neutral stimulus in the second session and vice versa. In each session, the experimenter is "blind" to the tachistoscopic stimulus content. Because the subject is also unaware of the stimulus (it is subliminal), the procedure may be termed *double blind.* The evaluation of pathological manifestations is also carried out blindly.

In the earliest studies, the primary interest was in investigating various clinical formulations derived from psychoanalytic theory. This usually involved stimulating pathogenic (rather than adaptation-enhancing) components of unconscious fantasies. In numerous studies, when subliminal stimuli designed to activate derivatives of conflictual unconscious wishes were compared with neutral stimuli, they were found to intensify characteristic behaviors of several different subject populations, including adult male schizophrenics (e.g., Litwack, Wiedemann, & Yager, 1979; Lomangino, 1969; Silverman & Silverman, 1967; Silverman & Spiro, 1968), stutterers (Silverman, Bronstein, & Mendelsohn, 1976; Silverman, Klinger, Lustbader, Farrell, & Martin, 1972), male homosexuals (Silverman *et al.,* 1976,; Silverman, Kwawer, Wolitzky, & Coron, 1973), and depressives (Dauber, 1980; Miller, 1973; Rutstein & Goldberger, 1973).* The data from these studies were consistent with psychoanalytic formulations concerning the relationship between oral-agressive wishes and ego pathology in schizophrenics, anal wishes and stuttering, incestuous wishes and male homo-

* The experimental effects were typically short lived. See Silverman (1977) for a full discussion of ethical issues in this research. These effects did not occur when the same stimuli were presented supraliminally. This is consistent with the psychoanalytic view that once a conflictual wish becomes conscious, its status as a contributor to psychopathology may be compromised (Lomangino, 1969; Silverman & Spiro, 1967).

sexuality, and aggressive wishes and depression. One of these studies (Silverman *et al.*, 1976) demonstrated the specificity of the relationships between these particular wishes and the characteristic behaviors of each of these groups.

A more recent series of studies relates more specifically to the subject matter of this chapter—the role played by certain unconscious fantasies in enhancing adaptation. The earliest of these studies was stimulated by several clinical reports that there was often an abatement of symptoms in schizophrenics when symbiotic-like wishes were gratified (e.g., Limentani, 1956; Searles, 1965). In order to study this phenomenon in the laboratory, a stimulus intended to activate a symbiotic-like gratification fantasy was devised. This stimulus consisted of the words "Mommy and I are one," either presented alone or accompanied by a picture of a man and woman joined together at the shoulders. When presented subliminally to male schizophrenic subjects utilizing the procedure described, this stimulus reduced thought disorder and/or nonverbal behavioral pathology (when compared with a control stimulus) in over a dozen studies (e.g., Bronstein & Rodin, 1983; Fribourg, 1981; Leiter, 1982; Mendelsohn, 1981; Silverman & Candell, 1970; Spiro, 1975). However, this well-replicated finding was subject to the following qualification: The reduction in pathology was found only in schizophrenics who could be characterized as "relatively differentiated from their mothers" (i.e., 50–80% of hospitalized schizophrenic populations).

These findings were understood in the following way. Symbiotic-like gratification fantasies are presumed to provide a number of gratifications and to meet a number of defensive needs. These include the provision of a sense of nurturance and sustenance, the restoration of narcissistic equilibria, the maintenance of feelings of well-being, protection against loss of the primary relationship, and protection against destructive wishes. However, these fantasies may at certain times and for certain individuals (i.e., less differentiated schizophrenics) be poorly tolerated; in particular, fantasies of merging may be feared as leading to an undifferentiated state, and thus they threaten the existence of the self (Silverman, 1970). Further data supporting the view that there could be negative as well as positive outcomes when such fantasies are activated were provided in one study (Silverman, 1970) where the stimulus "I am mommy," implying *no* distinction between self and mother, produced significant *increases* in psychopathology even among relatively differentiated schizophrenics. It was thus concluded that for schizophrenics, symbiotic-like gratifications are most likely to be ameliorative if they are limited so that sense of self can be preserved. Results from a recent study (Mendelsohn, 1981) in which it was found that the therapeutic effectiveness of a symbiotic-like gratification stimulus was enhanced when it was modified in a way that simultaneously reassured schizophrenic subjects against boundary loss are consistent with this formulation.

From a series of further studies carried out with schizophrenics (reviewed in detail in Mendelsohn & Silverman, 1982; Silverman, Lachmann, & Milich, 1982), the following additional findings have emerged.

1. The adaptation-enhancing effects resulting from the activation of oneness fantasies in relatively differentiated schizophrenics do not appear when other gratifying fantasies or other internalization fantasies involving "Mommy" are activated. For example, the effects of "Mommy feeds me well," "Mommy is always with me," "Mommy and I are alike," and "Mommy is inside me" were no different than those of a control stimulus (Bronstein & Rodin, 1983; Kaplan, 1976).

2. Although "Mommy and I are one" is ameliorative for schizophrenic men, this is not the case for schizophrenic women (Cohen, 1977; Jackson, 1984). For female schizophrenics, on the other hand, the stimulus "Daddy and I are one" has led to pathology reduction, but this latter stimulus has not proven therapeutic for schizophrenic men (Jackson, 1983; Kaye, 1975).

More recently, it was asked whether the adaptation-enhancing effects of symbiotic-like gratification fantasies are limited to schizophrenics. A number of studies were undertaken with various clinical and nonclinical populations in order to address this question. The results of these studies indicate that adaptation-enhancing effects can be produced with many nonschizophrenics as well. And, parallel to what was found for schizophrenics, a sex difference emerged in these studies also; "Mommy and I are one" proved to be a more reliable ameliorative stimulus for men than for women.*

The most compelling findings bearing on the therapeutic potential of symbiotic-like fantasies in nonschizophrenics have come from what have been termed *treatment adjunct studies.* Unlike the laboratory experiments already described, these studies have involved multiple exposures of

* However, in contrast to the findings with schizophrenics where "Mommy and I are one" was not at all effective with females, there were a number of studies involving nonschizophrenic women in which the stimulus *was* effective. As is detailed elsewhere (Silverman, Lachmann, & Milich, 1982), whether "Mommy and I are one" enhances adaptive behavior in females seems dependent on the degree to which subjects are differentiated from their mothers, and it is safe to assume that there has been greater self–mother differentiation in nonschizophrenic than in schizophrenic women. Just as it was found that "Daddy and I are one" is ameliorative for schizophrenic women, for nonschizophrenic women a different oneness stimulus—"My lover and I are one"—has given indication of being more reliably ameliorative than "Mommy and I are one." Apparently, for women a oneness fantasy involving someone other than "mommy" best gratifies the need for oneness while preserving self-boundaries.

"Mommy and I are one" over a period of several weeks. Further, instead of a counterbalanced design, subjects were assigned either to an experimental or to a control group and were repeatedly exposed to either the oneness stimulus or a control stimulus, for example, "People are walking." Several of these studies have been carried out with students in academic settings. In some cases, the subliminal intervention was combined with classroom teaching and/or academic counseling in an attempt to determine if the activation of oneness fantasies enhanced academic performance. Parker (1982), in one such study, found that a group of college students exposed to "Mommy and I are one" received examination grades that were significantly higher than those of a matched control group. Similar results with different student groups were obtained by Ariam and Siller (1982), Hobbs (1983), and Zuckerman (1980). (Ariam and Siller's study was conducted in Israel, with the stimuli translated into Hebrew.*)

A further series of treatment adjunct studies has investigated whether the activation of symbiotic-like fantasies can enhance the effectiveness of psychological therapies. Linehan and O'Toole (1982) and Schurtman, Palmatier, and Martin (1982) have demonstrated this for college students in group counseling and for alcoholics in AA-type individual counseling, respectively. In four other studies, ones that bear most closely on the theses presented in this chapter, subliminal stimulation of symbiotic-like fantasies proved successful as an adjunct to various behavior therapies—systematic desensitization (Silverman, Frank, & Dachinger, 1974); behavior modification of obesity (Silverman, Martin, Ungaro, & Mendelsohn, 1978); rapid smoking (Palmatier & Bornstein, 1980), and assertiveness training (Packer, 1982). In each of these studies, when the behavioral intervention was accompanied by the subliminal oneness stimulus, it proved more effective than when accompanied by a subliminal neutral stimulus.

Experimental evidence attesting to the adaptation-enhancing effects of impulse sanction fantasies is considerably sparser than the evidence bearing on the role of symbiotic-like gratification fantasies. In one group of laboratory studies with college men engaged in competitive dart throwing, the effects of stimuli sanctioning or forbidding the expression of Oedipal impulses was explored. The subliminal exposure of the verbal stimuli

* Two related studies, investigating the effects of the oneness stimulus on academic achievement on adolescents in residential treatment, have been carried out. Bryant-Tuckett (1980) found improvement in reading ability as assessed on the California Achievement Test. Robertson (1982) failed to replicate this result but did find that "Mommy and I are one" increased field independence in her subjects as measured by a rod and frame test. These findings as well as others reported by Bryant-Tuckett indicate that exposure to the oneness stimulus can increase subjects' capacity for independent functioning—another possible adaptation-enchancing effect of activating the "Mommy and I are one" fantasy.

"Defeating dad is O.K.," "Beating dad is O.K.," and "Winning mom is O.K."(each accompanied by a congruent picture) was followed by more accurate dart throwing than after the stimuli "Defeating dad is wrong," "Beating dad is wrong," and "Winning mom is wrong" (again accompanied by congruent pictures) (Carroll, 1979; Glennon, 1983; Hayden & Silverstein, 1983; Lonski & Palumbo, 1978; Palumbo, 1980; Silverman, Ross, Adler, & Lustig, 1978).*

In three of the studies just cited, there were additional data supporting the specifically Oedipal interpretation of the results. In each of these, messages that were identical to those referred to previously but that did not contain a specific Oedipal element failed to affect the performance of the male subjects differentially. Thus, Palumbo (1980) did not find any difference in effect between "Beating him is O.K." and "Beating him is wrong," although he did find such a difference between "Beating dad is O.K." and "Beating dad is wrong." Lonski and Palumbo (1978) who also found a difference between the two "Beating dad" stimuli found no difference between "Beating mom is O.K." and "Beating mom is wrong." And Hayden and Silverstein (1983) who found a difference between the stimuli "Winning mom is O.K." and "Winning mom is wrong" (intended to address the libidinal rather than the aggressive side of the Oedipus complex) found no difference between "Winning dad is O.K." and "Winning dad is wrong."

Two of the treatment adjunct studies cited earlier as demonstrating that the activation of symbiotic-like fantasies can facilitate positive behavior change also yielded data indicating that the activation of sanction fantasies can do the same. One was the study of Zuckerman (1980) in which subliminal activation accompanied academic counseling of high school underachievers. A group receiving the message "My success is O.K." (as well as a group receiving "Mommy and I are one") received higher grades than did a control group receiving "People are walking." The second was the study of Packer (1982) in which subliminal stimulation served as an adjunct to an assertiveness-training program for women. In addition to one group receiving the "Mommy and I are one" stimulus (and a second serving as a control receiving "People are thinking"), a third received ex-

* In contrast to other subliminal psychodynamic activation studies where there have been many more reports of positive than of negative findings (see Silverman, 1983, for a comprehensive listing and discussion of these experiments), there have been almost as many reports of negative results using the dart paradigm as positive results. In contrast to the studies cited, nonreplications have been reported by Haspel (1979), Heilbrun (1980), Shaver (1979), Swanson (1980), and Winnett (1981). Carroll (1979) and Glennon (1983) have offered hypotheses to account for this variability in results. Further research in this area is clearly needed.

posures of "Defeating mom is O.K." (a sanctioned Oedipal gratification fantasy), and a fourth, "Defeating dad is O.K." (sanctioning competitive-aggressive impulses thought to be rooted in penis envy). The third stimulus condition yielded no significant results, but the group receiving "Defeating dad is O.K." showed increased assertiveness.

A final word is in order on the treatment adjunct studies—*dosage matters.* Fourteen studies have been completed to date, with 11 reporting positive results (Ariam & Siller, 1982; Hobbs, 1983; Linehan & O'Toole, 1982; Packer, 1982; Palmatier & Bornstein, 1980; Parker, 1982; Robertson, 1982; Schurtman *et al.*, 1983; Silverman *et al.*, 1978b; Zuckerman, 1980) and 3 reporting nonsignificant findings (Condon & Allen, 1981; Emmelkamp & Straatman, 1976; Ungaro, 1981). All of the latter involved low dosage (stimulation once or twice a week), whereas almost all of the former involved higher dosage (stimulation three to five times per week).* Moreover, in one of these studies (Packer, 1982), dosage was one of the independent variables studied and was found to be clearly relevant. All of Packer's subjects received behavior assertiveness training over a 3-week period accompanied by subliminal stimulation. All experimental and control subjects received the stimulation four sessions per week and all the controls were given the subliminal neutral stimulus during these four sessions. However, each of the experimental groups was divided into two subgroups, one receiving the experimental stimulus (either "Mommy and I are one," "Defeating mom is O.K.," or "Defeating dad is O.K.") for two of the weekly sessions and the neutral stimulus for the other two, whereas the other subgroup received the experimental stimulus in all four sessions. The latter subgroups showed stronger experimental effects than did the former.

What are the implications of these research findings for the hypotheses presented in this chapter? What light is shed on the role of unconscious fantasies in the behavior therapies? The data clearly indicate that the activation of certain unconscious fantasies can enhance the effectiveness of various treatment modalities, including behavioral treatments. Although *consistent* with the hypotheses presented earlier, these data, however, do not demonstrate that these fantasies are typically activated in the behavior therapies nor that they play a role in mediating therapeutic gains. In order to test these hypotheses, the following research strategies could prove useful.

1. Personality assessments of patients undergoing various behavioral

* As has been discussed elsewhere (Silverman, 1982b), the absence of effects in the Emmelkamp and Straatman (1976), Condon and Allen (1981), and Ungaro (1981) studies may also have been a function of two other factors. The first two of the three studies cited had methodological weaknesses, and all three used female subjects. As we noted earlier, the "Mommy and I are one" stimulus is less reliable for females than it is for males.

treatments could be carried out by administering projective tests prior to starting and following the conclusion of therapy to determine whether certain unconscious fantasies had been activated. Changes in patients' perceptions of the therapist (cf. Crisp, 1966) could be made part of the study. Data emerging from such a study would only be indirectly confirmatory, but the design has the advantage of permitting the study of within-subject personality changes following behavioral treatments.

2. Such a strategy could then be combined with the following: The treatment under consideration could be administered as was done in past studies. Subjects could be divided into matched groups—those receiving the treatment and a control stimulus, those receiving the treatment and a stimulus designed to activate the ameliorative fantasy, and a third group who received the treatment and a stimulus designed to *inhibit* or *counter* the supposed ameliorative fantasy. Thus, in the case of a study of systematic desensitization, the three conditions would be control, "Mommy and I are one," and a stimulus such as "I am wholly on my own." If the last of these stimuli *interfered* with the effectiveness of systematic desensitization (i.e., if subjects in this group fared more poorly than did control subjects), then the hypothesis that symbiotic-like gratification fantasies are activated in the treatment and mediate symptomatic improvement would be supported.

3. Finally, it would be of interest to establish the specificity of the unconscious fantasies mediating behavior change by varying key words in the subliminal stimuli (e.g., "Mommy and I are one" amended to read "Daddy and I are one" or "Mommy and I are two") and then comparing their effectiveness.

In summary, a rationale derived from the behavioral and psychoanalytic literature for considering alternative ways of accounting for behavior change in the behavior therapies has been presented, and the relevance of the construct *unconscious fantasy* to this problem has been discussed. Research data that bear on the adaptation-enhancing effects of activating unconscious fantasies have been reviewed. In the concluding sections, some implications of the preceding discussions for clinical training and practice and for the question of the integration of the behavior therapies and psychoanalysis will be presented.

CLINICAL APPLICATIONS

The activation of unconscious fantasies may be considered one of several psychodynamic influences on outcome in the behavior therapies. As noted earlier, given the origins and theoretical foundations of the behavior therapies, there has been a tendency to emphasize the mutative effects of therapeutic techniques and not to formulate clinical change in terms of dynamic or interpersonal processes. Yet, even among behaviorists there has always been some questioning of this bias. Poser (1967) cited a division among behavior therapists regarding training philosophy between those emphasizing the teaching of technical procedures and those stressing the accumulation of general clinical experience. The author maintained that behavior therapists, as opposed to technicians, had to be competent in both areas. Klein *et al.* (1969) commented on the clinical sensitivity of experienced behavior therapists and voiced concern that adequate training in interviewing and diagnostic skills was not being provided in behavior therapy training programs. Goldfried and Davison (1976) stressed the importance of recognizing and managing resistances (what they termed tendencies toward "countercontrol") in behavioral treatments, and Braff *et al.* (1976) warned of clinical failures if interpersonal dynamics are not attended to.

In relation to the more specific issue of unconscious fantasies activated in the behavior therapies, what implications can be drawn for clinical practice? How might behavior therapies utilize the concepts and findings presented here in their work with patients? Several preliminary suggestions can be offered.

1. Specific therapist behaviors and technical procedures will affect different patients in different ways. It would seem advisable for behavior therapists to develop informed hypotheses about the *meaning* of interventions for patients and to evaluate responses to therapeutic techniques in light of these hypotheses about patients' subjective experiences. This may be especially important when resistances are encountered or idiosyncratic responses occur.

2. Opportunities for intensive psychodynamic inquiry or detailed personality testing are ordinarily not available to the behavior therapist. Thus, a precise delineation of the salient unconscious fantasies likely to be activated in treatment will not be possible in the vast majority of cases. However, clinical sensitivity and the likelihood of therapeutic success may be enhanced if it is recognized that specific technical procedures, especially when accompanied by a congruent therapist "stance," are especially likely to activate certain unconscious fantasies. For example, based on the data presented in the third section, it may be especially likely that a symbiotic-like gratification fantasy will be activated in systematic desensitization treatments where relaxation is employed and where the therapist is calm, reassuring, nonintrusive, and nondemanding, whereas a sanctioned impulse gratification fantasy will likely be activated in an assertiveness-training program that is conducted by an active, encouraging, directive, and re-

assuring therapist. (Note that *reassurance* can have different connotations in different contexts.*)

3. Therapeutic outcomes may be enhanced by controlling for the differential effects of activating unconscious fantasies in different patients. In an earlier discussion of this issue, one of the authors of this chapter speculated that failure to expose and/or dispel certain distortions (presumably resulting from the activation of unconscious fantasies) during the course of nonanalytic therapies can interfere with positive effects (Silverman, 1974). Certain fantasies may prove beneficial for some patients although they may lead to negative effects for others. For example, certain therapist behaviors and/or technical procedures might activate a fantasy that the therapist is a powerful, controlling figure. Certain patients with passive-dependent orientations who tend to accept authority figures uncritically and attribute omniscience to them might respond with eager compliance and therapeutic gains to such a "controlling" therapist. On the other hand, certain patients with oppositional or paranoid features might, under the same circumstances, respond resistively or even drop out of treatment. Thus, it is not only important for behavior therapists to be aware of which unconscious fantasies are most likely to be activated in any given treatment but also to realize what it is they do to reinforce or inhibit such effects. They would then be in a position to alter their technique or stance when positive effects are not obtained.

4. In certain cases a limited but focused inquiry can be helpful in uncovering the dynamic bases of resistances. Such an inquiry could include asking the patient his or her thoughts and feelings about the therapeutic procedures. The patient might also be asked if his or her experience of the treatment was reminiscent of reactions to other significant experiences. If such inquiry suggests links between the resistance and activated unconscious fantasies, making a "limited interpretation" to the patient might sometimes prove helpful. Such an interpretation would involve alluding to the unconscious meaning or significance of the patient's misperception, but it would not address the underlying motivational basis for the distortion. Consider, for example, a patient in systematic desensitization who paradoxically becomes increasingly tense whenever he or she is asked to relax and whose thoughts about this reaction suggest that he or she experiences the instruction as a sexual seduction. The therapist might simply comment that people sometimes, without being quite aware of it, view instructions to relax as having sexual connotations, and this makes it dif-

* Although the two fantasies discussed here may be among the most frequently activated in the behavior therapies, the likelihood that other unconscious fantasies often play a role in mediating behavior change is great. Further research is needed to identify such fantasies.

ficult for them to comply with the procedure. The therapist would go no further in exploring the historical roots of this fear.

INTEGRATION

In closing, the implications of some of the points made earlier will be applied to the issue of integrating behavioral and psychoanalytic approaches.

Such integrations can be considered on the levels of both theory and technique. With regard to the latter, the following questions can be raised: (a) Can techniques derived from the behavior therapies be utilized successfully in primarily psychoanalytic treatments? (b) Can techniques derived from psychoanalysis be utilized successfully in primarily behavioral treatments? and (c) Can hybrid treatments be developed that are neither psychoanalysis nor behavior therapy but that are some mixture of the two?

Considered solely from this vantage point, the question to be addressed is whether or not such treatments are more helpful or more widely applicable than traditional approaches—a question that can only be answered by research and clinical trial. Some of the studies presented in the third section, specifically the "treatment adjunct" studies (where the symbioticlike gratification fantasy and the sanctioned impulse gratification fantasy were used to enhance the effectiveness of behavioral treatments), come close to—though are not identical with—one type of integration referred to here. In these cases, an intervention based on a psychoanalytic understanding of behavior change (though not a psychoanalytic intervention proper) was added to a traditional behavioral treatment and, under particular conditions, the effectiveness of the treatment was enhanced. These results are consistent with the notion that integration on the level of technique is possible and potentially beneficial, though further research is clearly called for.*

In predominantly psychoanalytic treatments, the introduction of a behavioral intervention (e.g., behavior rehearsal preceding an important job interview) may be viewed as similar in form to the introduction of other "active" interventions (e.g., setting a limit, counseling, reassurance, etc.). Extrapolating from considerations outlined some 30 years ago by Eissler (1953), the crucial questions to be considered in such a circumstance

* This should not be understood as an endorsement of the use of the subliminal technique by therapists. At this point, the most valid use of this method is to study clinical psychoanalytic theory and to clarify the role of activated unconscious fantasies in mediating behavior change. Delineation of its clinical usefulness awaits further research.

are as follows: Does the intervention produce a beneficial effect that could not be accomplished by a traditional psychoanalytic technique? Will the introduction of the intervention be "at a price"? That is, will it interfere with the psychoanalytic process? The answer to the latter question might depend largely upon whether or not the therapist and patient can arrive at an understanding of the unconscious *meaning* of the intervention to the patient. This, or course, is an empirical question, and because it is quite possible that no general answer exists, the effectiveness of this type of integration will have to be studied in a variety of clinical situations.

In predominantly behavioral treatments, the introduction of a psychoanalytic intervention—for example, a limited interpretation of a resistance to treatment—might proceed along the lines discussed by Wachtel (1977) or in the fourth section of this chapter. The crucial issues here would be the following: Does the intervention accomplish its goal—the overcoming of resistances to making effective use of the behavioral treatment? Is the intervention "at a price"—that is, will it limit the effectiveness of later behavioral interventions? For example, it is possible that with some patients, the interpretation would be experienced as a kind of caring that would, in turn, engender wishes for further interpretive comments that would deflect the treatment away from its intended focus.

Finally, several hybrid treatments of the type described previously have been developed (Birk & Brinkley-Birk, 1974; Feather & Rhoads, 1972a, 1972b; Stampfl & Levis, 1967). With regard to these, the relevant question to be asked is whether they are more effective than traditionally "pure" psychoanalytic or behavioral treatments.

The integration of psychoanalysis and the behavior therapies can also be considered on the level of theory. Here, two levels of analysis can be considered. The first involves integrating the operational concepts of each school with those of the other with the goal of increasing the effectiveness of each approach. Examples of such integrations might include (a) the study of the conditioning and reinforcing properties of particular interventions during psychoanalytic treatment, or (b) consideration of the possibility that insight in psychoanalytic treatments is mutative because it involves deconditioning the fear that libidinal or aggressive impulse expression will lead to punishment (cf. Silverman, 1984). Similarly, within the realm of the behavior therapies, the possibility could be studied that one aspect of what is mutative in systematic desensitization is the opportunity for desensitization of conflictual unconscious impulses (cf. Feather & Rhoads, 1972a, 1972b; Weitzman, 1967). Or, as has been proposed in this chapter, the role of activated unconscious fantasies in mediating behavior change in the behavior therapies can be studied. To be true integrations the analyses proposed here should go beyond being mere translations of the language of one field into that of the other and should yield a system that incorporates viewpoints from both fields (cf. Ryle, 1978). For example, the theses presented in this chapter could, if carried further, be developed into a theory of behavior change in the behavior therapies that incorporates the principles of S–R learning theory (e.g., the reinforcing and deconditioning effects of various techniques) and psychoanalysis (e.g., the mutative effects of activating unconscious fantasies).

The second level of theoretical integration involves reconciling the basic assumptions of the behavior therapies and psychoanalysis. These assumptions include significantly divergent views about (a) the kinds of data and observational methods relevant to formulating clinical understanding; (b) personality development, including the etiology of psychopathology; and (c) the process of behavior change. Integration on this level of theory poses numerous difficulties. Comparisons between psychoanalysis and the behavior therapies indicate that different behaviors are sampled, different investigative methods are applied, and divergent assumptions about how behaviors develop and change are maintained. Moreover, therapeutic goals and criteria for assessing outcome may not only be different but may, in fact, be incompatible (cf. Messer & Winoker, 1980).

Finally, another aspect of the integration issue should be noted. This involves what may be termed *convergence* rather than integration proper. As psychoanalysis and the behavior therapies have developed, the difficulties that have been encountered in understanding and treating psychological disorders have led workers in each field to be concerned about the limitations of their therapeutic approaches (cf. Applebaum, 1975; Marks, 1978). Perhaps as an outgrowth of such concern, there has been an almost natural tendency to expand the focus of each field of study to include domains that in the past were primarily associated with the other. This process is more aptly termed *convergence* rather than integration because (a) the impetus for such expansion may not directly arise from the findings of the other school, and (b) the end product may involve an expanded field rather than the combining of two different systems. Examples of developments in psychoanalysis that may be seen as reflecting convergence with areas more traditionally associated with the behavior therapies and behavioral analysis include the studies of "here-and-now" determinants of transference reactions (Gill, 1982), the study of the treatment setting and its role in the therapy process (Langs, 1973), the study of the *stimulus value* of the therapist (Wachtel, 1977,* the study of everyday events that trigger unconscious

* These reflect a growing appreciation of the role of current experience, including the actual behavior of the therapist, in activating "transference" reactions. The analysis of such reactions takes in the immediate precipitating circumstances in addition to infantile antecedents.

conflict and psychopathology (Silverman, 1972), and the development of strategies and techniques suited to short-term treatment (Schafer, 1973). Examples of convergence that involve expansion of the domain of the behavior therapies to include phenomena previously associated more exclusively with psychoanalysis include the study of cognitive mediation in cognitive behavior therapy (Murray & Jacobson, 1978) and the development of technical recommendations concerning the reduction of resistances (Goldfried & Davison, 1976). The usefulness of modifications in psychoanalytic or behavioral treatments arising from their convergence is a matter for empirical study.

Acknowledgments

The authors wish to express their gratitude to Ann Appelbaum, Kenneth Barish, and Howard Hunt for their helpful comments about an earlier draft of this chapter.

AUTOBIOGRAPHICAL STATEMENTS

My interest in the integration issue is as a clinician and researcher. Over the past 9 years, I have had an opportunity to work in acute and long-term inpatient settings and in private practice with persons with psychotic conditions and severe character disorders. The clinical work, although usually conceptualized along psychodynamic and interpersonal lines, has—especially for hospitalized patients—required a flexible technical approach. I have often found it useful and necessary to provide teaching, counseling, and opportunities for rehearsal and *cognitive restructuring,* and to encourage and facilitate desensitization in the face of debilitating and persistent phobic/avoidant behavior. At times I have incorporated techniques similar to those described in the behavior therapy literature into essentially psychodynamically oriented expressive or supportive psychotherapies. In hospital work especially, there are numerous examples of what technically constitute departures from "neutrality," including limit-setting interventions and administrative decisions that the psychotherapist directly or indirectly participates in making. In most of these instances, whether the intervention is the introduction of a behavioral technique, a proscription, or an administrative decision, the goal is either to promote symptomatic or adaptational improvement or to limit harmful acting out and thus protect the patient and/or the setting. When such techniques are used, I try to assess their meaning to the patient and to me, though only in an expressive psychotherapy is this assessment systematic and explicit. I have found that the more successful psychotherapies tend to be those in which such interventions can be more thoroughly examined and their effects worked through. However, I am not sure if a causal relationship is operative.

Among the clinicians I have learned from, Ann Appelbaum and Howard Hunt have especially stressed the application of multiple perspectives to the resolution of clinical problems. Appelbaum, a psychoanalyst, is expert in devising milieu treatment strategies for severely disturbed patients. These programs of activities, structured interpersonal interactions, and opportunities for self-care are designed to control acting-out tendencies, to provide symbolic gratifications and thereby reduce the need for symptoms, and to provide opportunities for exercise of function. Developing these programs necessarily involves the application of multiple perspectives, usually including psychodynamic, interpersonal, and behavioral perspectives to the resolution of psychopathology. In reflecting upon patients' responses to such milieu programs, especially when these are combined with intensive psychotherapy, I have been impressed with the importance of providing patients with opportunities to develop and practice alternative means of problem solving as an adjunct and, in many cases, as a precursor to the development of insight. The opportunity to behave in more adaptive ways seems to me to be a crucial element in modifying essentially negatively toned self-representations.

Hunt, who is primarily a behaviorist, has written about and taught the usefulness of applying psychodynamic theory to the understanding of how certain behaviors develop and are maintained. He has pointed out that although behavioral techniques are often effective in promoting symptomatic or adaptational improvements, the reason for these effects is often not known. In his view, the meanings of interventions to patients—many of these meanings are quite personal and idiosyncratic—are important in determining the success or failure of a therapeutic regime.

As regards my research interests, and as Silverman and I describe in our chapter, one application of the subliminal psychodynamic activation method has been to study some of the unconscious fantasies that may be mediating symptomatic improvement in the behavior therapies. In particular, we have been interested in the effects of activating a "oneness" fantasy and, more recently, a sanctioned gratification fantasy as an adjunct to standard behavioral treatments. The generally positive results have reinforced my interest in conceptualizing the change process in the behavior therapies in terms derived from psychoanalytic theory.

ERIC MENDELSOHN, PH.D.

My interest in participating in ventures such as this has developed from a growing conviction that the great majority of scholars in the psychoanalytic and behaviorist communities have been operating under the mistaken assumptions that their observations, inferences, and formulations are sufficient for elucidating psychopathology and that their methods are adequate for overcoming such pathology. A position that I suspect is considerably closer to what future research will reveal is that the approaches of both groups as well as those operating out of other frames of reference are needed if our theoretical understanding is to be reasonably complete and our therapeutic methods consistently effective.

Let me make clear that it is not an indiscriminate eclecticism that I am advocating nor is it one that is based on clinical impressions alone, but rather, it is an eclecticism informed by systematically collected data from well-controlled research studies. Although some of the necessary data are currently available, the bulk of what is required is not, and its procurement remains the task of the future.

What have been the experiences that I view as having been most influential in shaping this vision of the future? First, I have observed an interesting paradox through the years. On the one hand, there is compelling evidence from an increasing number of well-controlled laboratory studies (cf. Fisher & Greenberg, 1979; Kline, 1981; Silverman, 1976, 1983) that many key psychoanalytic propositions are valid, particularly those propositions that link psychopathology to unconscious conflict. (These propositions clearly will have to be embodied in the encompassing eclectic view of the future.) On the other hand, evidence is lacking that the results of psychoanalytic treatment are more effective than those of other therapies. Although the absence of confirmatory evidence that psychoanalytic treatment is more effective is not the same as disconfirmation of that premise, I have felt inclined to entertain the possibility that psychoanalytic treatment is, in fact, no more effective, despite the soundness of some of its key premises. If this is indeed the case, I would assume that psychoanalytic understanding will have to integrate other theoretical ideas and/or its treatment procedures will require technique innovations before psychoanalytic treatment becomes substantially more effective.

As a point of information, what I have referred to previously has taken place to some extent already within the psychoanalytic community. With regard to theoretical integrations, consider for example, the integrations of psychoanalytic theory with gestalt psychology by Rapaport (1960), with anthropology by Erikson (1962), with cognitive psychologies by Klein (1970), with information theory by Peterfreund and Franceschini (1973), and with nonpsychoanalytic motivation theories by Holt (1976). Similarly, promising treatment innovations have been proposed in recent years by Gedo (1980), Gill (1972), and Kohut (1977). With regard to treatment, although it is possible to find some interesting links between these proposals and particular nonpsychoanalytic therapies (see, for example, Stolorow's 1976 paper on the similarities between Kohut's treatment recommendations and those of Carl Rogers), these proposals were not offered as instances of integrating psychoanalytic and nonpsychoanalytic approaches. On the other hand, Weitzman's 1967 paper "Behavior Therapy and Psychotherapy," Feather and Rhoad's 1972a,b "Psychodynamic Behavior Therapy," and Wachtel's 1977 book *Psychoanalysis and Behavior Therapy* do represent such instances. Although I have reservations about some of the technique recommendations proposed, I have been struck by the richness of possibilities that each of these writings offers with regard to theoretical understanding and treatment approaches.

These are some of the influences that have stimulated me to want to partake in efforts like the current one.

LLOYD H. SILVERMAN, PH.D.

REFERENCES

Appelbaum, S. The idealization of insight. In R. Langs (Ed.), *International Journal of Psychoanalytic Psychotherapy*, 1975, *4*, 272–302.

Ariam, S., & Siller, J. Effects of subliminal oneness stimuli in Hebrew on academic performance of Israeli high school students: Further evidence on the adaptation enhancing effects of symbiotic fantasies in another culture using another language. *Journal of Abnormal Psychology*, 1982, *91*, 343–349.

Bandura, A. Self-efficacy mechanism in human agency. *American Psychologist*, 1982, *37*(2), 122–147.

Birk, L., & Brinkley-Birk, A. W. Psychoanalysis and behavior therapy. *American Journal of Psychiatry*, 1974, *131*(5), 499–509.

Braff, D. L., Raskin, M., & Geisinger, D. Management of interpersonal issues in systematic desensitization. *American Journal of Psychiatry*, 1976, *133*(7), 791–794.

Bronstein, A. & Rodin, G. An experimental study of internalization fantasies in schizophrenic men. *Psychotherapy: Theory, Research and Practice*, 1983, 20(4), 408–416.

Bryant-Tuckett, R. *The effects of subliminal merging stimuli on the academic performance of emotionally handicapped students*. Unpublished doctoral dissertation, New York University, 1980.

Carroll, R. *Neurophysiological and psychological mediators of response to subliminal perception: The influence of hemisphericity and defensive style on susceptibility to subliminally presented conflict-laden stimuli*. Unpublished doctoral dissertation, St. John's University, 1979.

Cohen, R. *The effects of four subliminally introduced merging stimuli on the psychopathology of schizophrenic women*. Unpublished doctoral dissertation, Columbia University, 1977.

Condon, T. J., & Allen, G. J. The role of psychoanalytic merging fantasies in systematic desensitization: A rigorous methodological examination. *Journal of Abnormal Psychology*, 1980, *89*, 437–443.

Crisp, A. H. "Transference," "symptom emergence," and "social repercussion" in behavior therapy: A study of 54 treated patients. *British Journal of Medical Psychology*, 1966, *39*, 179–196.

Dauber, R. *An investigation of guilt, loss, and the separation-individuation process in depression*. Unpublished doctoral dissertation, Loyola Universtiy of Chicago, 1980.

Davison, G. C., & Wilson, G. T. Critique of "desensitization: social and cognitive factors underlying the effectiveness of Wolpe's procedure." *Psychological Bulletin*, 1972, *78*(1), 28–31.

Eissler, K. R. The effects of the structure of the ego on psychoanalytic technique. *Journal of the American Psychoanalytic Association*, 1953, *1*, 104–143.

Emmelkamp, P. M., & Straatman, H. A psychoanalytic reinterpretation of the effectiveness of systematic desensitization: Fact or fiction? *Behavior Research and Therapy*, 1976, *14*, 245–249.

Erikson, E. *Childhood and society*. New York: Norton, 1962.

Feather, B. W., & Rhoads, J. M. Psychodynamic behavior therapy: I. Theory and rationale. *Archives of General Psychiatry*, 1972, *26*, 496–502. (a)

Feather, B. W., & Rhoads, J. M. Psychodynamic behavior therapy: II. Clinical aspects. *Archives of General Psychiatry*, 1972, *26*, 503–511. (b)

Fisher, C. Dreams and perception. *Journal of the American Psychoanalytic Association*, 1954, *2*, 389–445.

Fisher, C. Dreams, images, and perception: A study of unconscious-preconscious relationships. *Journal of the American Psychoanalytic Association*, 1956, *4*, 5–48.

Fisher, S., & Greenberg, P. R. *The scientific credibility of Freud's theories and therapy*. New York: Basic Books, 1977.

Franks, C. M., & Wilson, G. T. Systematic desensitization, flooding, symbolic and participant modeling, cognitive restructuring, and assertion training. In C. M. Franks & G. T. Wilson (Eds.), *Annual review of behavior therapy and practice.* New York: Brunner/Mazel, 1976.

Fribourg, A. Ego pathology in schizophrenia and fantasies of merging with the good mother. *Journal of Nervous and Mental Disease,* 1981, *169,* 337–347.

Friedman, H. J. Patient-expectancy and symptom reduction. *Archives of General Psychiatry,* 1963, *8,* 61–67.

Gelder, M. G., Bancroft, J. H. J., Gath, D. H., Johnston, D. W., Mathews, A. M., & Shaw, P. M. Specific and nonspecific factors in behavior therapy. *British Journal of Psychiatry,* 1973, *123,* 445–462.

Gill, M. M. The analysis of the transference. In S. Slipp (Ed.), *Curative factors in dynamic psychotherapy.* New York: McGraw-Hill, 1982.

Gedo, J. *Advances in clinical psychoanalysis.* New York: International Universities Press, 1980.

Glennon, S. *The effect of hemispherity on the subliminal activation of residual oedipal conflicts.* Doctoral dissertation, New York University, 1983.

Goldfried, M. R., & Davison, G. L. *Clinical behavior therapy.* New York: Holt, Rinehart & Winston, 1976.

Gomes-Schwartz, B., Hadley, S. W., & Strupp, H. H. Individual psychotherapy and behavior therapy. In M. R. Rosenzweig & L. W. Porter (Eds.), *Annual review of psychology,* 1978, *29,* 435–471.

Grunbaum, A. The placebo concept. *Behavior Research and Therapy,* 1981, *19,* 157–167.

Haspel, K. *The effects of priming and subliminal oedipal stimulation on competitive behavior of college males.* Unpublished master's thesis, University of Rhode Island, 1979.

Hayden, B., & Silverstein, R. The effects of tachistoscopic stimulation on competitive dart throwing. *Psychological Research Bulletin,* 1983, *23*(1), 1–12.

Heilbrun, K. Silverman's subliminal psychodynamic activation: A failure to replicate. *Journal of Abnormal Psychology,* 1980, *89,* 560–566.

Hobbs, S. *The effects of the subliminal stimulation of oedipal and symbiotic fantasies on prejudiced attitudes.* Doctoral dissertation, New York University, 1983.

Holt, R. R. Drive or wish? A reconsideration of the psychoanalytic theory of motivation. In (M. Gill & P. Holtzman, Eds.), *Psychology versus metapsychology: Psychoanalytic essays in memory of George S. Klein* (Psychological Issues Monograph 36). New York: International Universities Press, 1976.

Ingram, R., & Goldstein, B. Role of expectancy factors in behavioral self-control therapies: An experimental inquiry. *Psychological Reports,* 1978, *42,* 535–542.

Jackson, J. The effects of fantasies of oneness with mother and father on the ego functioning of male and female schizophrenics. *Journal of Nervous and Mental Disease,* 1983, *171,* 280–289.

Kahn, M., & Baker, B. Desensitization with minimal therapist contact. *Journal of Abnormal Psychology,* 1968, *73*(3), 198–200.

Kaplan, R. *The symbiotic fantasy as a therapeutic agent: An experimental comparison of the effects of three symbiotic elements on manifest pathology in schizophrenics.* Unpublished doctoral dissertation, New York University, 1976.

Kaye, M. *The therapeutic value of three merging stimuli for male schizophrenics.* Unpublished doctoral dissertation, Yeshiva University, 1975.

Kazdin, A. E., & Wilcoxon, L. A. Systematic desensitization and nonspecific treatment effects: A methodological evaluation. *Psychological Bulletin,* 1976, *83*(5), 729–758.

Klein, G. S. *Perceptions, motives, and personality.* New York: Knopf, 1970.

Klein, M. H., Dittman, A. T., Parloff, M. B., & Gill, M. M. Behavior therapy: Observations and reflections. *Journal of Consulting and Clinical Psychology,* 1969, *33*(3), 259–266.

Kline, P. *Fact and fantasy in Freudian theory* (2nd ed.). New York: Methuen, 1981.
Kohut, H. The restoration of the self. New York: International Universities Press, 1977.
Langs, R. *The technique of psychoanalytic psychotherapy* (Vol. 1). New York: Jason Aronson, 1973.
Laplanche, J., & Pontalis, J.-B. *The language of psychoanalysis.* New York: Norton, 1973.
Leiter, E. The effects of subliminal activation of aggressive and merging fantasies in differentiated and nondifferentiated schizophrenics. *Psychological Research Bulletin,* 1982, *22*(7), 1–21.
Lick, J. Expectancy, false galvanic skin response feedback, and systematic desensitization in the modification of phobic behavior. *Journal of Consulting and Clinical Psychology,* 1975, *43*(4), 557–567.
Limentani, D. Symbiotic identification in schizophrenia. *Psychiatry,* 1956, *19,* 231–236.
Linehan, E., & O'Toole, J. The effect of subliminal stimulation of symbiotic fantasy on college students' self-disclosures in group counseling. *Journal of Counseling Psychology,* 1982, *29,* 151–157.
Litwack, T. R., Wiedemann, C. F., & Yager, J. The fear of object loss, responsiveness to subliminal stimuli, and schizophrenic psychopathology. *Journal of Nervous and Mental Disease,* 1979, *167,* 79–90.
Lomangino, L. *Depiction of subliminally and supraliminally presented aggressive stimuli and their effects on the cognitive functioning of schizophrenics.* Unpublished doctoral dissertation, Fordham University, 1969.
Lonski, M., & Palumbo, R. *The effects of subliminal stimulation on competitive dart throwing performance.* Unpublished manuscript, Hofstra University, 1978. (Available from senior author at Elmhurst Outpatient Department of Creedmore Psychiatric Center, 37-10 114th Street, Corona, N.Y. 11373.)
Luborsky, L., Singer, B., & Luborsky, L. Comparative studies of psychotherapy. *Archives of General Psychiatry,* 1975, *32,* 995–1008.
Mahler, M. S., Pine, F., & Bergman, A. *The psychological birth of the human infant.* New York: Basic Books, 1975.
Marcia, J. E., Rubin, B. M., & Efran, J. S. Systematic desensitization: Expectancy change or counterconditioning? *Journal of Abnormal Psychology,* 1969, *74*(3), 382–387.
Marks, I. Behavioral psychotherapy of adult neurosis. In S. L. Garfield & A. E. Bergin (Eds.), *Handbook of psychotherapy and behavior change: An empirical analysis* (2nd ed.). New York: Wiley, 1978.
Marks, I., & Gelder, M. G. Common ground between behavior therapy and psychodynamic methods. *British Journal of Medical Psychology,* 1966, *39*(11), 11–23.
Mendelsohn, E. The effects of stimulating symbiotic fantasies on manifest pathology in schizophrenics: A revised formulation. *Journal of Nervous and Mental Disease,* 1981, *169*(9), 580–590.
Mendelsohn, E., & Silverman, L. H. The effects of stimulating psychodynamically relevant unconscious fantasies on schizophrenic psychopathology: A review of research findings. *Schizophrenia Bulletin,* 1982, *8*(3), 532–547.
Messer, S. B., & Winokur, M. Some limits to the integration of psychoanalytic and behavior therapy. *American Psychologist,* 1980, *35*(9), 818–827.
Meyer, V., & Chesser, E. S. *Behavior therapy in clinical psychiatry.* New York: Science House, 1970.
Miller, J. *The effects of aggressive stimulation upon young adults who have experienced death of a parent during childhood and adolescence.* Unpublished doctoral dissertation, New York University, 1973.
Morris, R. J., & Magrath, K. H. Contribution of therapist warmth to the contact desensitization treatment of acrophobia. *Journal of Consulting and Clinical Psychology,* 1979, *47*(4), 786–788.
Morris, R. J., & Suckerman, K. R. The importance of the therapeutic relationship in systematic desensitization. *Journal of Consulting and Clinical Psychology,* 1974, *42*(1), 148–156. (a)

Morris, R. J., & Suckerman, K. R. Therapist warmth as a factor in automated systematic desensitization. *Journal of Consulting and Clinical Psychology,* 1974, *42*(2), 244–250. (b)

Murray, E. J., & Jacobson, L. I. Cognition and learning in traditional and behavioral therapy. In S. L. Garfield & A. E. Bergin (Eds.), *Handbook of psychotherapy and behavior change.* New York: Wiley, 1978.

Packer, S. B. *The effect of subliminally stimulating fantasies aimed at gratifying symbiotic and sanctioning competitive strivings on assertiveness difficulties in women.* Unpublished doctoral dissertation, New York University, 1982.

Palmatier, J., & Bornstein, P. The effects of subliminal stimulation of symbiotic merging fantasies on behavioral treatment of smokers. *Journal of Nervous and Mental Disease,* 1980, *168,* 715–720.

Palumbo, R. *The fear of success in adult males: The effects of subliminal messages derived from two theoretical models.* Unpublished doctoral dissertation, Hofstra University, 1980.

Parker, K. A. The effects of subliminal merging stimuli on the academic performance of college students. *Journal of Counseling Psychology,* 1982, *29,* 9–28.

Peterfreund, E., & Franceschini, E. On information, motivation, and meaning. In B. B. Rubinstein (Ed.), *Psychoanalysis and contemporary science* (Vol. 2). New York: Macmillan, 1973.

Poser, E. G. Training behavior therapies. *Behavior Research and Therapy,* 1967, *5,* 37–41.

Rapaport, D. *The structure of psychoanalytic theory: A systematizing attempt* (Psychological Issues Monograph 6). New York: International Universities Press, 1960.

Rhoads, J. M., & Feather, B. W. Transference and resistance observed in behavior therapy. *British Journal of Medical Psychology,* 1972, *45,* 99–103.

Robertson, S. *The effects of activated oneness fantasies on field dependence.* Unpublished doctoral dissertation, New York University, 1982.

Rose, G. Fusion states. In P. L. Giovacchini (Ed.), *Tactics and techniques in psychoanalytic therapy.* New York: Science House, 1972.

Rosen, G. M. Therapy set: Its effects on subjects' involvement in systematic desensitization and treatment outcome. *Journal of Abnormal Psychology,* 1974, *83*(3), 291–300.

Rosen, G. M. Subjects' initial therapeutic expectancies and subjects' awareness of therapeutic goals in systematic desensitization: A review. *Behavior Therapy,* 1976, *7,* 14–27.

Rutstein, E. H. & Goldberger, L. The effects of aggressive stimulation on suidical patients: An experimental study of the psychoanalytic theory of suicide. In B. Rubinstein (Ed.), *Psychoanalysis and contemporary science* (Vol. 2). New York: Macmillan, 1973.

Ryan, V. L., & Moses, J. A., Jr. Therapist warmth and status in the systematic desensitization of test anxiety. *Psychotherapy: Theory, Research and Practice,* 1979, *16*(2), 178–184.

Rycroft, C. *A critical dictionary of psychoanalysis.* New York: Basic Books, 1968.

Ryle, A. A common language for the psychotherapies? *British Journal of Psychiatry,* 1978, *132,* 585–594.

Schafer, R. The termination of brief psychoanalytic psychotherapy. *International Journal of Psychoanalytic Psychotherapy,* 1973, *2*(2), 135–148.

Schurtman, R., Palmatier, J. R., & Martin, E. S. On the activation of symbiotic gratification fantasies as an aid in the treatment of alcoholics. *International Journal of the Addictions,* 1982, *17*(7), 1157-1174.

Searles, H. *Collected papers on schizophrenia and related subjects.* New York: International Universities Press, 1965.

Shapiro, A. K., & Morris, L. A. The placebo effect in medical and psychological therapies. In S. L. Garfield & A. E. Bergin (Eds.), *Handbook of psychotherapy and behavior change.* New York: Wiley, 1978.

Shaver, P. Personal communication, 1978.

Silverman, L. H. An experimental approach to the study of dynamic propositions in psychoanalysis: The relationship between the aggressive drive and ego regression—Initial studies. *Journal of the American Psychoanalytic Association,* 1967, *15,* 376–403.

Silverman, L. H. Further experimental studies on dynamic propositions in psychoanalysis: On the function and meaning of regressive thinking. *Journal of the American Psychoanalytic Association,* 1970, *18,* 102–124.

Silverman, L. H. An experimental technique for the study of unconscious conflict. *British Journal of Medical Psychology,* 1971, *44,* 17–25.

Silverman, L. H. Drive stimulation and psychopathology: On the conditions under which drive-related external events evoke pathological reactions. In R. R. Holt & E. Peterfreund (Eds.), *Psychoanalysis and contemporary science.* New York: Macmillan, 1972.

Silverman, L. H. Some psychoanalytic considerations of nonpsychoanalytic therapies: On the possibility of integrating treatment approaches and related issues. *Psychotherapy: Theory, Research and Practice,* 1974, *11,* 298–305.

Silverman, L. H. On the role of laboratory experiments in the development of the clinical theory of psychoanalysis: Data on the subliminal activation of aggressive and merging wishes in schizophrenics. *International Review of Psychoanalysis,* 1975, *2,* 43–64.

Silverman, L. H. Psychoanalytic theory: "The reports of my death are greatly exaggerated." *American Psychologist,* 1976, *31,* 621–637.

Silverman, L. H. *Ethical considerations and guidelines in the use of subliminal psychodynamic activation.* Unpublished manuscript, Research Center for Mental Health, New York University, 1977.

Silverman, L. H. The unconscious symbiotic fantasy as a ubiquitous therapeutic agent. *International Journal of Psychoanalytic Psychotherapy,* 1978, *7,* 562–585.

Silverman, L. H. Two unconscious fantasies as mediators of successful psychotherapy. *Psychotherapy: Theory, Research and Practice,* 1979, *16,* 215–230.

Silverman, L. H. The unconscious fantasy as a therapeutic agent in psychoanalytic treatment. In S. Slipp (Ed.), *Curative factors in dynamic psychotherapy.* New York: McGraw-Hill, 1982. (a)

Silverman, L. H. A comment on two subliminal psychodynamic activation studies. *Journal of Abnormal Psychology,* 1982, *91,* 126–130. (b)

Silverman, L. H. The subliminal psychodynamic activation method: Overview and comprehensive listing of studies. In J. Masling (Ed.), *Empirical studies in psychoanalysis* (Vol. 1). Hillsdale, N.J.: Erlbaum, 1983.

Silverman, L. H. Beyond insight: An additional necessary step in redressing intrapsychic conflict. *Psychoanalytic Psychology,* 1984, in press.

Silverman, L. H., & Candell, P. On the relationship between aggressive activation, symbiotic merging, intactness of body boundaries and manifest pathology in schizophrenics. *Journal of Nervous and Mental Disease,* 1970, *150,* 387–399.

Silverman, L. H., & Silverman, S. E. The effects of subliminally presented drive stimuli on the cognitive functioning of schizophrenics. *Journal of Projective Techniques,* 1967, *31,* 78–85.

Silverman, L. H., & Spiro, R. H. Some comments and data on the partial cue controversy and other matters relevant to investigations of subliminal phenomena. *Perceptual and Motor Skills,* 1967, *25,* 325–338.

Silverman, L. H., & Spiro, R. H. The effects of subliminal, supraliminal and vocalized aggression on the ego functioning of schizophrenics. *Journal of Nervous and Mental Disease,* 1968, *146,* 50–61.

Silverman, L. H., Klinger, H., Lustbader, L., Farrell, J., & Martin, A. The effect of subliminal drive stimulation on the speech of stutterers. *Journal of Nervous and Mental Disease,* 1972, *155,* 14–21.

Silverman, L. H., Kwawer, J., Wolitzky, C., & Coron, M. An experimental study of aspects of the psychoanalytic theory of male homosexuality. *Journal of Abnormal Psychology,* 1973, *82,* 178–188.

Silverman, L. H., Frank, S., & Dachinger, P. Psychoanalytic reinterpretation of the effectiveness of systematic desensitization: Experimental data bearing on the role of merging fantasies. *Journal of Abnormal Psychology,* 1974, *83,* 313–318.

Silverman, L. H., Bronstein, A., & Mendelsohn, E. The further use of the subliminal psychodynamic activation method for the experimental study of the clinical theory of psychoanalysis: On the specificity of relationships between manifest psychopathology and unconscious conflict. *Psychotherapy: Theory, Research and Practice,* 1976, *13,* 2–16.

Silverman, L. H., Martin, A., Ungaro, R., & Mendelsohn, E. Effect of subliminal stimulation of symbiotic fantasies on behavior modification treatment of obesity. *Journal of Consulting and Clinical Psychology,* 1978, *46,* 432–441. (a)

Silverman, L. H., Ross, D., Adler, J., & Lustig, D. A simple research paradigm for demonstrating subliminal psychodynamic activation. *Journal of Abnormal Psychology,* 1978, *87,* 341–357. (b)

Silverman, L. H., Lachmann, F., & Milich, R. *The search for oneness.* New York: International Universities Press, 1982.

Sloane, R. B., Staples, F. R., Cristol, A. H., Yorkston, N. J., & Whipple, K. *Psychotherapy versus behavior therapy.* Cambridge, Mass.: Harvard University Press, 1975.

Spiro, T. *The effects of laboratory stimulation of symbiotic fantasies and bodily self-awareness on relatively differentiated and nondifferentiated schizophrenics.* Unpublished doctoral dissertation, New York University, 1975.

Stampfl, T. G., & Levis, D. J. Essentials of implosive therapy: A learning-theory-based psychodynamic behavioral therapy. *Journal of Abnormal Psychology,* 1967, *72*(6), 496–503.

Stolorow, R. Psychoanalytic reflections in client-centered therapy in the light of modern conceptions of narcissism. *Psychotherapy: Theory, Research and Practice,* 1976, *13,* 26–29.

Stolorow, R. D., & Lachmann, F. M. *Psychoanalysis of developmental arrests.* New York: International Universities Press, 1980.

Strupp, H. A psychodynamicist looks at modern behavior therapy. *Psychology: Theory, Research and Practice,* 1979, *16*(2), 124–131.

Stuart, R. B. Weight loss and beyond: Are they taking if off and keeping it off? In P. O. Davidson & S. M. Davidson (Eds.), *Behavioral medicine: Changing health lifestyles.* New York: Brunner/Mazel, 1980.

Swanson, R. *The effects of oedipally related stimuli in the subliminal psychodynamic activation paradigm: A replication and an extension.* Unpublished doctoral dissertation, Loyola University of Chicago, 1980.

Ungaro, R. *The therapeutic effects of subliminal stimulation of symbiotic fantasies on behavior modification treatment of obesity.* Unpublished doctoral dissertation, Adelphi University, 1981.

Wachtel, P. L. Psychodynamics, behavior therapy, and the implacable experimenter: An inquiry into the consistency of personality. *Journal of Abnormal Psychology,* 1973, *82*(2), 324–334.

Wachtel, P. L. *Psychoanalysis and behavior therapy.* New York: Basic Books, 1977.

Walen, S., Hauserman, N. M., & Lavin, P. J. *Clinical guide to behavior therapy.* Baltimore: Williams & Wilkins, 1977.

Weitzman, B. Behavior therapy and psychotherapy. *Psychological Review,* 1967, *74*(4), 300–317.

Wilkins, W. Expectancy of therapeutic gain: An empirical and conceptual critique. *Journal of Consulting and Clinical Psychology,* 1973, *40*(1), 69–77.

Wilson, G. T., & Evans, I. M. Adult behavior therapy and the therapist–client relationship. In C. M. Franks & G. T. Wilson (Eds.), *Annual review of behavior therapy and practice.* New York: Brunner/Mazel, 1976.

Wilson, G. T., Hannon, A. E., & Evans, W. I. M. Behavior therapy and the therapist–patient relationship. *Journal of Consulting and Clinical Psychology,* 1968, *32*(2), 103–109.

Winnett, R. L. *The comparative effects of literal and metaphorical subliminal stimulation on the activation of oedipal fantasies in dart-throwing performance and word recall tasks.* Unpublished doctoral dissertation, University of Montana, 1981.

Wolf, E. Learning theory and psychoanalysis. *British Journal of Medical Psychology,* 1966, *39,* 1–10.

Wolitzky, D. L., & Wachtel, P. L. Personality and perception. In B. B. Wolman (Ed.), *Handbook of general psychology.* Englewood Cliffs, N.J.: Prentice-Hall, 1973.

Zuckerman, S. *The effects of subliminal symbiotic and success-related stimuli on the school performance of* high school underachievers. Unpublished doctoral dissertation, New York University, 1980.

9

Activation of Unconscious Fantasies

Commentary on Eric Mendelsohn and Lloyd H. Silverman

ALAN E. KAZDIN

Mendelsohn and Silverman suggest the unconscious fantasies play a critical role in the process of therapeutic change. Unconscious fantasies are defined as "an organized configuration of unconscious ideas and images, motivated (to varying degrees) by libidinal and aggressive wishes, anxieties, defensive operations, and adaptive strivings." The unconscious fantasies are considered to be activated inadvertently in behavior therapy and, indeed, in therapy in general. Neither the therapist nor the patient is aware of the activation. The activation of fantasies is considered to produce a general effect on diverse facets of behavior and functioning. The broad impact is attributed to the overriding psychodynamic wishes (e.g., Oedipal strivings) from which the diverse behaviors are derived.

Support for the role of unconscious fantasies is derived from a large number of laboratory-based investigations using a technique referred to as "subliminal psychodynamic activation" (Silverman, 1976, 1982). The paradigm consists of presenting material (e.g., the sentence "Mommy and I are one") subliminally via a tachistoscope. The paradigm has been investigated with diverse clinical problems, including anxiety, obesity, smoking, assertiveness training, and with a number of nonclinical behaviors (academic performance as well).

ALAN E. KAZDIN • Western Psychiatric Institute and Clinic, University of Pittsburgh School of Medicine, Pittsburgh, Pennsylvania 15261.

The difficulties associated with subjecting propositions from psychoanalytic theory to empirical scrutiny have long been recognized. Consequently, the programmatic work reviewed by Mendelsohn and Silverman represents a remarkable effort that stands in its own right. The work has served as the basis for arguing that unconscious fantasies may be responsible for behavior change among alternative forms of psychotherapy. Reliance on research to advance the argument stands in sharp contrast to many armchair treatises about the putative common processes operative in psychoanalytic, behavioral, and other therapies.

The research to date has consistently demonstrated that the presentation of stimulus material that is considered to activate unconscious processes leads to changes on a variety of different measures for diverse populations. This research represents an exceedingly important step to make the case that fantasy activation accounts for therapeutic change in the usual practice of treatment. However, to make the case, much research is needed.

First, studies need to demonstrate that such fantasies are activated in routine applications of treatment. How or what unconscious fantasies are activated without the explicit introduction of special experimental content or stimuli in the sessions is unclear. Although the laboratory paradigm reflects a process considered to be operative in ordinary treatment, the hiatus from what is done in the experiments and in actual psychotherapy or in behavior therapy is great.

Second, measures of the processes that are activated need to be developed so that processes that are considered to mediate therapeutic change can be assessed independently, that is, with separate operations, from that change. Developing measures may also help test the specific constructs that are proposed. An initial requirement of the assessment devices is to establish that specific unconscious fantasies are assessed. Construct validation of the measures will be important to identify further the actual processes responsible for changes.

Third, the extent to which inadvertent or explicit manipulations enhance therapy outcome remains to be studied. The impact of fantasy activation has been demonstrated in a few "therapy adjunct" studies with clinical populations, as reviewed by Mendelsohn and Silverman. Yet, the evidence that explicit introduction of the experimental manipulation exerts important clinical impact is not clear. The implications of the research on treatment outcome have been given less priority than treatment process at this point.

The research on unconscious fantasy makes an important conceptual contribution to understanding therapeutic processes. The programmatic series of studies is impressive in showing what can happen under special laboratory arrangements. Whether the processes investigated in laboratory research mimic the processes in treatment where tachistoscopically introduced material is not presented is an entirely different matter. Finally, clinical trials of the use of fantasy activation will be needed eventually to evaluate whether the processes can be exploited, so to speak, to improve therapy outcomes. A major contribution of the work reviewed by Mendelsohn and Silverman is that the preceding questions have been placed in the arena of empirical research. Such efforts can only be applauded.

REFERENCES

Silverman, L. H. Psychoanalytic theory: "The reports of my death are greatly exaggerated." *American Psychologist*, 1976, *31*, 621–637.

Silverman, L. H. The subliminal psychodynamic activation method: Overview and comprehensive listing of studies. In J. Masling (Ed.), *Empirical studies in psychoanalysis* (Vol. 1). Hillsdale, N.J.: Erlbaum, 1982.

9

A Rejoinder to Alan E. Kazdin

LLOYD H. SILVERMAN AND ERIC MENDELSOHN

The proposals that Kazdin offers for further investigating the effects of unconscious merging and sanction fantasies on treatment outcome are excellent. We fully agree that "considerably more research is needed . . . to make the case that [unconscious] fantasy activation accounts for therapeutic change in the usual practice of treatment." We think that his first two recommendations in particular—for studies demonstrating "that such fantasies are activated in routine application of treatment" and for "measures of the processes that are activated"—are crucially needed, though these recommendations would not be easy to implement. However, we believe that implementation would be much more possible if we could secure the collaboration of behavior therapists. Thus, we would like to spell out one proposal for implementation in the hope that it might tempt some behavior therapists to join us in a collaborative effort.

We propose a study in which patients entering behavior therapy are given a short battery of projective tests—specifically, a Rorschach and Thematic Aperception Test (TAT—with the same battery being repeated at the end of treatment. With the first battery as a baseline, the second could be examined for the degree to which there is evidence that unconscious merging and/or sanction fantasies have been activated in treatment. We believe that scoring systems could be devised for assessing the degree

LLOYD H. SILVERMAN • New York Veterans Administration Regional Office, New York, New York 10001 and Department of Psychology, New York University, New York, New York 10003. ERIC MENDELSOHN • The New York Hospital-Cornell Medical Center, Westchester Division, White Plains, New York 10605.

to which each type of fantasy is present and that these scores then could be correlated with ratings of how successful the treatment had been in reducing pathology. The prediction following from the thesis we offered earlier is that the more successful the treatment, the greater will be the evidence for the activation of unconscious merging and/or sanction fantasies.

In order to give the reader an understanding of how the activation of unconscious fantasies could be inferred from projective test material, let us make reference to a case study that recently appeared in the literature by Wachtel and Arkin (1980). These investigators reported on the systematic desensitization treatment of a woman with a dog phobia in which the phobia dissipated after six sessions. The point of their article was to consider whether this very favorable outcome from the vantage point of symptom remission was matched by positive changes on another level—that reflected in Rorschach responses and TAT stories. Their conclusion was that this, indeed, was the case. When the pre- and posttreatment TATs and Rorschachs were compared, there were, according to Wachtel and Arkin, more signs of mental health in the second set of tests. This, the authors argue, justifies the inference that the positive changes brought about by the systematic desensitization were not superficial and were not an instance where symptomatic improvement could be said to be accompanied by negative personality changes.

The projective test variables that Wachtel and Arkin looked at do not deal with unconscious fantasies. However, because they presented the pre- and post-Rorschach and TAT protocols verbatim in their article, we had the opportunity to examine the material from that standpoint. From that examination we conclude that there is evidence that merging fantasies were indeed activated by the treatment process, though these seem to be fantasies of merging with the "powerful father" of childhood rather than the fantasies discussed in Mendelsohn and Silverman (Chapter 9) of merging with the "good symbiotic mother." As one of us had detailed (Silverman, 1982, p. 212), fantasies of merging with the powerful father also can facilitate treatment, though we have not yet sought laboratory data that bear on this proposition.

The evidence that was most convincing to us of the activation of these fantasies in Wachtel and Arkin's patient were two highly unusual Rorschach responses that she gave during the second testing. One was of "someone standing . . . with arms raised, like [in] an orchestra leader's position—a conductor's position (Card 1)." The other was "like an old man pointing down directing thunder and lightning, like the myth of a storm. . . . The hands are extended to bolts of lighting" (Card IX). These responses, we suggest, support the formulation that the patient had internalized the therapist (an older male) who was unconsciously perceived as the powerful (phallic) father. This resulted in unconscious fantasies in which his power and control were now hers. These fantasies, in our view, served as a mediating variable that played a role in the therapeutic improvement.

Any behavior therapists who wish to join us in a large scale test of our hypothesis might (understandably) want to withold judgment on the plausibility of our thesis. All that we are requesting is that the therapists collect Rorschach and TAT protocols from patients when they enter behavior therapy and then again when the treatment is completed and that they supply us with these protocols. We would then develop measures for assessing the degree to which the kinds of unconscious fantasies that we have considered have been activated in treatment. Our collaborators would simultaneously assess each patient for treatment outcome variables. They would withold from us these ratings until ours were completed, at which time we would examine together the relationship between the two sets of ratings. As indicated previously, our prediction would be that the greater the indications that unconscious merging and sanction fantasies have been activated during treatment, the better the therapeutic outcome.

Of course, if the hypothesized relationship is borne out, it would not necessarily mean that the fantasy activation *caused* the favorable outcome. However, in the context of our laboratory findings that clearly did indicate a cause-and-effect relationship, it would seem more likely than not that such a relationship exists during normally conducted treatment. If the same projective test responses that we interpret as reflecting the activation of merging and sanction fantasies during successful behavior therapy are found to emerge in laboratory studies after the subliminal exposure of our experimental stimuli—that is, the stimuli designed to activate these very fantasies—this would perhaps seal the case.

We would be happy to discuss this proposal further with any behavior therapists who might be interested in such a collaborative study.

REFERENCES

Silverman, L. H. The unconscious fantasy as therapeutic agent in psychoanalytic treatment. In S. Slipp (Ed.), *Curative factors in dynamic psychotherapy.* New York: McGraw-Hill, 1982.

Wachtel, P., & Arkin, A. Projective test responses before and after behavioral therapy. *Comprehensive Psychotherapy,* 1980, *1,* 1–12.

10

Psychoanalysis and Behaviorism

The Yin and Yang of Determinism

MICHAEL J. MAHONEY

When I first sat down to write this chapter, I found myself half consciously drawn to the lowest shelf of a nearby bookcase. On that shelf, I have some treasured textbooks from my early training in behavior modification. I can remember with great warmth the energy that seemed to pervade behavior therapy in the middle and late 1960s. Although I am sure that a significant portion of my memory must be colored by the associated personal phases in my life, I do not think that historians of behavior modification would disagree with the assertion that the 1960s were expansive and exciting times. We were onto the "laws of learning." We were in search of the "principles of human behavior," and it seemed only a matter of time before we would be relieving millions of people of their unnecessary sufferings and self-limitations.

It was not all that easy to be a behavior therapist in the 1960s. When I attended my first meeting of the Association for the Advancement of Behavior Therapy, I think there were fewer than 400 members in the organization. Almost a decade later, that organization had grown tenfold and had become one of the most active organizations of applied clinical researchers in the world. I was proud to be a member of such a rapidly growing and ostensibly progressive group of scientists and practitioners. We were, after all, opposed to the archaic and inhumane "medical model,"

MICHAEL J. MAHONEY • Department of Psychology, Pennsylvania State University, University Park, Pennsylvania 16802.

and we had scientific respectability that had been purchased at the dear price of ignoring private processes. When I look back on the excitement of those times, I can vividly recall the sense of inspiration I felt when I read some of the more affirming statements of pioneer behavior therapists. Patriotic quotes were easy to find in the writings of such people as Skinner, Wolpe, and Eysenck. We were assured that the science of behavior would lead us out of the darkness of speculative inference and into the daylight of data:

> All behavior, as we can now discern it, is composed of variations on a few basic themes. For the first time in mankind's saga, these themes are open to all who wish to see them in the steady light of science, rather than by the rare illuminations of intuitive minds. We are on the frontier of an enormous power; the power to manipulate our own behavior scientifically, deliberately, rationally. (Keller & Schoenfeld, 1950, p. 401)

Many of the more emancipative statements were directed against the ruling authority of psychoanalysis and its associated medical model. It was in some half-conscious recollection of that early behavioral defiance that I found myself drawn to the lowest shelf of my bookcase that contained a yellow-leafed and well-thumbed copy of Andrew Salter's ground-breaking book *Conditioned Reflex Therapy,* which was published in 1949. As I thumbed through the telltale artifacts of underlining, I was struck by several sentences that had brought many a chuckle during my graduate training:

> It is high time that psychoanalysis, like the elephant of fable, dragged itself off to some distant jungle graveyard and died. Psychoanalysis has outlived its usefulness. Its methods are vague, its treatment is long drawn out, and more often than not, its results are insipid and unimpressive. (p. 1)

But times change. It is now two decades since I first read those words and chuckled at their impertinence. I was a bit impertinent myself in those days. It was hard not to be, given the fervent intoxication of a budding paradigm. Having now weathered many more seasons as a therapist, theorist, and aspiring teacher, I no longer find those words quite as amusing as before. I do not think this can be explained by any loss in my sense of humor, nor—as I hope to show in this chapter—is there any warrant for claiming that I have somehow dropped the sterile scientistic banner of behavior therapy and picked up the furrowed-brow emblem of psychoanalysis. I have never considered myself an orthodox anything (including a behavior therapist), and I fail to see the importance of what label should be most appropriately applied to my work.

Let me return for a moment to the quotation from Andrew Salter. Why is it, in the wake of such oppositional sentiment, that we are now experiencing a resurgence of interest in rapprochement between psychoanalysis and behavior therapy (e.g., Feather & Rhoads, 1972; Goldfried, 1982; Marmor & Woods, 1980; Messer & Winokur, 1980; Wachtel, 1977, 1982)? Why are we beginning to witness the emergence of more than occasional articles on the theme of convergence? There are now several scholarly volumes addressed to the possibility of resuming the quest for convergence that was last energized by John Dollard and Neil Miller (1950). What is it that we might learn about psychotherapy and its development as a science from this apparent—yet clearly controversial—attempt to explore the possibility of a theoretical coalition? It is my opinion that the present interest in a convergence between psychoanalysis and behavior therapy reflects several possible influences. To begin with, I would be surprised to learn that most contemporary psychoanalysts, behavior therapists, or indeed, mental health practitioners of any ideology are enthusiastically satisfied with their current understanding and facilitation of human change processes. In a recent survey of influential behavior and cognitive therapists (Mahoney, 1979), both groups rated the adequacy of their current understanding as very modest. I do not know what the corresponding estimation would be among psychoanalysts, but I doubt that the leading figures in the field would be overly enthusiastic about the adequacy of their current knowledge. In other words, I think that contemporary behavior therapists and psychoanalysts are each operating from a position of partially acknowledged theoretical inadequacy. Both paradigms are struggling amid the throes of internal revolutions and a differentiation into subspecialties that has continued to dissipate power and decentralize the locus of paradigm directions. Likewise, I think that there is sufficient integrity and dedication to human service in both disciplines (as well as their less muscular siblings), such that at least part of their motivation for even a delicate interface is itself an expression of their own desire for personal and professional growth. It would not be the first time in the history of science that two ostensibly incompatible schools of thought have engaged one another for the primary purpose of energizing their own development. Contrast is an integral part of the learning process.

There may likewise be some political motives behind the recent interest in rapprochement. The recent economic and sociocultural crises have had their impact on the therapist as well as the client. Humans tend to band together when they are in a state of perceived danger. There might thus be some sense in which psychoanalysis and behavior therapy would prefer "hanging together" rather than "hanging separately." But I am not convinced that this is the most viable or powerful explanation of the move toward convergence. When I search my own mind about this phenomenon, one of the first queries is whether or not there is a phenomenon to be explained. That is, is there really all that much interest in psychoanalysis and behavior therapy getting together? The answer is clearly yes and no. There has been much more interest in this possibility in the last few years than we have witnessed in the prior four decades. Yet, such interest is probably an expression of a very small minority of writers and thinkers in these fields. It is clear, for example, that Paul Wachtel's (1982) excursions into behavior therapy were not met with the most open of psychoanalytic arms. The same has been true of those few behavior therapists who have attempted to establish communication between behaviorism and psychoanalysis. At a national convention of behavior therapists in 1980, for example, the program committee and current president of the organization were publicly chastised by one of the more orthodox "elders" for having invited an eminent psychoanalyst to present his views on therapy. There may or may not be a phenomenon to explain, depending on one's criteria for a "genuine and popular interest in convergence."

A more interesting and perhaps more pertinent question is, "Is it possible and/or desirable for psychoanalysis and behavior therapy to converge?" This is the essential question that underlies the present volume, and it invites a careful appraisal of the most fundamental aspects of each perspective. What does psychoanalysis have to offer behavior therapy and vice versa? And, to put the question in balance, what is behavior therapy now willing to learn from psychoanalysis and vice versa? I believe that both approaches have some important insights, conjectures, and techniques to share with the larger community of psychotherapists. There is, for example, a growing appreciation for the therapeutic importance of resistance, dreams, graduated behavioral performance, self-perceptions of personal efficacy, the therapeutic alliance, and so on (cf. Burton, 1976; Mahoney, 1980a,b; Wachtel, 1982). Recent increases in conceptual and technical eclecticism also suggest that there may be some deep structure shifts underway in our basic approaches to life counseling (Garfield & Kurtz, 1976, 1977). It is the nature and direction of these shifts that may be most enlightening, and it is for this reason that my ensuing remarks will focus on elucidating one apparent sign of an evolution in our thinking.

By way of preview, I will be suggesting that one candidate for making sense out of the current courtship between psychoanalysis and behavior therapy is the possibility that we are witnessing yet another crisis in the survival of deterministic metatheories of change. I will be arguing that psychoanalysis and behaviorism represent the two strongest versions of deterministic theory in the social sciences and that their current paradigmatic problems are forcing them toward a reflective reappraisal of some very basic assumptions. The current faltering of determinism—if that is what we are witnessing—may itself represent an omen of an evolution in our conceptualization of causation (cf. Liotti & Reda, 1981; Locke, 1980).

It should be noted that I do not believe that this conceptual evolution is the *only* one reflected in attempts toward rapprochement. In a recent paper on the contacts of behaviorism with Adlerian psychology, I have also elaborated on the conjecture that the centuries-old dualism between idealism and realism appears to be undergoing major reappraisal (Mahoney, 1982). Finally, lest my comments suggest otherwise, I will be commenting on (a) the wisdom of respecting psychoanalysis and behaviorism as two archetypal forms of determinism in their purest forms, and (b) the simultaneous and timely imperative that we explore and harvest the conceptual mutations to which they have contributed. Let me therefore move on to some prefatory reflections on our metatheories of change, which will set the stage for the current courtship between psychoanalysis and behavior therapy.

METATHEORIES OF DEVELOPMENT, STABILITY, AND CHANGE

All approaches to psychotherapy contain and convey implicit assumptions about the nature of reality, the nature of humanness, and the basic processes of development, stability, and change. It is not my intention to delve into the intricacies of metatheory that are afforded by the voluminous literatures on psychoanalysis and behavior therapy. I will instead offer a few brief comments on the respective presumptions in some of these areas. It is noteworthy, to begin with, that similarities between behaviorism and psychoanalysis are readily apparent. Both approaches draw heavily upon a metatheory that involves deterministic causation, hedonistic motivation, and a conflict-based model of psychological movement. On this last dimension, the conflict is explicit in psychoanalytic theory and early drive-reduction behavioral theories. In operant theory (e.g., Skinner, 1969), the conflict is between responses competing for selective retention. For the most part, then, psychoanalysis and behavior therapy agree on several major dimensions of reality and causality. They posit very different levels of mechanisms in their causal theories, of course, and they focus their theoretical attention on very different expressions of hedonistic determinism.

One noteworthy point of distinction between psychoanalysis and behaviorism has to do with their tacit assumptions about human nature. As Maurice Friedman (1967, 1974) so aptly noted in his valuable works on tacit assumptions in our psychological theories, there is always a "hidden human image" in our theoretical constructions. In the case of psychoanalysis, for example, it is clear that Freud's assumptions are quite distant from those thinkers who have been termed "vitalists" because of their basic affirmation of a value in human existence. Not only did Freud explicitly claim an objective detachment from the social and cultural rules that were so often the object of his attack, but he explicitly outlined what many readers would consider to be an essentially negative and pessimistic view of the human being. This picture is explicitly stated in *Civilization and Its Discontents* (Freud, 1958):

> The bit of truth behind all of this—one so eagerly denied—is that men are not gentle, friendly creatures wishing for love, who simply defend themselves if they are attacked, but that *a powerful measure of desire for aggression has to be reckoned as a part of their instinctual endowment.* The result is that their neighbor is to them not only a possible helper or sexual object, but also a temptation to them to gratify their aggressiveness on him, to exploit his capacity for work without recompense, to use him sexually without his consent, to seize his possessions, to humiliate him, to cause him pain, to torture and to kill him. (p. 61)

It would appear that Freud did not concur with the more romantic pictures drawn by such writers as Bergson and Rousseau (Russell, 1945). It is only fair to note, however, that Freud's existential pessimism remains a matter of both interpretation and translation. In his excellent critique of the crude and apparently misrepresentative translations of Freud's writings into English, for example, Bruno Bettelheim (1982) has recently lamented American psychoanalytic views:

> The English translations cleave to an early stage of Freud's thought, in which he inclined toward science and medicine, and disregard the more mature Freud, whose orientation was humanistic, and who was concerned mostly with broadly conceived cultural and human problems and with matters of the soul. (p. 63)

On this last point, Bettelheim believes that "of all the mistranslations, not one has hampered our understanding of Freud's humanistic views more than the elimination of his references to the soul" (p. 84). In my own admittedly limited exposure to European and American renditions of psychoanalysis, I have likewise sensed a perceptible difference in the overall "flavor" of the meanings and intentions attributed to Freud. Nevertheless, I believe that Friedman (1967) and others have been accurate in depicting Freud as leaning toward a form of negative naturalism that conveyed a deep mistrust of the ambivalent and potentially destructive tendencies of the human mind. This theme is likewise apparent in Bettelheim's defense and in his ultimate concession that "recognition of the worst possibilities—the destruction of all mankind—led Freud to his tragic view of life" (p. 93).

Behaviorism did not take quite as strong a stand on the issue of human value. Watson (1913, 1924), who probably came closer to commenting on the issue than did Skinner (1953, 1959, 1974), seemed to view the human being as a very pliable container of conditioned associations. The impression that one gets from his writing as well as from that of Skinner is basically one of rationalized abstention. When there are lapses in this intentional avoidance of value statements regarding human nature, they tend to be somewhat less negative than those offered by Freud. In *Beyond Freedom and Dignity* (Skinner, 1971), for example, Skinner laments some of the "reactions to a scientific conception of man" and offers a rare glimpse of his own expectations about natural processes in human development:

> The traditional conception of man is flattering. . . . It was designed to build up the individual as an instrument of counter-control, and it did so effectively but in such a way as to limit progress. We have seen how the literatures of freedom and dignity, with their concern for autonomous man, have perpetuated the use of punishment and condoned the use of only weak nonpunitive techniques, and it is not difficult to demonstrate a connection between the unlimited right of the individual to pursue happiness and the catastrophies threatened by unchecked breeding, the unrestrained affluence which exhausts resources and pollutes the environment, and the imminence of nuclear war. (p. 213)

There is thus a hint of at least moderate pessimism about natural tendencies and a corresponding emphasis on the centrality of control in behavioristic theory and practice.

Their views of human nature are not the most salient dimension along which to differentiate psychoanalysis and behavior therapy, however. More relevant to my present thesis is the shared presumption of causal determinism that permeates their theoretical assertions. Determinism is, of course, a prevalent assumption in many different ideological approaches; its representation is not restricted to these two major viewpoints. On the other hand, deterministic ideas have been powerfully and persuasively preserved in these two major systems. Likewise, as I shall elaborate in a moment, they may both be suffering from clinical/empirical confrontations with the limited and diminishing returns of a theory of causality that is inadequate for complex systems—like human beings.

On a philosophical basis, it is interesting to note that the assumption of determinism is one that has received extensive speculative attention, and yet its everyday impact has been rarely appreciated. Although there have been numerous philosophical inquiries into causality and determinism, there have been no real attempts to translate these investigations into practical implications. Thus, the field of psychology and indeed the social sciences in general continue to be dominated by an essentially tacit assumption that shapes not only their theories and hypotheses but also their instrumentation and methodology. Because most philosophers and physicists have long since abandoned naive determinism, it is not surprising that they might occasionally decry its continued power in our fields. In commenting on the impact that the doctrine of associationism has had on our thinking, for example, philosopher Karl Popper made it clear that deterministic thinking is anything but a benign necessity:

> [It] is the most terribly misleading doctrine which has emerged from Cartesian dualism under the influence of later parallelistic ideas. Nothing, I suggest, can be further from the truth. (Popper & Eccles, 1977, p. 194)

Associationism is, of course, a direct and inevitable corollary of naive determinism. The basic ideas underlying a deterministic philosophy have to do with (a) the viability and wisdom of separating objects of experience into classes or discrete events, and (b) the contention that certain classes are existentially dependent upon others. These themes can be traced throughout the many analyses of determinism (e.g., Hook, 1958; Hume, 1748/1902).

Many classical discussions of determinism have been muddied by excursions into the more personally relevant issues of choice, freedom, and individual responsibility. It is in the heated emotional context of some of these debates that we find otherwise intelligent writers arguing that indeterminism is equivalent to personal freedom and that the unpredictability of particulars is necessarily reflective of causal indeterminism. Without belaboring technical points in the free-will/determinism debate, I will simply emphasize that the problem seems to have stemmed in part from a begging of the question. With its penchant for dualistic dichotomies, the doctrine of determinism has encouraged many thinkers to unnecessarily bifurcate in their analyses of a very complicated phenomenon. The concept of *control*, for example, is often treated as a unidimensional construct that can be polarized into "present" and "absent" statuses. "Causes" and "effects" are presumed to be perfectly separable categories. Such a conceptualization invites speculation on a putative locus of control and on relative concentrations of control being internal (within the agent) or external (cf. Lefcourt, 1976; Rotter, Chance, & Phares, 1972). In classical determinism, of course, the phenomenon is further complicated by dividing experience into discrete categories of thought, feeling, action, and so forth. Each distinct event in these categories is said to have been caused by the summation of past and present influences. (This focus on temporal dimensions is interesting in that its reflects one of the more central and tacit predicaments of any scientific analysis of change [cf. Prigogine, 1980]). With aspirations toward a precision similar to that found in the physical sciences, the social scientist tends to view human experience as a challenge that is most aptly met with the higher order vector analyses of a very active pool table. Hence, the popular term *billiard ball determinism*.

The tenacity of billiard ball determinism in our analyses is not accidental. Indeed, the fact that most "common sense" thinking reflects a deep appreciation for this kind of causation is perhaps the best illustration of its inherent attractiveness during natural selection processes. The problem, however, is that deterministic perspectives fare much more poorly in the realm of explanation than they do in the realm of description. As David Hume (1748/1902) so aptly noted, we must be careful not to confuse our descriptions of *sequence* with our attempts to explain *consequence*. The desire to predict and control the particulars of experience is an understandably human one, but there are quite different sequelae associated with different approaches to the issues of knowledge and power. Likewise, it is quite apparent that different levels of analysis may be more useful for different classes of phenomena. Newton's physics builds better bridges than Einstein's, and yet there is little doubt that their relative usefulness is quite different in the areas of high-energy theoretical physics (Zukav, 1979). The issue here is not whether different rules of causation are operating so much as the level of complexity in the systems under study. Indeed, this is one of the main points that Popper has so beautifully elucidated in his essay "Of Clouds and Clocks" (Popper, 1972). Billiard balls, of course, represent one of the simplest conceptions of causal schema—with uniform events and linear, two-dimensional exchanges of energy. The situation becomes infinitely more complex at the organic and animate levels.

I realize that I am belaboring a somewhat technical point there, but I feel that it has important implications that merit our reflection. Let me therefore pursue this theme a step further and share some impressions on the costs of our continued faith in naive determinism and what the current alternative appears to be. On the first point, I would venture the theme that contemporary psychology remains preoccupied with the prediction and control of particulars as if such investigations are most helpful in the development of our understanding. One of the most persistent *problems* in psychological research, of course, is that of *individual differences.* Human billiard balls are undeniably variable in their responses to and interactions with their contexts. We are likewise enamored with the idea that our approaches to psychotherapy would be best served by a powerful program of research directed at answering the factorial question of the outcome researcher:

> The ultimate question to be answered in . . . research [is]: What treatment, by whom, is most effective for this individual, with that specific problem, under which set of circumstances, and how does it come about? (Paul, 1969, p. 62)

The essence of this classic question is not simply the commendable intention of "How best can we help?" but also an explicit affirmation of a tacit faith in the powers of particulate causality. The assumption is that if we simply gather enough information on the particulars and their matrices of covariation, we will acquire the necessary knowledge. And, in true Baconian fashion, there is the additional (and hopefully warranted) assumption that "knowledge *is* power" (Bacon, 1620/1960).

The problems of particulate causation are much too extensive and far afield for the present discussion. I will therefore conclude this section with a reference to Hayek's (1964) classic essay "The Theory of Complex Phenomena." He cogently argues that we cannot ever hope to achieve a more powerful or precise class of theories than those that will be restricted ultimately to the descriptions and explanations of certain *classes* of phenomena that potentiate certain *patterns* of experience. In other words, we cannot—logically or pragmatically—hope to achieve a science of complex phenomena that is capable of any respectable degree of particulate prediction. Just as nuclear physicists had to confront the failure of their old paradigm (basically, Newtonian mechanics) in the face of early 20th-century evidence, it would appear that the contemporary social sciences must anticipate a parallel self-confrontation with their deterministic and associationistic presumptions about human behavior. Not only have we been naive in many of our notions about the nature of experience, but we have been clearly remiss in appraising and advancing our ideas about how best to study ourselves. As Hayek's article indicates, it is clear that we have much to be hopeful about in our attempts to organize and understand the phenomena of interest. Our theories, however, will have to take a very different form than what we may have anticipated. Our theories may have to be, in Hayek's terminology, "algebraic" in the sense that "we are in fact unable to substitute particular values for the variables." The implications of this for our conception and enactment of scientific process are noteworthy, and they are best expressed in Hayek's (1964) own words:

> It would then appear that the search for the discovery of laws is not an appropriate hall-mark of scientific procedure but merely a characteristic of the theories of simple phenomena . . . and that in the field of complex phenomena the term "law" as well as the concept of cause and effect are not applicable without such modifications as to deprive them of their ordinary meaning. It would probably have saved much confusion if theoretical science had not . . . come to be identified with the search for laws in the sense of a simple dependence of one magnitude upon another. (p. 42)

SURFACE AND DEEP DETERMINISM

I do not think I need to spend much time documenting the deterministic substructure of both psychoanalytic and behavioristic thinking. What is more intriguing is their apparent expression of a shared metatheory of causality, which I have elaborated in the preceding section. For purposes of the present treatise, I shall argue that psychoanalysts have endorsed a *deep* form of determinism as their rallying point, whereas behaviorists have chosen a diametrically contrasting *surface* form of determinism. The analogy to linguistic terminology is not accidental here, but I do not require that we push it to an isomorphism.

Let us begin with a discussion of the primary locus of change in psychoanalysis and behaviorism. In psychoanalysis, it is apparent that the primary dynamic is a transformation of unconscious expressions of energy. "Where id was, there shall ego be" is a fairly direct assertion that important psychological change tends to be focalized in the more central and core dimensions of personal functioning. For Freud, of course, these were unconscious, and we continue to associate *deep structures* with unconscious ones. More recent advances in clinical science and some of its associated psychobiology have suggested that the more central and core features of our nervous system tend to precede and potentiate our conscious experience in such a way that they would be more aptly termed "metaconscious" rather than "unconscious" (Hayek, 1978; Weimer, 1977, 1982). The former does not refer to a repository of either impulses or experiences but to interdependent preconscious processes that limit the range and nature of potential experience. In traditional psychoanalytic thought, however, it is clear that the locus of change is not that of the surface particulars, but it is rather at some level of experience and personal organization that is far removed from both signs and symptoms.

In contrast, the locus of change for behaviorism is explicitly confined to the level of the observable particular. This contention is variously represented as a metaphysical one in radical behaviorism (Watson, 1924) or an epistemological one in methodological behaviorism (Skinner, 1950). In the latter, the existence of a mediating organism is at least grudgingly admitted, if not openly welcomed:

> A small part of [one's] inner world can be felt or introspectively observed, but it is not an essential part, . . . and the role assigned to it has been vastly overrated. . . . It is impossible to estimate the havoc [that theories about internal states and processes] have wreaked . . . [upon] effort(s) to describe or explain human behavior. (Skinner, 1974, pp. xii–xiii)

The early behaviorist assumed that the most parsimonious, efficient, and scientific way to study regularities in human behavior was to focus on the surface of its expressions—that is, those aspects that were publicly observable—and to restrict theoretical analyses to descriptive covariance statements regarding the relationship between inputs and outputs. As has been argued extensively in the last decade, it would appear that the inadequacies of "surfacism" and its associated two-dimensional models are becoming increasingly apparent (Bever, Fodor, & Garrett, 1968; Bolles,

1972; Brewer, 1974; Dulany, 1968; Estes, 1971; Mahoney, 1974; McKeachie, 1974).

If I were asked to speculate on the more "progressive" trends in our theoretical development, I would have to say that there appears to be a growing interest in depth psychology and an increasing dissatisfaction with "surfacistic models." This is certainly reflected in the "cognitive revolution" (Dember, 1974) that is being witnessed most generally in the social sciences and most ironically in the very heart of behaviorism. As I have noted previously (Mahoney, 1980a), I have some concerns about the current focus and unbridled zeal of this most recent wave of cognitivism. Rather than belabor those concerns again, however, I shall move to yet another dimension on which these two representatives of determinism may yet be differentiated.

The second dimension has to do with mechanisms of change. At one level of analysis, psychoanalysis and behavior therapy are quite compatible in their conceptualization of change processes. Both tend to be relatively mechanical in their metaphors, with analysts preferring a hydraulic model of energy exchange and behaviorists preferring a linear movement metaphor. Both presume that the organism is pushed and pulled through a lifelong sequence of hedonistic conflicts. There is a tinge of disagreement as to the implicit goal of therapy, however. The analysts appear to be arguing that the goal of one's psychological project is to attain some equitable degree of balance among the opponent processes, whereas the behaviorists appear to be hinting that the wise organism is one that (a) learns to identify the contingencies of consequent effect, that (b) efficiently minimizes the output necessary to satisfy those contingencies, and that (c) somehow "beats the system" by a rigorous and logical manipulation of it (Skinner, 1969, 1971, 1974). There is at least one respect in which the question of mechanisms of change overlaps with the issue of locus. Bandura's (1969) classic defense of central nervous system processes as being more important than peripheral ones in behavior change is an example. Behaviorists have had a long and revered tradition of opting for the periphery of the system in their pursuit and particulars. That is, of course, where the particulars lie. Freud and his followers, on the other hand, have been much more inclined toward the infinite abyss of the human psyche and its reflective attempts to attain a clearer glimpse of first principles.

Thus far I have argued that psychoanalysis and behaviorism—although sharing the basic assumption of determinism—have been different in their expressions of its theoretical and practical implications. The behaviorist has tended to adopt a more "surfacistic" (or, if we can avoid the excess meaning, "superficial") approach to deterministic analyses and has simultaneously preferred a linear vector model of physical causation. The psychoanalysts, on the other hand, have exhibited a preference for central and less observable dimensions of experience as their locus of change, and they have more frequently employed hydraulic models of energy dissipation instead of the simpler linear ones.

The third dimension on which one can differentiate these two representatives of determinism has to do with the activity or passivity of the individual in response to the more fundamental issues of causation. As I see it, psychoanalysis represents a relatively passive form of determinism and behaviorism is distinctively more active. This is not so much a commentary on their hypothesized processes of human learning and development so much as it is a reflection of their respectively different invocations to practical action. Stated more simply, analysts have historically adopted a relatively passive and pessimistic approach to human behavior, implying that one's current experiential reality is something that has been brought into existence by a long series of tacit and often temporally distant events. Indeed, I think it could be argued that the gradual revolution that has been taking place within psychodynamic conceptualizations (almost since their inception at the turn of the century) has been focused upon the relative activity and responsibility of the organism in shaping and responding to both its internal and external environments. Many of the more progressive "neoanalytic" thinkers have protested the pessimism and passivity that seem to have dominated orthodox psychoanalytic formulations. It is thus not surprising that we have been witnessing a shift in the directions of *ego psychology* and what might be called *behavioral activism* and *corrective emotional experiences* in the more liberal psychodynamic approaches.

Behaviorists began from the same basic premise of determinism but have drawn a very different conclusion about its implications for human behavior. Freud left us not only with the impression that "the child is father of the man" but also that our relative powers of conscious choice and active regulation are quite limited. This may well be a tragic misrepresentation as Bettelheim (1982) has argued, but it is still the tacit metatheory of thousands of contemporary psychoanalysts. But for individuals like John Watson, B. F. Skinner, and their followers, the clearest implication of physical determinism was basically a bold invitation to enter *into* the causal sequence. Thus, we have Skinner (1959) asserting that "the simple fact is that man is able, and now as never before, to lift himself by his own bootstraps. In achieving control of the world of which he is a part, he may learn at last to control himself" (p. 4). The redemption from complete determinism is accomplished by inserting ourselves into the deterministic system as one of the "master switches" (Popper, 1972). This basic bootstrapping strategy was the explicit raison d'être of the pioneering attempts to incorporate self-control procedures into the behavioral armamentarium:

> The procedures to be discussed center around the position that behavior . . . is described by a functional relation between . . . [an organism and its environment]. More technically, given a specified behavior B and a specified environmental variable *x*, a lawful relation can be found, such that B = f(*x*), under certain empirical constraining conditions *c*. This implies that when the constraints *c* are set up, and *x* is set up at a stipulated value, then B will have a stipulated value, given by the value of B = f(*x*). When the experimenter sets *x* at that value, *he* will get the B stipulated. This defines the experimental control of behavior which has been demonstrated repeatedly in operant and other laboratories. When the subject himself sets *x* at that value, *he* will get his own B, as stipulated. This defines self-control. (Goldiamond, 1965, p. 853)

I have argued elsewhere that the emergence of research interest in self-control and private processes may represent an important historical turning point in the development of behaviorism as a coherent paradigm (Mahoney, 1974; Mahoney & Arnkoff, 1978). These two areas seem to have led the behaviorist into the domains of reciprocal causation, choice, and a whole variety of cognitive processes that had been intentionally eschewed by pioneering writers in that area. But the historiography of behaviorism's recent movement away from peripheralist analyses and in the direction of central processes is far afield from my intent for this essay. Let me therefore return to the theme of differences in activity/passivity between psychoanalytic and behavioral interpretations of physical determinism.

My main point here is that psychoanalysis and behavior therapy represent two of the most powerful contemporary interpretations of the age-old doctrine of particulate determinism. As I mentioned in the last section, this kind of determinism remains a problem due to its theoretical and empirical inadequacies. Where the psychoanalyst has come to believe that we are the unwaivering products of psychologically determined events and experiences, the behaviorist has contended that we are simply a medium of (albeit complicated) exchange with a physically determined environment. In the end, both psychoanalysis and behavior therapy admit and assert that we are the product of our experience. We are determined effects in an elaborate causal sequence, and our behavior and inner experience—whether classified as a "symptom" or a "sign" (Mischel, 1968)—may be analyzed as a composite of perfectly determined components. We are, in Popper's terminology, organisms whose behavior is likened to that of a mechanical clock (i.e., "highly regular, orderly, and more or less predictable") as contrasted with the unpredictable mutability of a cloud system. The practical import of this assumption is one that receives differential interpretation by the analysts and behaviorists. For Freud and his more orthodox followers, the apparent implication of psychological determinism was a relatively helpless and primarily passive reactivity to the hydrodynamics of energy shifts. Indeed, I would not be the first commentator to suggest that orthodox psychoanalysis may have sacrificed much of its potential power by its marriage to a relatively impotent and inert strategy for the use of that knowledge.

The behaviorist has traditionally been in favor of a much more active utilization of deterministic principles. Thus, the pragmatic import may appear to be diametrically opposed in the behavioral formulation. Applied behaviorism has come to be associated with practical problem solving and the strategic structuring of environmental contingencies. In essence, then, what we seem to have is a contrast primarily along the dimension of active participation in versus passive assimilation of environmental influences. In oversimplification, practitioners of dogmatic psychoanalysis might say "you are the end product of your experience." The lack of an explicit prescription for action is as close as one gets to the passive philosophy that is being offered here. In behaviorism, on the other hand, the statement is extended to: "You are a product of your experience; therefore, participate in the production." My hunch is that Freud's later writing reflected a shift in this direction and that the contrast I have created here must be criticized by the reflective reader as an oversimplification of a very complicated historico-developmental sequence (cf. Bettelheim, 1982; Goldfried, 1982).

Although behaviorism has been a more activistic perspective than psychoanalysis, it would be misleading to conclude that it has therefore offered a "better" model of human experience. For my part, the practical energetics and tacit optimism of behaviorism are valuable assets. Notwithstanding its relative pessimism and passivity, however, psychoanalysis continues to reap a more fertile theoretical harvest than its behavioral neighbor. Contemporary theorists are generally more indebted to analytic insights than to those offered by behavioral analyses. The point here is that *any* binary evaluations of these two perspectives must be necessarily oversimplifying ones. In my opinion, psychoanalysis and the depth psychology from which it developed (cf. Ellenberger, 1970) have offered valuable and heuristic ideas regarding the structure of personality, the dynamics of a developmental consciousness, and the reflection of central ordering processes in the pattern of surface particulars. Behaviorism, on the other hand, has been a major force in the grounding of speculation in empirical accountability, the study of technique in the restructuring of experience, and the role of active participation in significant personal change. I see no need to assign these contributions differential significance in any absolute sense.

ON DIVERGENCE AND DINOSAURS

What I will attempt in this brief section is to pull together some of the themes I have been developing. Recall that we began with a query into the resurgence of interest in some kind of collaboration, if not convergence, between psychoanalysis and behavior therapy. The modest magnitude of the phenomenon to be explained should again be noted. Current interest in rapprochement is greater than it has been in years and appears to be increasing; yet, it may describe a relatively small segment of the ideologies involved. Likewise, much of the interest in this phenomenon has been voiced by individuals who would probably be classified as progressive and liberal in their respective domains (Feather & Rhoads, 1972; Goldfried, 1982; Marmor & Woods, 1980; Messer & Winokur, 1980; Wachtel, 1977, 1982). As mentioned earlier, I believe that the interest in rapprochement is most likely a reflection of multiple influence processes and that it would be naive and misrepresentative to look for a single "billiard ball" of causation. At least some of the motivation for collaboration or convergence seems to be coming from a sense of maturity and a desire for stimulation. At the same time, however, it is clear that both fields have been encountering problems in the preservation of their orthodoxy in light of current experimental research.

It is interesting to note that Andrew Salter's (1949) statement that "psychoanalysis has outlived its usefulness" (p. 1) has recently been (perhaps unconsciously?) paraphrased in reference to behavior therapy. In his relatively defiant statement of emancipation from behavior therapy, Arnold Lazarus has recently suggested that "behavior therapy [has] outlived its usefulness" (Lazarus, 1977, p. 550). This statement is an ironic one coming from one of the pioneering clinicians in the area (cf. Wolpe & Lazarus, 1966) and has—not surprisingly—invited some rather lively responses from the behavioral "old guard" (e.g., Wolpe, 1978). The continuing controversy about the role of cognitive processes in personal change and, more critically, their role in a behavioral approach to therapy is something that has clearly generated quite a bit of heat, if not much light (cf. Ledwidge, 1978; Mahoney & Kazdin, 1979). The point here, of course, is that both psychoanalysis and behaviorism have been described as moribund movements by some of their own former adherents. Their diminishing returns as theoretical systems is, I believe, a reflection on their need to embrace a more adequate view of causality.

This is neither the time nor place to expound on alternatives to billiard ball determinism and the more adequate conceptualizations that are loosely subsumable under the rubric of *determinate order.* I believe that the implications of our possible shift in thinking on the issue of determinism may be much more far-reaching than we can now anticipate. They have relevance, for example, for how we conceptualize our interventions and for specific aspects of the therapeutic endeavor. More importantly, they influence both our conceptualization and conduct of scientific inquiry. Because these issues have been touched upon more adequately by previous writers and are only now being given their due in terms of theoretical and empirical attention, I will simply offer references to these resources as well as a parting comment on their significance for our continuing development as a discipline (cf. Barrett, 1967; Guidano & Liotti, 1982; Hayek, 1967, 1978; Mahoney, 1976, 1982; Popper, 1972, 1982; Popper & Eccles, 1977; Prigogine, 1980; Russell, 1945; Weimer, 1982; Zukav, 1979). My comment is basically this: If we are to develop an adequate theory of human experience and the rules that describe its development, stability, and change, it is clear that we must move beyond the original straitjacket of billiard ball determinism. The issue is no longer an esoteric philosophical autopsy of a linguistic or semantic enigma (Ryle, 1949). We must, if we aspire to a scientific (as opposed to scientistic) approach to the matter, confront the paradoxical fact that we are both causes and effects in our dynamic exchanges with external as well as internal realities. I therefore believe that one of the most pressing issues for the coming years in psychology will be a reappraisal of some of our most basic assumptions about the human experience and its most appropriate methods of study. Likewise, I think it is inevitable that our theories and data will bring us into progressively closer confrontation with the complexities of the human nervous system and the irreducible facticity of unpredictable particulars. Finally, I think that such a reappraisal, when combined with the growing pressure of theoretical heuristics and empirical embarrassments, will force us to devote more serious and respectful attention to such areas as choice, will, intentionality, and expectancy (Mahoney, 1983b).

The essence of my remarks on the current interest in rapprochement between psychoanalysis and behavior therapy might be summarized as follows. I believe that the interest in such rapprochement is itself a possible reflection of more significant issues in the metatheories involved. In this chapter, I have talked primarily about the principle of determinism and its differential expression in classical psychoanalytic theory and orthodox behaviorism. (It would be tempting to venture some parallel speculations about the current reappraisal of tacit views of human nature by these two perspectives.) But I have yet to be explicit about the possibility and desirability of convergence. Let me therefore address this issue directly.

I do not believe that psychoanalysis and behavior therapy could accomplish a theoretical integration that would in any way preserve their original identities as models of human functioning. The reasons for this should be apparent from some of what I have already said. For the most part, I do not think that psychoanalysis and behaviorism will ever reconcile their differences regarding the locus and nature of significant change processes—especially in terms of the idealism/realism dichotomy and the centralist/peripheralist bifurcation. Likewise, I think that there is a generally pessimistic overtone to psychoanalysis that is incompatible with some of the more activistic dimensions of behavioral philosophy. And finally, I think that these two perspectives are of a bascially different genus. Their metatheoretical chromosomes are incompatible. Orthodox behaviorism continues to waive the banner of *realism* and to assert that there is an objective external reality that is, in principle, completely separable from the subjective perceiver. Psychoanalysis, on the other hand, remains deeply committed to a form of *idealism* that its critics consider seclusive and far removed from the realm of present particulars. This incompatibility does not challenge the value of dialectical exchange, however, nor should it blind us to the possibility that both behaviorism and psychoanalysis are contributing to the evolution of a more adequate paradigm. It is in this sense that it might be more accurate to talk about *emergence* rather than convergence. We are now witnessing what may be a much more exciting development than the simple integration of two parochial contenders for therapeutic power. In other words, I think we are participant observers in a significant metatheoretical evolution. The current movements within and alongside psychoanalysis and behavior therapy are a reflection of this evolution.

I should perhaps add that I do not join with either Salter (1949) or Lazarus (1977) in their respective invitations for the dinosaurs of psychoanalysis and behaviorism to "drag themselves off to some jungle graveyard and die." It would be impossible to estimate from this vantage point in time and theory the contributions that could be rightfully claimed by these two ostensive dinosaurs. Nor do I believe that either has totally finished with its growth and contributions to the dialectics of science. Thus, I would not only argue for their preservation in light of historical respect but also for their continuing contribution via an established tradition of inquiry. The popular theories and therapies that annually present themselves in a seemingly endless progression will have to make many significant steps in order to go beyond the territory already covered by the first and second "forces" in psychological theory.

The controversies will, of course, continue. There will be debates about the debates and significant shifts of opinion. I do not remove myself from the dynamics of those dialectics, and, indeed, I anticipate them with a strong sense of intellectual excitement. As to whether the psychoanalytic lamb will ever lie with the behavioristic lion, one cannot honestly claim to know. I have voiced my own fallible opinion in this chapter and have used it as an opportunity to share some impressions about larger themes of theoretical evolution in psychology and psychiatry. Whatever the ultimate directions of our development, I hope that we can continue to recognize the value of volumes like this one and the critical importance of dialectical exchange in the nurturance and encouragement of theoretical progress. It is from the crucible of such exchanges that our most promising ideas are most likely to emerge.

ACKNOWLEDGMENTS

I would like to thank Gianni Liotti, Mario Reda, and Edwin Locke for sending me their own previous works on this topic; special thanks are due Walter B. Weimer for his conceptual copyediting and support.

AUTOBIOGRAPHICAL STATEMENT

A number of historical and conceptual themes have bearing on my interest in the issue of rapprochement. When I began my undergraduate studies, I was interested in becoming a writer. I then took my first psychology course and was inspired by the material and the humanness of my instructor. She encouraged me to consider psychology as a career, but by then, philosophy and medicine were also vying for my attention. I continued taking courses in psychology—most of which were psychodynamic in flavor—until it was time to decide. I can remember that summer most vividly—it was between my sophomore and junior years, and I had transferred to Arizona State University. I was still not sure whether I wanted to pursue a career in writing or psychology. Having saved enough money for one session of professional counseling, I decided to take a risk and get an expert opinion on the matter. From the Phoenix yellow pages I somehow arrived at one unknown counselor to consult. I still do not understand everything that was said during that counseling session in 1967, but I declared psychology as my major the next week. It would be years later before I realized that the wise, gentle old man who had counseled me was more than just a random pick from the Phoenix phone book. I still feel a warm sense of appreciation for Milton Erickson and his subtle nudge.

My two years at Arizona State University were exciting. At the time the Department of Psychology there was very Skinnerian; the faculty included Arthur Bachrach, Frederick Keller, Thomas Verhave, and Lee Meyerson. Two new assistant professors, David Rimm and John Masters, had just graduated from Stanford. Rimm became my adviser and helped me steer a path toward broader horizons. Although I had been impressed with the empirical leanings of the Skinnerians, I had been disappointed in their occasionally dogmatic avoidance of "private processes" and the whole issue of self-development. My graduate years at Stanford offered me valuable time and opportunities to pursue some of my nascent interests in *self-control* and *cognitive behavior modification.* In addition to my valuable apprenticeship with Albert Bandura, I was influenced by my interactions with Gerald Davison, Walter Mischel, David Rosenhan, Carl Thoresen, Gordon Bower, and Daryl Bem.

I joined the faculty at Pennsylvania State University in 1972, eager to pursue further studies in personal change processes. By 1974 I was aware that my interest in *systemic* aspects of personal belief systems was taking me into such areas as epistemology, sociology of knowledge, the psychology of science, and the psychology of belief. My clients were also teaching me some lessons that were unavailable in the laboratory and library, and I found myself becoming increasingly less encumbered by any single approach to therapy. Since the mid-1970s, I have focused my attention on basic patterns and processes in human change, both "inside" and "outside" psychotherapy. My hunch has been that enduring and popular forms of counseling often reflect some valuable wisdom and that our understanding of fundamental change processes might be aided by an appreciation of the "invariance within the variance"—the principles and phenomena that are robust enough to shine through each of the divergent sets of theoretical bifocals. Although I do not believe that psychoanalysis and orthodox behavior therapy can or should "merge" into a unified approach, I think that the dialectics we are now witnessing are a clear reflection of a major paradigm reappraisal and evolution.

My chapter is a conjectural commentary on the demise of naive dualistic determinism in contemporary models of human behavior. As such, it touches upon old and embedded themes in our thinking. I hope it is apparent in the chapter that my intent is to harvest the paradigmatic implications of the psychoanalytic-behavioral interface, not to discourage it. For those of us who have watched the field of psychotherapy undergoing such dramatic change in the past two decades, the current interest in convergence is a welcome and exciting "new twist" in our continuing struggles to understand and to serve the mystery of individual human development better.

MICHAEL J. MAHONEY, PH.D.

REFERENCES

Bacon, F. *Novum organum.* New York: Bobbs-Merrill, 1960. (Originally published, 1620.)

Bandura, A. *Principles of behavior modification.* New York: Holt, Rinehart & Winston, 1969.

Barrett, W. *The illusion of technique.* New York: Doubleday, 1967.

Bettelheim, B. Freud and the soul. *New Yorker,* March 1, 1982, pp. 52–93.

Bever, T. G., Fodor, J. A., & Garrett, M. A formal limit of associationism. In T. R. Dixon & D. L. Horton (Eds.), *Verbal behavior and general behavior theory.* Englewood Cliffs, N.J.: Prentice-Hall, 1968.

Bolles, R. C. Reinforcement, expectancy, and learning. *Psychological Review,* 1972, *79,* 394–409.

Brewer, W. F. There is no convincing evidence for operant or classical conditioning in adult humans. In W. B. Weimer & D. S. Palermo (Eds.), *Cognition and the symbolic process.* Hillsdale, N.J.: Erlbaum, 1974.

Bugental, J. F. T. *The search for authenticity: An existential-analytic approach to psychotherapy.* New York: Holt, Rinehart & Winston, 1965.

Bugental, J. F. T. *Psychotherapy and process: The fundamentals of an existential-humanistic approach.* Reading, Mass.: Addison-Wesley, 1978.

Burton, A. (Ed.). *What makes behavior change possible?* New York: Brunner/Mazel, 1976.

Dember, W. N. Motivation and the cognitive revolution. *American Psychologist,* 1974, *29,* 161–168.

Dollard, J. & Miller, N. E. *Personality and psychotherapy: An analysis in terms of learning, thinking, and culture.* New York: McGraw-Hill, 1950.

Dulany, D. E. Awareness, rules, and propositional control: A confrontation with S–R behavior theory. In T. R. Dixon & D. L. Horton (Eds.), *Verbal behavior and general behavior theory.* Englewood Cliffs N.J.: Prentice-Hall, 1968.

Ellenberger, H. F. *The discovery of the unconscious.* New York: Basic Books, 1970.

Estes, W. K. Reward in human learning: Theoretical issues and strategic choice points. In R. Glaser (Eds.), *The nature of reinforcement.* New York: Academic Press, 1971.

Feather, B. W., & Rhoads, J. M. Psychodynamic behavior therapy. *Archives of General Psychiatry,* 1972, *26,* 496–511.

Freud, S. *Civilization and its discontents.* New York: Doubleday, 1958.

Friedman, M. *To deny our nothingness: Contemporary images of man.* Chicago: University of Chicago Press, 1967.

Friedman, M. *The hidden human image.* New York: Dell, 1974.

Garfield, S. L., & Kurtz, R. Clinical psychologists in the 1970's. *American Psychologist,* 1976, *32,* 1–9.

Garfield, S. L., & Kurtz, R. A study of eclectic views. *Journal of Consulting and Clinical Psychology,* 1977, *45,* 78–83.

Goldfried, M. R. (Ed.). *Converging themes in psychotherapy: Trends in psychodynamic, humanistic, and behavioral practice.* New York: Springer, 1982.

Goldiamond, I. Self-control procedures through personal behavior problems. *Psychological Reports,* 1965, *17,* 851–868.

Guidano, V. V., & Liotti, G. *Knowledge organization and emotional disorders: A structural approach to psychotherapy.* New York: Guilford, 1982.

Hayek, F. A. The theory of complex phenomena. In M. Bunge (Ed.), *The critical approach to science and philosophy: Essays in honor of K. R. Popper.* New York: Free Press, 1964.

Hayek, F. A. *Studies in philosophy, politics, and economics.* Chicago: University of Chicago Press, 1967.

Hayek, F. A. *New studies in philosophy, politics, economics, and the history of ideas.* Chicago: University of Chicago Press, 1978.

Hook, S. *Determinism and freedom in the age of modern science.* New York: Collier, 1958.

Hume, D. *An inquiry concerning human understanding.* Oxford: Clarendon Press, 1902. (Originally published, 1748.)

Keller, F. S., & Schoenfeld, W. N. *Principles of psychology: A systematic text in the science of behavior.* New York: Appleton-Century-Crofts, 1950.

Kuhn, T. S. *The structure of scientific revolutions.* Chicago: University of Chicago Press, 1962.

Kuhn, T. S. Logic of discovery or psychology of research? In I. Lakatos & A. Musgrave (Eds.), *Criticism and the growth of knowledge.* Cambridge: Cambridge University Press, 1970.

Lazarus, A. A. Has behavior therapy outlived its usefulness? *American Psychologist,* 1977, *32,* 550–554.

Ledwidge, B. Cognitive behavior modification: A step in the wrong direction? *Psychological Bulletin,* 1978, *85,* 353–375.

Lefcourt, H. M. *Locus of control.* Hillsdale, N.J.: Erlbaum, 1976.

Liotti, G., & Reda, M. Some epistemological remarks on behavior therapy, cognitive therapy, and psychoanalysis. *Cognitive Therapy and Research*, 1981, *5*, 231–236.

Locke, E. A. Behaviorism and psychoanalysis: Two sides of the same coin. *The Objectivist Forum*, 1980, *1*, 10–15.

Mahoney, M. J. *Cognition and behavior modification.* Cambridge, Mass.: Ballinger, 1974.

Mahoney, M. J. *Scientist as subject: The psychological imperative.* Cambridge, Mass.: Ballinger, 1976.

Mahoney, M. J. Cognitive and noncognitive views in behavior modification. In P. Sjoden, S. Bates, & W. S. Dockens (Eds.), *Trends in behavior therapy.* New York: Academic Press, 1979.

Mahoney, M. J. Psychotherapy and the structure of personal revolutions. In M. J. Mahoney (Ed.), *Psychotherapy process: Current issues and future directions.* New York: Plenum Press, 1980. (a)

Mahoney, M. J. (Ed.). *Psychotherapy process: Current issues and future directions.* New York: Plenum Press, 1980. (b)

Mahoney, M. J. Psychotherapy and human change processes. In J. H. Harvey & M. M. Parks (Eds.), *Psychotherapy research and behavior change.* Washington, D.C.: American Psychological Association, 1982.

Mahoney, M. J. Behaviorism and Individual Psychology: Contacts, conflicts, and future directions. In A. Reinelt (Ed.), *The encounter of Adlerian psychology with other schools of therapy.* Munich: Verlag Ernst Reinhardt, 1983. (a)

Mahoney, M. J. *Personal change processes: Notes on the facilitation of human development.* New York: Basic Books, 1983. (b)

Mahoney, M. J., & Arnkoff, D. B. Cognitive and self-control therapies. In S. L. Garfield & A. E. Bergin (Eds.), *Handbook of psychotherapy and behavior change* (2nd ed.). New York: Wiley, 1978.

Mahoney, M. J., & Kazdin, A. E. Cognitive behavior modification: Misconceptions and premature evacuation. *Psychological Bulletin*, 1979, *86*, 1044–1049.

Marmor, J., & Woods, S. M. (Eds.). *The interface between the psychodynamic and behavior therapies.* New York: Plenum Press, 1980.

Maslow, A. H. *The farther reaches of human nature.* New York: Viking, 1971.

Messer, S. B., & Winokur, M. Some limits to the integration of psychoanalytic and behavior therapy. *American Psychologist*, 1980, *35*, 818–827.

McKeachie, W. J. The decline and fall of the laws of learning. *Education Researcher*, 1974, *3*, 7–11.

Mischel, W. *Personality and assessment.* New York: Wiley, 1968.

Paul, G. L. Behavior modification research: Design and tactics. In C. M. Franks (Ed.), *Behavior therapy: Appraisal and status.* New York: McGraw-Hill, 1969.

Popper, K. R. Of clouds and clocks. In K. R. Popper (Ed.), *Objective knowledge: An evolutionary approach.* London: Oxford University Press, 1972.

Popper, K. R. *The open universe: An argument for indeterminism.* Totowa, N.J.: Rowman & Littlefield, 1982.

Popper, K. R., & Eccles, J. C. *The self and its brain: An argument for interactionism.* New York: Springer, 1977.

Prigogine, I. *From being to becoming: Time and complexity in the physical sciences.* San Francisco: W. H. Freeman, 1980.

Rotter, J. B., Chance, J. E., & Phares, E. J. (Eds.). *Applications of a social learning theory of personality.* New York: Holt, Rinehart & Winston, 1972.

Russell, B. *A history of western philosophy.* New York: Simon & Schuster, 1945.

Ryle, G. *The concept of mind.* New York: Barnes & Noble, 1949.

Salter, A. *Conditioned reflex therapy.* New York: Capricorn, 1949.

Skinner, B. F. Are theories of learning necessary? *Psychological Review*, 1950, *57*, 93–216.
Skinner, B. F. *Science and human behavior.* New York: Macmillan, 1953.
Skinner, B. F. Freedom and the control of men. In B. F. Skinner, *Cumulative Record.* New York: Appleton-Century-Crofts, 1959. (Originally published in *The American Scholar*, 1955–1956.)
Skinner, B. F. *Contingencies of reinforcement: A theoretical analysis.* New York: Appleton-Century-Crofts, 1969.
Skinner, B. F. *Beyond freedom and dignity.* New York: Knopf, 1971.
Skinner, B. F. *About behaviorism.* New York: Knopf, 1974.
Wachtel, P. L. *Psychoanalysis and behavior therapy: Toward an integration.* New York: Basic Books, 1977.
Wachtel, P. L. (Ed.). *Resistance: Psychodynamic and behavioral approaches.* New York: Plenum Press, 1982.
Walsh, R. N., & Vaughan, F. (Eds.). *Beyond ego: Transpersonal dimensions in psychology.* Los Angeles: J. P. Tarcher, 1980.
Watson, J. B. Psychology as the behaviorist views it. *Psychological Review*, 1913, *20*, 158–177.
Watson, J. B. *Behaviorism.* Chicago: University of Chicago Press, 1924.
Weimer, W. B. A conceptual framework for cognitive psychology: Motor theories of the mind. In R. Shaw & J. Bransford (Eds.), *Perceiving, acting, and knowing.* Hillsdale, N.J.: Erlbaum, 1977.
Weimer, W. B. Hayek's approach to the problems of complex phenomena: An introduction to the theoretical psychology of *The Sensory Order.* In W. B. Weimer & D. S. Palermo (Eds.), *Cognition and the symbolic processes* (Vol. 2). Hillsdale, N.J.: Erlbaum, 1982.
Wolpe, J. Cognition and causation in human behavior and its therapy. *American Psychologist*, 1978, *33*, 437–446.
Wolpe, J., & Lazarus, A. A. *Behavior therapy techniques.* Oxford: Pergamon Press, 1966.
Zukav, G. *The dancing Wu Li masters: An overview of the new physics.* New York: Morrow, 1979.

10

In Search of Substitutes for Binary Models

Commentary on Michael J. Mahoney

THOMAS E. SCHACHT

Reading and digesting Michael Mahoney's far-ranging chapter was both a difficult and rewarding experience. The difficulties were due in part to the inherently formidable subject matter (fundamental issues of causality and determinism), and in part to an apparent paradox in the chapter's argument. The rewards, as usual, came from struggling with the difficulties.

Mahoney adopts a commendably catholic perspective on the current interest in bringing psychoanalysis and behaviorism together. Thus, rather than emphasizing the concrete particulars of each approach, he attempts, in broad strokes, to place rapprochement (convergence, collaboration, etc.) into a wider historical and intellectual perspective. A central organizing theme behind the chapter is the question Why *now* for rapprochement? In answering, Mahoney refers to:

1. Apparent theoretical and empirical failures or limitations of both approaches
2. Avoidance motivations in the form of protection against common economic and sociocultural dangers (cf. "hanging together" rather than "hanging separately")

THOMAS E. SCHACHT • Center for Psychotherapy Research and Department of Psychology, Vanderbilt University, Nashville, Tennessee 37240.

3. Approach motivations in the form of a "desire for stimulation," a "sense of maturity," and a hope for a positive unification
4. Rapprochement as a side effect or epiphenomenon of a broader shift in the modern metatheoretical **zeitgeist** away from the simplistic "straitjacket" of "billiard ball determinism" and toward a deeper and more pluralistic view of causality. This last topic—determinism—is the central focus of the chapter.

In brief, Mahoney argues that behaviorism and psychoanalysis are both mired in the anachronistic swamp of outdated "billiard ball" theories of determinism. Furthermore, so long as both psychologies remain under the umbrella of such theories, they will likely appear incompatible. Thus, Mahoney asserts that differences between behaviorism and psychoanalysis are irreconcilable at several major levels, including: (a) theoretical models of behavior, (b) views regarding the locus and nature of significant change processes, and (c) philosophical dimensions of "idealism" versus "realism," "existential pessimism" versus "optimism," and "centralism" versus "peripheralism."

Mahoney's pessimism about prospects for rapprochement or unification is tempered, however, by his optimistic expectation that the residual pluralism is a positive force in the search for knowledge. Along these lines, he pokes fun at "patriotic" allegiance to any theoretical orthodoxy. He also seeks to "decentralize" the "locus of paradigm directions" (on the implicit premise that more directions are better), and he explicitly values contrasts and controversy as factors through which behaviorism and psychoanalysis mutually "energize their own development."

Although I am in substantial agreement with much of the chapter, I believe the overall persuasive power of the arguments is regrettably reduced by repeated and self-defeating oversimplifications. The most frequent oversimplifications involve an incorrect portrayal of psychoanalysis as a "mechanical," "hydraulic," and, "energy" model. At best, this characterization is outdated. Modern psychoanalysis has clearly moved away from Freud's Newtonian metapsychology in favor of alternatives that abandon physicalistic space–time assumptions about the mind (cf. Schafer, 1976) and that view behavior as structured via information rather than energy (cf. Peterfreund & Schwartz, 1971).

There is also an interesting conceptual problem. Although Mahoney repeatedly stresses various inadequacies of binary or dualistic comparisons of behaviorism and psychoanalysis, the chapter almost exclusively offers exactly such comparisons. Thus, "deep" determinism is contrasted with "surfacistic" determinism; "active" stances with regard to causality are contrasted with "passive" ones; "optimistic" values and world views are contrasted with "pessimistic" ones; "idealism" is contrasted with "realism"; "centralism" is contrasted with "peripheralism"; "billiard ball determinism" is contrasted with its unnamed alternative; and even the chapter title implies a dualism of "yin" versus "yang". Mahoney himself acknowledges this conceptual self-sabotage at one point by observing that "the [binary] contrast I have created here must be criticized by the reflective reader as an oversimplification of a very complicated historico-developmental sequence."

My own suspicion is that the problem may stem from an incompatibility between the pluralistic, nonlinear, nonreductionistic model of causality that Mahoney espouses and the traditional model of causality within which he constructs his argument. Specifically, although he views the future as transcending simplistic binary conceptions, he also envisions scientific progress as a "dialectic." However, a dialectic, by definition, embodies a dualistic perspective because it pits binary antitheses against each other to achieve a new synthesis. A binary perspective is attractive, of course, because of its logical elegance and because it adds great power to the reasoning process within the structure of a dialectical argument. But is there a paradox, perhaps, in Mahoney's vigorous use of binary constructs to pursue an argument whose major point is that binary constructs are inadequate? Could a shift to a new model of determinism also imply that we must find alternatives to the dialectic as a model for knowledge advancement? If this is so, then Mahoney's belief that a rapprochement of psychoanalysis and behaviorism is dependent upon shifts in broader metatheoretical issues could not be more correct.

Unfortunately, the chapter stops short of elucidating any clear metatheoretical options to traditional linear causality. Mahoney asserts that different rules for causation are appropriate to phenomena of differing levels of complexity. He views "cause" and "effect" in complex behavior as reciprocal and logically interchangeable. He also awards a central position to the concept of "emergence" as a counterpoint to simple linear causality. All this seems to verge on embracing general systems theories, (cf. Buckley, 1968) as philosophical models for the determinism of the future. This would certainly be a position that has won broad support in recent years. But, the chapter does not tell us concretely how a new determinism falls specifically into place with regard to behaviorism and psychoanalysis. Many of the points touched upon early in the chapter seemed very promising; for this reason, I felt somewhat teased by Mahoney's concluding statement that "this is neither the time nor the place to expound on alternatives to billiard ball determinism." I look forward to an occasion when it *is* the time and place to expound such alternatives.

REFERENCES

Buckley, W. (Ed.). *Modern systems research for the behavioral scientist: A sourcebook for the application of general systems theory to the study of human behavior.* Chicago: Aldine, 1968.
Peterfreund, E., & Schwartz, J. T. *Information, systems, and psychoanalysis: An evolutionary biological approach to psychoanalytic theory.* New York: International Universities Press, 1971.
Schafer, R. *A new language for psychoanalysis.* New Haven: Yale University Press, 1976.

10

A Rejoinder to Thomas E. Schacht

MICHAEL J. MAHONEY

Thomas Schacht's commentary on my chapter is a welcome and rather pithy invitation to reiterate what I had hoped to have made clearer in the chapter itself. His lament that the persuasive power of my arguments, for example, "is regrettably reduced by repeated and self-defeating oversimplifications" stands out as one of the more provocative invitations. Because one of the main points of the chapter was its cautionary overtones regarding oversimplification and artificial dichotomization, it would seem that some clarification is in order.

Rather than proceed to a point-by-point commentary or rebuttal, I will try to address myself briefly to some of the more obvious misunderstandings and ambiguities in Schacht's reading of my admittedly crude rendition. To begin with, his reference to my poking fun at patriotic allegiance to any theoretical orthodoxy should be qualified by an appreciation of the important role played by orthodoxy and commitment in any scientific paradigm. This point was made in my reference to some of Thomas Kuhn's work and my own previous writings in the areas of philosophy and psychology of science.

The issue regarding loyalty to a paradigm is not a simplistic one. All theoretical perspectives require the allegiance of their staunch supporters, and I concur with Kuhn and others on the vital role of such loyalty and dedication in the progress of science. Thus, in my remarks about the decentralization of paradigm directions, I am not—as Schacht suggests—

MICHAEL J. MAHONEY • Department of Psychology, Pennsylvania State University, University Park, Pennsylvania 16802.

endorsing or conveying "the implicit premise that more directions are better." Even a cursory review of the ongoing Kuhn-Popper debate in the philosophy of science would reveal that the only person endorsing such a premise in contemporary epistemology is Paul Feyerabend (1970). Feyerabend's call to anarchy and others' incantations toward "revolutions in permanence" fail to recognize that a revolution necessarily entails changing and unchanging dimensions (Weimer, 1979). The decentralization of power and control in science is, in my opinion, a progressive direction toward which we should move (Mahoney, in press), but it is hardly accurate to translate this statement into the contention that the absolute quantity of competing paradigms is the critical variable in scientific progress.

A second nit that Schacht has chosen to pick has to do with my allegedly frequent "oversimplifications involv(ing) an incorrect portrayal of psychoanalysis as a 'mechanical,' 'hydraulic,' 'energy' model." He goes on to point out that "modern psychoanalysis has clearly moved away from Freud's Newtonian metapsychology in favor of alternatives that abandon physicalistic space–time assumptions about the mind." One of the points that I tried to emphasize in my chapter was its focus upon *orthodox* psychoanalysis and orthodox behaviorism, as contrasted with the more contemporary and revisionary renditions of these two perspectives. I am well aware of the more sophisticated dimensions of the "systems approaches" that are becoming increasingly popular in many quarters, but these were not the guiding schemata underlying the original writings of Freud, Watson, or any of the other pioneering contributors in these areas. The caveat of anachronism applies only if one is misrepresenting past as present; my intent has been to reflect on how that past (orthodoxy) has differentiated and evolved toward our contemporary situation.

Perhaps the most central and, in some ways, most insightful comment by Schacht has to do with his question, "Is there a paradox, perhaps, in Mahoney's vigorous use of binary constructs to pursue an argument whose major point is that binary constructs are inadequate?" This comes on the heels of his having listed a series of pairs of dualities that permeate the chapter. He likewise argues that "a dialectic, by definition, embodies a dualistic perspective because it pits binary antitheses against each other to achieve a new synthesis." This rendition of dialectics is, of course, accurate only for those who would confine dialectics to the writings of Hegel. Such conceptual constriction is rare in contemporary epistemology and rhetoric. *Dialectics* need not be restricted to a dyadic or dualistic competition, and the term is enjoying increasing usage as a reference to the multiple exchange processes involved in any rhetorical confrontation among differing perspectives.

The self-contradictory aspect of using binary constructs to challenge their own utility is equivocal, but I shall not dwell here on some of the technicalities that its clarification would entail. By way of passing, however, let me say that it is reminiscent of the argument leveled against William Bartley (1962) when he first demonstrated—by means of logic—that logic itself is not and cannot be an absolute authority in settling scientific (or nonscientific) knowledge claims. If one has challenged the power of logic by using that logic to demonstrate its own limitations, is that self-contradictory? One of the main themes of my chapter was the extensive use of contrasts and polarities in all contemporary theories of personality, learning, and motivation. I have, indeed, argued that contrasts, polarities, and discrepancies serve important roles in human nervous system functioning. The identification of anchor points (polar opposites) of a continuum does not deny the existence of the continuum; nor does it imply that binary concepts are somehow misleading, oversimplifying, or otherwise without value in our analyses. Just as Bartley cannot communicate without relying on the very logic that he criticizes, it would be difficult for me to challenge the naivete of "excluded middle" dichotomies without at least referring to the anchor points—the "ends"—by which we define that middle.

Finally, Schacht states that I have attempted to contrast "billiard ball determinism" with an "unnamed alternative" and laments my failure to elucidate "any clear metatheoretical options to traditional linear causality." The unnamed alternative he is referring to is called *determinate order,* and—from my reading, at least—it receives substantial attention in my discussion of Popper's essay "Of Clouds and Clocks" and Hayek's discussion of complex phenomena. As I may have repeated too often in my chapter, there *are* alternatives to particulate determinism and the references that I suggest are a good starting place for anyone interested in exploring their heuristics.

Let me close this brief response by reiterating the importance of this kind of exchange of ideas. Schacht and I, in our respective chapters, commentaries, and responses, have apparently touched upon some themes that are both familiar and unfamiliar, persuasive and perplexing. Our interpretations, scaffoldings, and emphases have varied, and there are signs of both agreement and disagreement. The highest priority in all of this must be the invaluable role played by such exchanges in our deepening understanding of the principles of human change and development.

It should be obvious that I believe we are in a state of active transition in our profession (both within and among paradigms). The emergence of a single, monolithic metatheory is, I believe, unlikely. At the same time,

I do not endorse Feyerabend's call to anarchy and the idea that we can progress in our understanding simply by rejecting competing paradigms as quickly as they emerge. There is almost a century of embedded wisdom in the theory and practice of both psychoanalysis and behaviorism. I would like to think that that embedded wisdom can be harvested in whatever new perspectives emerge, and I look forward to being a participating observer in that harvest.

REFERENCES

Bartley, W. W. *The retreat to commitment.* New York: Knopf, 1962.

Feyerabend, P. K. Consolations for the specialist. In I. Lakatos & A. Musgrave (Eds.), *Criticism and the growth of knowledge.* Cambridge, England: Cambridge University Press, 1970.

Mahoney, M. J. Scientific publication and epistemic progress. *American Psychologist,* in press.

Weimer, W. B. *Notes on the methodology of scientific research.* Hillsdale, N.J.: Erlbaum, 1979.

11

Psychoanalysis and Behavior Therapy

LEON SALZMAN

Therapy, which is broadly defined as the remedial treatment of bodily disorders, can be specifically classified in many ways, depending upon one's prejudices and preconceptions. There is *etiological therapy,* in which the cause of the disorder has been definitely established. In contrast to this is *symptomatic therapy,* which is designed to alleviate specific discomforts associated with a disorder. The former is the case when isoniazid is used to kill the tubercule bacillus, whereas, in the latter, codeine may be administered to relieve the distressing and disabling cough that accompanies tuberculosis. Thus, some therapies are *palliative* and do not destroy the underlying disorder, whereas others are *ameliorative* because they undermine and eliminate the causal factor.

Such a significant distinction may be distorted by false claims when etiology is unknown, disputed, or still in the process of being established. This is the case in psychiatry with all but a fraction of the organic disorders of the brain. Who, today, would have the consummate arrogance to assign a specific cause of schizophrenia? Who would presume to flatly claim that schizophrenia is one disease and not a cluster of related disorders? A similar dilemma exists with the neuroses because our definitions and classifications are based either on ill-defined etiological factors or behavioral manifestations that may be interpreted in many ways.

LEON SALZMAN • School of Medicine, Georgetown University, Washington, D.C. 20037.

Our therapeutic approaches, therefore, tend to be both palliative and ameliorative; we cannot separate those factors at this time because current knowledge of causation is so sparse. Pharmacotherapy has the distinct advantage of having known targets and relatively clear effects. Whether it is palliative only, rather than etiological, is an open question. Psychoanalysis is still based on so many unproven and poorly demonstrated hypotheses that it is difficult to demonstrate a clear relationship between the therapeutic process and the alleviation of the disorder. It is also difficult to isolate those elements in the process that are ameliorative in contrast to those that are purely palliative.

Webster defines psychotherapy as "a treatment designed or serving to bring about social adjustment." This definition is unfortunately a very limited one and fails to describe the goals of therapy adequately. Psychotherapy strives to eliminate the causes of psychological disorders and to improve adaptive capacities, rather than to serve the social adjustment of the patient. Utilization of our total capacities and the elimination of impediments toward that goal should be the role of psychotherapy or other therapeutic modalities whose aim is to advance the functioning of the individual beyond mere adjustment. Any approach that attempts to achieve this end should be considered as significant as any other.

The prevailing classification of therapy, beyond the descriptive level of etiologic or symptomatic, conveys value judgments. It expresses the prejudices or preconceptions of the classifier, implying what to him or her is correct or incorrect, true or false, deep and basic, or superficial and secondary therapy. How else are we to interpret the labels of deep versus superficial therapy, adjuvant or subsidiary therapy versus psychotherapy, or a situation in which all approaches other than the classically defined psychoanalytic techniques are classified as psychotherapy? Often, the term *psychotherapy* is used to describe what is thought of as a second-class approach that is nonetiological and therefore, not truly ameliorative. This reflects a view of therapy in hierarchical terms. Psychoanalysis, or etiological therapy, is at the top, and all the lesser, nonetiological, and therefore symptomatic approaches are on the bottom. Although seemingly attractive and certainly seductive, this viewpoint is destructive and irrational because all valid therapeutic programs reflect varying goals and expectations. There are not simply *pure* versus *alloyed* methods of treatment. There are a group of descriptive labels that identify the technical processes, such as active versus passive, expressive versus suppressive, and directive versus nondirective approaches. I will not be concerned with these different techniques in this chapter.

Despite ignorance about the ultimate causes of many neurotic and psychotic disorders, we are not entirely in the dark about psychological processes in human beings, along with their development, history, distortions, and alterations. Some therapies attempt to explore causes, whereas others are entirely symptom oriented, even though there is no consensus about how symptoms develop. If we incorporate the concept of *character* in human functioning into theory, we assume that behavior may be a direct expression of inner need or motivation or a defense against an underlying character process rather than a simple stimulus–response action. We can also be fairly certain that some modalities of therapy that claim to be etiological—whether primal scream, scientology, encounter experiences, or weaning traumata, and the like—are minor pieces in a great puzzle, if they belong at all. We can be sure in some instances of the irrelevancy of those approaches that are completely irrational, unscientific, or simply not based on any neurophysiological possibilities. For example, the human brain is incapable of storing all those "engrams" the scientologists require, and a single trauma is *not* capable of causing the enormous personality complications described by the "scream" therapists.

Because of the epochal contributions of Freud, psychodynamics seems to have cornered the market in therapy and to have claimed the greatest validity and probity. Some of the existing definitions of therapy are derived from the framework of its theoretical propositions, and all deviations are labeled less pure and worthy. In this atmosphere, there has been a prevalent tendency to denounce all psychotherapeutic ventures as secondary, derivative, and superficial, no matter how useful they might be. Some spurious rationalizations of extreme analytic theorists are offered to support this position, which involves the notion that unless the deep, basic etiological factors are resolved, the symptoms will return and the disorder might even be aggravated. Their fallacious reasoning is based on unproven hypotheses that there are deep basic etiological biological factors involved. They view symptoms as manifest response to an underlying malfunction, an overreactive adjustment, or an adaptation to an alteration in the organism. Such symptoms can be altered or changed or eliminated, but unless the underlying stimulus is removed, the argument goes, new symptoms or maladaptive responses will occur.

However, removal or alteration of a symptom may also induce altered patterns of behavior that then act as an impetus for further constructive personality changes. For example, the removal of a phobia of public places may be the stimulus to encourage greater socializing and more risk taking in other ventures even though the underlying obsessional personality that accounted for the phobias may remain. At times, the behavioral changes may be critical and may initiate and sustain personality reorganization that will bring about basic characterological changes.

Most of the arguments for and against psychoanalysis or behavior therapy are either too defensive or simplistic (e.g., Apfelbaum, 1981; Ellis, 1981). We can, however, approach this matter on a serious, scientific basis. There are many points of agreement between behavior modification approaches and those therapeutic approaches that emphasize characterological alteration. First, it is possible to change behavior by a variety of techniques that include conditioning, hypnosis, suggestion, and the like. Second, the process of maturing in animals and humans is greatly influenced by conditioning processes. This was clearly established by Pavlov and has become a part of all valid theories of personality development. Third, there is a clear and demonstrable relationship between the alteration of behavior patterns through the psychotherapeutic process and conditioning (Frank, 1961; Masserman, 1955; Salzman, 1968). Many behavioral scientists have long been aware of the need to integrate learning theory into the psychoanalytic process (e.g., Marmor, 1964). Learning theory can account for how distorted patterns of behavior may cause disturbed relationships. In addition, it can show how distorted patterns of behavior are the consequences of either a malevolent atmosphere or set of experiences. Learning theory also accounts for how such distorted patterns of behavior may persist. The process of therapy can be viewed as one of relearning or reexperiencing, which is aided by insight into the origin of the faulty behavior pattern, although this is not always essential. It is necessary, however, to have an awareness of the presence and function of these faulty patterns.

There are also some important points of difference between therapies emphasizing conditioning and those emphasizing character alteration. Animal and human behavior have been differentiated during 14 million years of evolution. In animals, conditionability provided a way to deal with dangers and threats to physical survival and may have involved fear. *Anxiety,* however, relates to a threat to one's psychological well-being and is a human attribute. It implies a capacity for foresight and an awareness of one's ultimate dissolution and demise. It is related to intimacy, the need for relationships involving trust, affection, and acceptance. Anxiety is an awareness of being disapproved by significant others. We have no knowledge of its existence in other than human beings or late anthropoids. Thus, we cannot make a simple analogy between fear in animals and anxiety in humans, as the learning theorists do. Human beings have the capacity to symbolize and communicate with language and to be aware of themselves as functioning beings. Although learning in man may be similar to animal learning in many respects, it cannot be viewed as identical or even parallel without accounting for an indefinite number of intervening variables that relate to humans' capacity to experience foresight and hindsight and to be influenced by factors beyond physiological survival such as goals, values, and standards (Masserman, 1955; Rado, 1969; Sullivan, 1953). Learning theorists do not acknowledge these differences except in the concepts of "second signal" systems or "stimulus generalization hypotheses." Their concepts apply to simple, human, behavioral manifestations instead of addressing themselves to the human as complex individuals, who are motivated by many complicated factors.

The addition of a cortex and a psychology based on the need for contact, relationship, communication, and avoidance of loneliness has required the development of an overriding economical character structure in humans to manage their security needs. It is through the agency of our character structure that much of our behavior must be viewed, rather than through the stimulus–response reaction, which is a more primitive preservative mechanism.

The ability to control the variables in animal studies, in contrast to the indefinite and largely uncontrollable variables in studies of men and women, has given the behaviorist a pseudoscientific objectivity in equating experimental neuroses in animals with neuroses in humans. This is a serious defect in applying the results of animal studies to ourselves.

Behaviorists like Wolpe, Eysenck, and others arrogate to themselves a scientific "objectivity" when they equate "experimental neurosis" in animals with neurosis in humans because they see some similarities. They define "neurosis" in humans as behavior that either parallels or resembles neurotic behavior in animals, as if they were identical in origin. In so doing, they define neurosis as being due to faulty conditioning. However, fear reactions that can be identified in animals are *not* the same as phobias in men and women, even if we superfically define phobias in man as *fear reactions.* The crucial question is whether the phobia is a simple, conditioned response, or whether it is a complicated, psychological avoidance technique that is designed to deal with a situation or object that threatens the person with loss of control and humiliation. This aspect of the avoidance reaction cannot be identified in animals; yet, it is consistently demonstrated in human phobias. In humans, a phobia is *not* a specific response to a specific stimulus or to one's physiological integrity, but it is a defensive reaction to some threat or danger to one's self-esteem system. This response prevents the person from facing a symbolic situation that will cause him or her to lose control. It can occur in any characterological type, but it is particularly notable in the obsessional defense system in which control is the key element.

This view was implicit in the earliest formulations of Freud and the subsequent research on phobias that, in recent years, include the research studies of Sullivan (1953), Salzman (1968, 1980), and others. It implies that the experienced anxiety that results in avoidance responses is not a fear of physical danger but a psychological dread of losing control, which in most instances means "going crazy." Such reactions are viewed as weak, humiliating, and shameful, and they are to be avoided at all costs. The response is generally in terms of the symbolic significance of the threat, such as tunnels, bridges, closed spaces, and open spaces. This is equally true when the phobic avoidance may be to a specific object such as a snake, a particular color, or an event. These specifics, on further inquiry, symbolize events or occasions when one has lost control and which may occur again if the object is encountered. This matter was dealt with in detail in my article on obsessions and phobias (Salzman, 1968).

Behavior therapy has been described as the treatment of "bad habits," not as the treatment of neuroses. Wolpe (1958) insists that all neuroses are really bad habits. Although this view is not acceptable to all behavioral therapists, it does, in fact, underlie their therapeutic programs. Most psychiatrists distinguish between bad habits and obsessional, schizoid, manic, and hysterical behaviors. Maladaptive behavior does not necessarily imply neurosis. It can be one feature of a neurosis, or it can occur without neurosis and be due to faulty conditioning, ignorance, limited psychological capacities, or the contradictory demands of the culture.

There is little doubt that behavior therapy can alter behavior patterns, particularly by deconditioning those aspects of behavior that were originally caused by conditioning. However, manifest behavior is only a small part of a patient's problem that is imbedded in the organization and functioning of character structure. Behavioral therapy is therefore most clearly indicated when the problem may be only some manifest behavioral difficulty, such as stuttering, compulsive behavior, or a phobia in which the avoidance prevents further activity, as in agoraphobia.

The evidence for the assumption of an underlying character structure lies in the perduring patterns of reaction under various circumstances and in response to varied stimuli. Although the manifest behavior is the visible spectrum of the underlying character and may be maladaptive and therefore require correction, when we alter the behavior we notice we have not altered the related characteristics that are still operating within the character structure. For example, the obsessive-compulsive character structure that includes a complex collection of traits—namely, perfectionism, procrastination, indecision, emphasis on intellectualization, and multiple behavioral or mentative rituals, to mention but a few—is not altered when some rituals are eliminated through behavior modification. Rituals are a piece of the characterological attempt at certainty, control, and absolutism. They can be eliminated, although the focus on perfectionism, meticulousness, and procrastinating behavior remain. The elimination of the rituals may be extremely beneficial to the functioning of that individual. However, perfectionism and avoidance of commitment may still produce serious discomforts in the patient's life. Thus, the concept of *character,* which is an effective way of understanding behavior, does not reduce the significance of behavioral changes. It only emphasizes the need to be aware of the multiple facets of which one item may be extreme and maladaptive.

In recent years, there has been considerable effort to deal with compulsive rituals through behavior modification approaches. The research efforts of Foa and Goldstein (1978) and Rachman Cobb, Greys, McDonald, Sartory, and Stern (1979) have demonstrated the value of these approaches in reducing or eliminating some disturbing rituals like hand washing and other cleansing rituals. They have spent much time in organizing and classifying such rituals as if they were distinctive etiological syndromes. In this sense, they conceptualize the ritual as a disease entity, and when it is treated, they see it as "curing" the compulsive disorder. At times they avoid this issue by eliminating the words "disease" or "cure"; however, in essence, they only focus their research efforts on these isolated behavioral phenomena, no matter if they are phobic avoidance, ritualistic behavior, or obsessive thought instrusions—as if these constituted disease entities. In my opinion, this harkens back to an earlier medical epoch when fevers were diseases and the treatment was the same for all fevers, namely, blood letting or hot or cold herbal therapies. We now know that fever is a symptom, which is present in many diseases where a noxious agent is disturbing the physiology and is producing inflammation or cell destruction, with consequent efforts at restitution. We still treat fever with behavioral or pharmacological agents, but we also determine the underlying etiology in order to deal with the disease that is associated with fever as one of its symptoms. The present-day preoccupation with intricate, detailed, statistical comparison studies of various behavioral modification approaches to symptoms like avoidance phenomena or ritualistic behaviors is a return to the "fever" approach. In the studies of Foa and Goldstein (1978) and Rachman *et al.* (1979), whether it is stated explicitly or not, the symptom is dealt with as if it was the disease. These researchers should only speak of altering ritualistic behavior, rather than stating that they are treating compulsive behavior disorders.

A person's character structure manifests itself in a broad range of activity in autonomous and somatic manifestations, or in gross behavioral terms that extend to all areas of living. Some of it may be contradictory and maladaptive, transient or enduring. And it is almost always symbolic rather than a direct expression of interest, desire, or adaptive potential. The actual behavior is often a small part of the problem. This is especially apparent in the obsessional states where the manifestations may be entirely subjective, disruptive, and produced by factors outside the person's awareness. Although we can forbid an obsessional or compulsive bit of behavior, we obviously do not alter its underlying basis. I am not referring here to the issue of substitution of symptoms but to the treatment of a symptom—for example, a cough rather than the tuberculosis that causes it. Nor am I implying that we should allow the cough to continue untreated until we have eliminated the tubercule bacilli. We simply have not cured the illness by alleviating the cough with codeine. This is analogous to behavior therapy, even though we have not yet arrived at a consensus of the causes of neuroses or mental illnesses. To say the symptom *is* the disease, as some behaviorists do, is to deny 2000 years of scientific growth in all disciplines and to return to the prescientific era of description and the primitive tendency to identify single elements as total disease processes instead of recognizing that clusters of symptoms are often involved in single disease processes.

For example, I once treated a patient who had multiple phobias about signing her name, eating in public, being in high places, being closed in subterranean places, being out of doors in a crowd, being indoors with one or two people, and avoiding small parties and large gatherings. She also presented a wide variety of symptoms relating to her frigidity, her demands for perfection, her inability to get along with her husband, her tendency to be unemotional in her relationship with her children, her feeling that she was not functioning as effectively as she should, and an endless variety of psychosomatic complaints in her day-to-day life. At what point would we begin to impose a deconditioning process? Would it be for her handwriting problem, her weight problem, her frigidity, her tendency to be unexpressive, or the general area of failing to live up to her expectations? Her anxiety was manifest everywhere in her living, and she herself could not set any priorities.

This patient was a 45-year-old woman whose major problem was a writing phobia that had its beginning when she had to sign her name to a contract in the presence of other people. She was in the spotlight and began to get uneasy about the possibility of losing her composure and shaking visibly, which would have been very humiliating for her. By pleading illness, she was able to avoid the actual trial, but thereafter she could not sign her name at banks, department stores, or even at home in the presence of strangers or friends. Her pride prevented her from informing anyone except her husband and one close friend about her incapacity. The major focus in this phobia was the issue of displaying a tremor that would betray her nervousness. The writing phobia gradually extended to a phobia about socializing wherever drinks were to be served. This included luncheons, teas, dinners, and the like. Her social life became very restricted and the agitation and preoccupation in anticipation of such engagements became very great. The phobias served a vital purpose in her life, but they were entirely unacceptable to her; she felt ashamed and disappointed in herself for not being able to overcome these weaknesses. She was a very bright person who could not tolerate any situation in which she was second best or less well informed than another. Aside from the tremors, socializing was difficult because she never knew in advance whether she would measure up to her own standards with all the people she might encounter. She felt that she must know everything, or else others would find her dull and uninteresting. Her emphasis was entirely on intellectual achievement and, though she recognized the impossibility of competing with everyone about everything, she actually expected this of herself. She recognized that she demanded the impossible of herself; yet she felt that anything less than this was unacceptable. To be less than perfect meant that one was ordinary, and this was humiliating. Although she wanted her phobias eliminated, she did not wish to alter her perfectionistic goals and her omniscient requirements. The phobias directly intervened at times when she felt she was in danger of appearing human and therefore limited and imperfect. Her obsessional problems were manifest not only in her demands for perfection, control, and guarantees of the future but in specific matters as well, such as her meticulous concern for her own person and affairs and her obsessional ruminations and preoccupations.

The treatment consisted of weekly sessions, 40 weeks a year for 2 years, and was entirely psychotherapeutic, focusing on her obsessional and compulsive tendencies toward absolute control in all her affairs. The themes of her requirements for perfection, guarantees, unwillingness to take risks, and make commitments repeatedly became manifest and were explored. Encouragement and support for more spontaneous activities, in which perfection and certainty could not be guaranteed, followed on the insights that accounted for her phobic and compulsive behavior. Treatment was concluded when her anxieties were alleviated and when new, venturesome activities were more frequent. Her phobias had almost completely disappeared, and her obsessional personality traits were no longer an ongoing source of concern and intimidation. She became more social, initiated a new career, and her depression lifted. Fifteen years later, she reported a more active and happy marriage, with a broadening of all her experiences. She has had no new phobias and has participated in group activities with only a minimum of discomfort.

My patient suffered a typical obsessive-compulsive neurosis in which phobias were in evidence. Deconditioning may, indeed, have had a valid role, but it was unnecessary because the phobic problem was only a small piece of the symptomatology. The writing problem could have been easily treated by a deconditioning procedure. But what about the rest of the symptomatology? Do we treat each manifestation separately, or do we see it all as reflective of a character disorder in which there is a marked compulsive need to be absolutely free from anxiety in all situations? Such a concept of character represents the total picture and could account for every single aspect of her phobic and obsessive life. Grasping the significance of this unfortunate woman's character structure enabled one to work with the compulsive defenses and their organization. As psychotherapy proceeded, her phobic avoidances and the whole set of anxiety manifestations began to disappear. Yet, we never focused on any single phobic symptom. The symptoms became unnecessary as the obsessional character structure of the patient was altered. This is the general experience of psychotherapists. In my experience, phobias can come and go without any special focus on them, *except for those phobias that have become the central pillar of support for the compulsive structure itself.* These *do* require direct behavioral intervention because they may interfere with productive activity. In fact, conditioning approaches may be most useful here in overcoming such major obstacles when the obsessional intrusions interfere with a patient's work life. We must tackle these predominant symptoms before we can make any further moves in directing the patient's focus to the significant events in his or her life that are the instigating agents in producing the obsessional thoughts or compulsive rituals. However, we focus on the misdirected emotional reactions or distorted expectations or goals rather than on the rituals. We can do this by relieving the distress through the reduction of the rituals and obsessions. This is clearly demonstrated in the avoidance rituals as well as "doing" rituals like handwashing or cleaning. Here, the compulsive and inescapable need to avoid anxiety prevents any attempts to observe or assess other areas in the patient's life. Through direct action on these symptoms, we can free patients sufficiently to allow them to investigate other issues in their lives. Drugs or conditioning techniques can often do this quickly, and thus become integral parts of the therapeutic process. The same therapist can prescribe drugs or conditioning techniques as well as psychotherapy. In this sense, psychoanalytic and behavior therapy can be integrated. One can accompany phobic patients on their deconditioning ventures as well as recommend or train thought-stopping or response prevention tactics without jeopardizing psychotherapeutic collaboration. In my opinion, these *ancillary* behavioral techniques strengthen and, in fact, may be essential for a therapeutic benefit to occur. At times, the reduction of anxiety by deconditioning tactics may be the motivating force in encouraging the patient to explore the psychological factors and develop insights into his or her defensive behavior (cf. Rhoads, Chapter 7, this volume).

Behavior modification techniques can and should be integrated into the therapeutic process when they will aid and implement the resolution of disordered mental functioning. If the symptoms are so severe as to incapacitate the individual and prevent him or her from earning a living or meeting minimal social demands, immediate steps need to be taken to alleviate the symptoms even when long-term therapy may be required to alter the total process. Drugs, conditioning techniques, and other ancillary approaches should be initiated. Rituals, for example, may so preoccupy the individual that he or she has neither the time nor the freedom to pursue other necessary tasks. Conditioning therapies may be used at the beginning of an integrated therapeutic program, or even later when a strong alliance has been built with the psychotherapist. This process can be carried out by the same therapist if his or her training encompasses both approaches. If the therapist lacks training in behavior therapy, the patient could be referred to a behavior therapist who would work jointly with the psychotherapist. Concurrent psychotherapy and behavior therapy can be achieved when mutual respect is sufficient to overcome prejudices about which theory or therapy is the best. This situation appears to be happening more often among enlightened practitioners whose goals are to relieve distress as well as to advance our understanding of human behavior. I believe that behavior therapy may be most useful when the problems are motoric or behavioral, rather than cognitive or ideational.

Many behavioral scientists believe that behavior is a manifestation of an underlying character structure, even though some aspects of behavior or personality may be simply conditioned as well. A neurosis consists of behavior that develops out of personality distortions and is not a simple, conditioned response to anxiety phenomena. It is significant that the paradigm for the behavioral therapist is the phobia or the ritual in which there is a direct relationship between the anxiety and the subsequent failure to function. However, behavior therapists are less successful when they try to deal with complex behavioral problems because they do not fit their theoretical pattern, no matter how strongly they insist upon the secondary elaborations of the initial conditioning process. Do they cure homosexuality, or do they, at times, alter homosexual behavior? The abandonment of homosexual behavior is not to be confused with the notion that its etiology has been clarified or the personality structure, of which the homosexual behavior is only a symptom, has been altered. Does behavior therapy advance our understanding of alcoholism when it alters compulsive drinking into compulsive nondrinking? Aversion therapy approaches may force the discontinuance of excessive drinking, as antabuse can, with unquestioned benefit to the individual, her or his family, and society. But if drinking is a symptom either of a biological dysfunction or a psychological malfunction, we have not advanced our understanding of the underlying factors in dealing with this disease.

Behavior therapy has proven to be effective in many situations, particularly with phobias and other symptoms in which the behavior can be directly traced to anxiety and can be manipulated by rewards or punishments. Even if it can affect behavior, it has had little success with diseases or disorders where the underlying causes are expressed symbolically, whether in thought or behavior. Behavior therapy can deal with specific behaviors, but it has had questionable success with disease entities. Thus, although it has had some success in dealing with rituals, it has had little success in dealing with obsessive-compulsive disorders. Beech and Vaughn (1978), following their extensive review of the behavioral treatments of obsessive states, concluded:

> Accordingly, in the light of our review of treatment evidence, we must reluctantly conclude that there is no conclusive evidence that behaviour modification offers a viable approach to the modification of abnormal thoughts in obsessionals. For the motor components of these conditions, however, the picture appears to be a little brighter—or at least to encourage a degree of cautious optimism. Here, flooding, modeling, and response prevention would seem to involve elements helpful to the patient, although it is important to say that these methods still require further careful, controlled experimental work. Nor of course, is there any convincing evidence about the mechanisms involved in these techniques and how they deal with the abnormalities of function to which they are directed. (p. 169)

According to behavioral theorists such as Eysenck and Wolpe, ideas, emotions, attitudes, and feeling play only a slight role in initiating, maintaining, or changing behavior. The psychodynamic or developmental view is seen as being soft and romantic. The behavior therapist's concepts are viewed as hard, realistic, and scientific. Actually, the reverse is closer to the truth. It is a hard, cruel fact that humans are complicated, and it is difficult to uncover the multiple factors that influence behavior. Scientific truths about humans do not come easy, not even with oversimplified formulas demanded by our propensity for quick results and magical transformations. Although some aspects of behavior *are* measureable, identifiable, and quantifiable, we cannot discard or overlook the role and influence of subjectivity because it is not now and may never be quantifiable.

It is unfortunate that some critics of psychoanalysis tend to use outmoded or disputed concepts as targets for attack. This is particularly true when Freud's description of the phobia in Little Hans is viewed as the last word in the psychoanalytic formulation of phobias. By so doing, otherwise valid objections are diluted, and we are left with the opinion that they are either uninformed, contentious, or blindly doctrinaire.

Behavior therapists such as Eysenck also use the categories of mental disorder (e.g., DSM-III) developed primarily by psychodynamically oriented psychiatrists. They use these categories in their outcome research and claim results in treating these diseases. Although I am not saying that this is right or wrong, I *am* saying that in using such a system, behavior therapists are perpetuating a way of thinking for which they criticize psychodynamically oriented therapists.

Further, by criticizing the most vulnerable and often outmoded formulations of psychoanalytic theory (e.g., Freud's libido theory and his views on masochism, female psychology, and depression), behavior therapists are able to erect a very flammable straw man. They (particularly Eysenck) amass voluminous data and use statistics about undifferentiated groups of symptoms, and they claim great success in overcoming disorders that are neither clearly identified nor defined. They also use medical classifications that they reject in their philosophical objections to dynamic personality theory.

A numbers game has become confused with scientific research. Although they gather data of doubtful entities from mixed sources, there is little searching exploration of the experimental design or definitions that have produced the data. Nor are there precise statements about the criteria used to determine the quality of improvement in these outcome studies. The categories of improvement are so arbitrary at times that it becomes questionable how much change has occurred. When the data suit their views, they seem to be accepted uncritically. Despite claims of precision, many behavior therapists persist in utilizing a single label for phenomena that may seem to be similar but, in fact, may be quite different. I am referring to the notion that all avoidance behavior is not phobic nor are all rituals part of the obsessional disorders. Anxiety has many causes, even though the manifestations may be identical. Addictive behavior may be influenced by aversive therapy, but the addictive agents can be very disparate, ranging from food to drugs. Until behavior therapists define concepts precisely and until there is general agreement that their terms are comparable to those used by others, we cannot compare results of therapy or even discuss etiology.

Psychoanalytic theory is neither monolithic nor universally accepted as fixed and unchanging. Most psychoanalysts would agree that behavior is not necessarily symbolic or representative of deeper unconscious needs. Although we can alter behavior by arranging reinforcers, we must concern ourselves with the dynamics of why, when, and how such behavior began. Psychoanalysis is a science in the making, and it is a unique science. It cannot be compared to or judged by the traditional criteria of the physical sciences. It is a psychological science with the inherent but unprecedented potentialities of subjectivity that make it unique. Psychoanalysis does have many limitations that may complicate its claim as a science in the classical sense. Not only is there difficulty collecting and quantifying data, but there is also a paucity of measuring instruments that permit validation of the generalizations that are made. Statistically, mass data that cannot be reduced, except at the risk of great distortion to the phenomena studied, prevent adequate control of the variables. The presence of multiple determinants to every psychological event geometrically aggravates the issue of causality. It is not particularly reassuring to say that we can overcome these deficiencies in the course of time. However, the problems of a science whose inherent elements are ones in which subjectivity is of the essence and in which determinism and causality are too broad in time and space to be quantifiable must be confronted. Because causality has a time and space configuration, the utilization of probability theory—not strict determinism—seems eminently appropriate. Furthermore, no concept of causality can have permanent validity because it must be dependent upon scientific contributions from all available sources that are yet to come.

Too much stress has been placed on the absence of statistical verification for the validation of psychoanalytic concepts. We forget that replicability, probability predictions, manipulation of controlling variables, and the production of anticipated results are also indications of the validity of scientific formulations. In psychoanalysis, replicability is possible only in a limited sense because we cannot reconstruct precisely what has passed. Yet, in a broad sense, we can repeat and verify concepts relevant to the life history of every human being. Simpson (1949) calls this the multiplication of relevant observations with the absence of negative instances. The statistical verification possible in the physical sciences may never be possible in the psychological sciences. But every individual's therapy is a novel experiment that validates the existence of trends or patterns of behavior. Completely accurate predictability depends on patterns of behavior and upon a knowledge of all the variables in personality development and human behavior. All of the variables can never be isolated, let alone be identified.

Most open-minded behavioral scientists recognize the validity of operant conditioning techniques in some therapeutic programs. We have long been aware of the need for integrating learning theory and the theory of the psychoanalytic process, being mindful of the need to be aware of the functions of distorted patterns of behavior. Only when this is clear can the individual experience relationships in a new light and avoid confirming and reinforcing previous patterns.

AUTOBIOGRAPHICAL STATEMENT

My interest in integration can be traced directly to my awareness that the modification of behavior must go beyond the process of illumination or reconstruction of the past and that it requires a determined, volitional process of replacing old established patterns of behavior. Franz Alexander, Sandor Rado, and Harry Stack Sullivan were significant influences in developing this point of view. The recognition of learning as a key issue in behavior was emphasized by Sullivan in his *Conceptions of Modern Psychiatry.* The clear relevance of behavior modification approaches to some mental dysfunctions and my convictions about the role of out-of-awareness factors in the adaptational process drew my interest to this issue.

LEON SALZMAN, M.D.

REFERENCES

Apfelbaum, B. Integrating psychoanalytic and behavior therapy. *American Psychologist,* 1981, *36,* 796–797.

Beech, H. R., & Vaughn, M. *Behavioral treatment of obsessional states.* New York: Wiley, 1978.

Ellis, A. Misrepresentation of behavior therapy by psychoanalysts. *American Psychologist,* 1981, *36,* 798.

Foa, E. B., & Goldstein, A. Continuous exposure and complete response prevention in the treatment of obsessive-compulsive neurosis. *Behavior Therapy,* 1978, *9,* 821–829.

Frank, J. *Persuasion and healing.* Baltimore: Johns Hopkins Press, 1961.

Marmor, J. Psychoanalytic therapy and theories of learning. *Science and Psychoanalysis,* 1964, *7,* 265–279.

Masserman, J. *The practice of dynamic psychiatry.* Philadelphia: W. B. Saunders, 1955.

Rachman, S., Cobb, J., Greys, S., McDonald, B., Mowson, D., Sartory, G., & Stern, R. The behavioral treatment of obsessive compulsive disorders with and without clomipramine. *Behavior Research and Therapy,* 1979, *17,* 467–478.

Rado, S. *Adaptational psychodynamics.* New York: Science House, 1969.

Salzman, L. Obsessions and phobias. *International Journal of Psychiatry,* 1968, *6,* 451–465.

Salzman, L. *Treatment of the obsessive personality.* New York: Aronson, 1980.

Simpson, G. G. *The meaning of evolution.* New Haven: Yale University Press, 1949.

Sullivan, H. S. *The interpersonal theory of psychiatry.* New York: Norton, 1953.

Wolpe, J. *Psychotherapy by reciprocal inhibition.* Stanford: Stanford University Press, 1958.

11

Psychoanalysis and a Behavior Therapy for 1983

Commentary on Leon Salzman

CYRIL M. FRANKS

Salzman's view of behavior therapy is not behavior therapy as it exists today. All that can be attempted in a few pages is a brief synopsis of what contemporary behavior therapy is about, leaving readers to draw their own conclusions. For Salzman, psychodynamic theory, in some form or another, represents the present best guess at truth, and behavior therapy is an occasionally useful tool to be judiciously deployed in a purely adjunctive capacity as the psychodynamic therapist thinks fit. Behavior therapy as described by Salzman appears naive, simplistic, and inappropriate for complex problems. Although it can play a limited role in the hands of the skilled clinician who appreciates the psychodynamic subtleties of the human psyche, behavior therapy can never function as an independent and mature therapeutic modality for anything beyond the simplest of problems.

To make his point, Salzman correctly argues that overt behavior is often a direct expression of inner needs or motivation rather than a simple S–R reaction and that we cannot make a simple analogy between fear in animals and anxiety in humans. Human learning has to take into account an indefinite number of intervening variables that relate to such complex human attributes as foresight, hindsight, goals, and values as well as sched-

CYRIL M. FRANKS • Graduate School of Applied and Professional Psychology, Rutgers University, Busch Campus, Piscataway, New Jersey 08854.

ules of reinforcement. His incorrect assumption is that most behavior therapists reject his contention and think in terms of a prescientific era of superficial description and a primitive tendency to identify single elements as total disease processes. If behavior therapy is of any independent value at all, it is, according to Salzman, in the limited treatment of such uncomplicated behavioral malfunctions as stuttering or certain phobias where the problems are motoric or behavioral rather than cognitive or ideational.

Salzman's position evidences two serious deficits: a lack of concern with the need for hard data and documentation (especially with respect to his belief system about what behavior therapy is and is not good for) and a lack of familiarity with contemporary behavior therapy. To appreciate the subtleties and intricacies of modern behavior therapy, it is essential to have a working and up-to-date knowledge of the current literature. Few or no 1983 behavior therapists would disagree with Salzman's description of human beings as exquisitely complex and subtle organisms for whom any form of conceptualization in terms of simple S–R conditioning derived from animal data is inadequate. None would contend that maladaptive behavior is necessarily all that there is to a neurosis, and no experienced behavioral clinician would uncritically accept a presenting or manifest complaint at face value or as a "disease entity." Much has been written about behavioral assessment and its evolution into the sophisticated process that it has now become. Behavioral assessment is an ongoing strategy for systematic monitoring and evaluation of intervention that recognizes the fact that assessment and therapy can never be totally independent. Both are dynamic processes that in no way resemble the limited portrait of behavior therapy drawn by Salzman. As indicated in my chapter, one key distinction between the behavioral and psychodynamic approaches lies in the closeness with which behavior therapists try to keep to the data and rely upon objective verification to strengthen the links between operationally defined intervening variables and behavior.

Behavior therapists no longer argue that "the symptom is the disease" or that it is not the disease, for that matter, because neither "symptom" nor "disease" form part of the conceptual system known as behavior therapy. Discussion of such matters as whether symptom substitution can or cannot occur and under what circumstances is totally superfluous and irrelevant to behavior therapy. Similar arguments apply to the notion of "transference." Both symptoms and transference have precise meanings within a psychodynamic context and none whatsoever in a behavior therapy context. Engagement in the psychodynamic versus behavior therapy debate about either symptom substitution or transference is a disheartening as well as futile activity that primarily reflects mutual lack of understanding of the fundamental differences between the two approaches. The *observation* that treatment of a particular deviant behavior or cognition is sometimes followed by the emergence of different problems *is* a legitimate subject for discussion and follow-up by either group. Explanation in terms of symptom substitution is meaningful only for psychodynamicists.

Behavior therapy, then, is neither a series of specific techniques nor a model for intervention in the treatment of specific symptoms. It is a broad-based learning theory approach whose strength lies in its methodology. As such, it has many roots and no authoritative founding figure or guiding school of thought. Social learning theorists, applied behavior analysts, Pavlovian conditioners, and ecosystem behavior therapists all have their places in the behavioral galaxy.

In the 1950s, behavior therapy was simplistic in its understandable focus upon specific responses and the treatment of circumscribed maladaptive behaviors. It was all we were able to deal with at that stage in our evolution. Early behavior therapists deliberately ignored cognitive processes and were ill-equipped to deal with complex social systems and configurations. The intervening years saw the advent of cognitive behavior therapy, on the one hand, and the extension of behavior therapy into the external environment by way of systems theory and community psychology, on the other. There was a growing recognition of the reciprocity of relationships between people and their environments and between inner processes and their outward manifestations.

It is false to think of behavior therapy as a unitary system whose proponents share a set of common beliefs. Philosophically, some behavior therapists espouse a radical behaviorism that rejects all forms of intervening variables: others advocate a methodological behaviorism and little more. Behavior therapists are similarly divided with respect to environmental and genetic influences and dimensions of personality (traits) as opposed to behavioral specificity. Free will, determinism, and the concept of the self are other issues about which behavior therapists are in friendly disagreement among themselves.

What, then, do contemporary behavior therapists have in common? To answer this question, it is helpful to think of behavior therapy as an approach that is based upon a set of methodological assumptions and strategies that are predicated loosely upon some form of learning theory rather than as either a compendium of techniques or a unitary system. Contrary to Salzman's implicit belief, a clinician versed only in the techniques of behavior therapy is not a behavior therapist at all. The hallmarks of behavior therapy are accountability, openness to behaviorally plausible alternatives, and appeal to evidence rather than authority. Current and historical determinants of behavior are emphasized, overt behavior change is the main criterion by which treatment is evaluated, basic research in psychology is a primary source of hypothesis generation, and specificity, objectivity, and replicability are the yardsticks to be used in defining, treating, and measuring target populations.

Contemporary behavior therapy is also characterized by "doing" as well as "talking," by a variety of multidimensional procedures rather than single treatments, by a focus on client responsibility, and by a cautious readiness to go beyond the confining straits of traditional conditioning for a data base as long as this progression is determined in orderly fashion rather than by caprice, whim, or the dictate of an authority figure. For behavior therapy, a theory is a servant, which is useful only until better theory and better therapy come along.

The strength of behavior therapy lies neither in the brevity of its procedures, the ease with which they can be accomplished, nor their greater effectiveness. The early days of behavior therapy were, indeed, characterized by an unfortunate but understandable I-am-better-than-you bravado in which we strived to prove our superiority. Alas, time and research indicated that, all too often, these alleged advantages were more in the realm of mythology than reality. As we know now, the potency of behavior therapy lies more in the advantages of a flexible methodology that enables us to pose and explore increasingly complex and sophisticated questions in an orderly fashion and apply them to all situations than in any tenuous superiority as therapy.

There is nothing that is sacrosanct within behavior therapy other than an allegiance to methodology and, as indicated in my chapter, even this is open to change. If the principles of conditioning, modeling, and learning theory are of major significance, contemporary behavior therapy is also free to draw upon objective data that are derived from other branches of psychology and from other disciplines. Private events—the cognitive mediators of behavior—are no longer beyond the psychological pale, and a major role is now attributed to vicarious and indirect learning processes.

The appeal, then, of modern behavior therapy is to those who prefer a coherent, disciplined, adaptable conceptual framework to a melange of intuition, anecdotal evidence, dogmatic assumptions, and personal preference. Whether this will evolve into a meaningful model of our species remains to be seen. Behavior therapy is still a young discipline, and it is premature to expect unifying theories in a relatively new field when physics and chemistry have failed in this respect after 2,000 years.

It is regrettable that it is still believed in certain circles that behavior therapists reject interpersonal relationships, that behavior therapy cannot encompass the complexities of human behavior, that behavior therapy is a naive treatment of symptoms, that behavior therapy is overly technique oriented, that behavior therapists are interested only in the presenting complaint, and that behavior therapy is generally limited in its applicability. Another serious misconception by many nonbehavioral clinicians is that behavior therapy is simple to do and that it requires little training, care, sophistication, or attention to detail. Most of these faulty perceptions are based upon inadequate knowledge of contemporary behavior therapy, and a little reading will go a long way toward their correction. *The Annual Review of Behavior Therapy* chronicles both progress and problems in behavior therapy over the years. The first seven volumes cover the years from 1973 to 1979. Later volumes, written by Franks, Wilson, Brownell, and Kendall, bring this series up to date. For additional reading in this area, see also Franks and Barbrack, cited in my chapter in this volume.

What is disturbing to me is that Salzman—an intelligent, sophisticated, otherwise well-informed and well-motivated professional—thinks, feels, and writes about behavior therapy as he does. Those of us who are behavior therapists have to ask ourselves what it is that we continue to do or not do that reinforces such false impressions of behavior therapy. Do certain behavior therapists still make bombastic statements? Do some behavior therapists still espouse antiquated notions of behavior therapy? To what extent do we practice what we preach? Are we promoting ourselves in a valid, honest, and effective fashion? Are we willing to engage, without fear of appeasement, in dialogue with psychodynamic and other therapists? Difficult as this may seem, have we tried hard enough to present our point of view in "their" journals? As behavior therapists, we should surely be able to modify our own behavior. But then, how much should we engage in these defensive interchanges at all? How far can such accommodating maneuvers go, and how much should we invest in these endeavors? As suggested, while striving to put our best public image forward, our main concern might well be with going about our own business, letting the "chips fall where they may" and, regardless of orientation, leaving each camp to ferret out "truth" as its adherents think fit. To recognize the fundamental and irreconcilable incompatability between the two systems at virtually all levels, it is essential to have a realistic and accurate appreciation of both approaches. I refer the reader to my chapter for arguments against the integration of psychoanalytic therapy and behavior therapy, and, hopefully, for possible correction of Salzman's outmoded and inconsistent notions about behavior therapy.

11

A Rejoinder to Cyril M. Franks

LEON SALZMAN

Franks's response to my presentation seems to be somewhat at odds with his dictum of a dialogue with psychodynamic theorists. On the one hand, he asserts that my piece did not characterize contemporary behavior therapy. However, although clarifying some errors, he fails to touch on the essential issues of "symptoms and diseases" that he denies but in fact continues to deal with in the therapeutic process. He makes no attempt to answer my specific concerns about behavioral theory's limited role in understanding and altering the complexities of human functioning. Franks is guilty of the psychoanalytic canard that denies any criticism on the grounds that the critic was not psychoanalyzed. He asserts that no one can truly understand behavioral therapy who is not a committed, practicing behaviorist.

I am a psychiatrist and psychotherapist who has a special interest in the obsessive-compulsive states, and my reading in behavioral therapy is admittedly limited in view of my extensive interests elsewhere. I was invited to participate in this volume as a psychotherapist of psychodynamic orientation and, in a collaborative fashion, I suggested areas of potential rapprochement and integration. I hardly expected my disagreement or criticism to be met with an intolerant approach to my presentation. Franks admits the possibility that "behavior therapists still espouse antiquated notions, that some may not practice what they preach." He pleads for opportunities to present his viewpoint in "their" journals. But if he responds to "us" in this way, what does he expect in return, and why does he not practice what he preaches?

LEON SALZMAN • School of Medicine, Georgetown University, Washington, D.C. 20037.

I have been interested in behavioral therapy for some time since I recognized the possibility of altering behavior as an intrinsic part of the psychotherapeutic discipline. Many behavioral therapeutic techniques can alter behavior rapidly and put into motion broader personality changes that can have far-reaching effects on the total functioning of the individual. However, I raised serious questions about its limitations, especially in the area of my competence and interest; namely, the obsessive state. I quoted a pair of highly qualified behavioral theorists from their book *Treatment of Obsessional States* (Beech & Vaughn, 1978) in an article reviewing over 200 articles, most of them by behavioral therapists (Salzman & Thaler, 1981). Beech and Vaughn stated in part that, "in the light of our evidence . . . we must reluctantly conclude that there is no conclusive evidence that behavioral modification offers a viable approach to the modification of abnormal thoughts in obsessionals," but they held out more hope for the motor components. Why does Franks avoid addressing this point? He can be lucid about many aspects of behavioral theory, but he neatly avoids all those findings that cast doubt on the potential for influencing some mental mechanisms by conditioning procedures.

Like Franks, I look forward to the day when a comprehensive theory of personality development, human behavior, and its adaptive failures will unfold. A unified theory is, in my opinion, still a long way into the future, and there must be an active pursuit and accumulation of data in all branches of the behavioral sciences with a tolerance for the discrepant and, at times, contradictory data we have with regard to the same phenomena. Unlike Franks, I cannot acknowledge a "fundamental and irreconcilable incompatability between the two systems at virtually all levels." Instead, I see an ultimate integration that will encompass the validities of all the relevant disciplines. It seems to me essential to have an accurate appreciation of all the tributaries, and it is also necessary to have an open mind that is optimistic, with a modest awareness of one's own human limitations. Authoritarian intolerance of opposing points of view will surely fulfill the prophecy that the future cannot add to the present inadequacies and that an integrative science of the mind is an impossible goal. Franks's response is a rigid, black-or-white approach in an area that is still largely gray. It is neither a frank, scientific exchange nor a humanistic challenge, and thus only serves to discourage dialogue.

REFERENCES

Beech, H. R., & Vaughn, M. *Behavioral treatment of obsessional states.* New York: Wiley, 1978.

Salzman, L., & Thaler, F. Obsessive-compulsive disorders: A review of the literature, *American Journal of Psychiatry,* 1981, *138,* 286–296.

12

The Integration of Psychoanalytic Therapy and Behavior Therapy

Summing Up

STANLEY B. MESSER

In setting out to edit this book, Arkowitz and I sought contributions from creative scholars and clinicians (and scholar-clinicians) who we knew could write substantive and stimulating essays on the prospects for therapeutic integration. Rather than assigning them specific topics, we allowed the authors maximum latitude to define the issues as they viewed them. The extent of our predetermined framework was to choose contributors—both psychologists and psychiatrists—who stood on different points along the ideological spectrum stretching from psychoanalysis to behavior therapy, yet who were not situated on the conceptual equivalent of the ultraviolet or infrared extremes.

With the individual chapters assembled, we are now in a position to provide the emergent "topic headings." Of course, each of us could think of rubrics other than those included under which to discuss the thorny theoretical and practical issues regarding rapprochement, but that is inherent in the elasticity of the subject matter. It surprised us, for example, that no one referred to the special case of treating children and adolescents and how the prospects for integration may be considerably greater in this population. The immature state of ego development in younger clients

STANLEY B. MESSER • Graduate School of Applied and Professional Psychology, Rutgers University, Busch Campus, Piscataway, New Jersey 08854.

requires modifications in psychoanalytic therapy that give it, at times, a cognitive-behavioral slant. There is more emphasis on clarification and information giving, less on the interpretation of transference, and more on the direct control of upsetting physiological and emotional states (Meeks, 1980). Similar arguments for integration could be applied to the treatment of very seriously disturbed adult patients.

Therapeutic integration as a field of inquiry presents many challenging issues regarding the nature of psychoanalytic therapy and behavior therapy: their respective views and image of people, the values they embody, their methodologies, their scientific status, and so on. The refreshing look that the authors take at one or both of these therapies, the questions they raise, and the direction in which they point are thought-provoking, aside from the specific answers offered to the question posed in the book's title. The attempt in this concluding chapter will be to extract major themes that run through the book and to bring them into high relief. It will focus most directly on the units by which psychoanalytic and behavior therapy are compared, on the various proposals for integration offered, and on the related issues and obstacles such proposals present.

UNITS OF ANALYSIS

Although "psychoanalysis," "psychoanalytic therapy" and "psychodynamic therapy" share many attributes, they are also quite different in several ways (see Gill, Chapter 7, this volume). The same can be said of "behavior modification," "rational-emotive therapy," and "cognitive-behavioral therapy" (see Kazdin, Chapter 5). The prospects for integrating psychoanalysis and behavior modification, most would agree, are substantially dimmer than the possibilities for integrating psychodynamic and cognitive-behavioral therapies. Thus, Wachtel (Chapter 2) makes it clear that it is in the latter instance and not the former that he sees real possibilities. Even these terms, however, lack specificity and require refinement of the exact units being compared or integrated. Schacht (Chapter 4) provides a comprehensive list of the units by which behavioral and dynamic therapies have been compared, ranging from the philosophical and metapsychological (e.g., teleology, reductionism, peripheralism) to the nitty-gritty of specific techniques (e.g., modeling, direct suggestion, desensitization). Comparing the different arguments and conclusions about integration is made more difficult by the diversity of units that have been employed. Schacht believes that the prospects for integration depend on the units chosen, with the more global units being the hardest to integrate. The essays in this book consider a range from more molar, abstract, and theoretical units—and the difficulties of integration that appear from that level—to molecular-sized units that lie in the more clinical, technical, and empirical stratum.

PROPOSALS FOR INTEGRATION

TRANSLATING THE CONCEPTS AND/OR LANGUAGE OF PSYCHODYNAMIC THERAPY AND THEORY INTO THOSE OF BEHAVIOR THERAPY AND THEORY OR VICE VERSA; TRANSLATING BOTH INTO A COMMON LANGUAGE (SCHACHT'S MODEL 2, KAZDIN'S CONCEPTUAL INTEGRATION)

In this model, a concept taken from one therapy is extended to include a related concept in the other therapy. To pick just one example, Mendelsohn and Silverman's approach to integration (Chapter 9) is to propose the psychoanalytic concept of "activated unconscious fantasies" to explain what is called in the language of behavior therapy "nonspecific effects," "cognitive mediation," "expectancies", and "relationship variables." That is, the therapeutic phenomena referred to by these terms can be understood by invoking the construct of unconscious fantasy. They describe experiments in which the deliberate evocation of specific unconscious fantasies (such as "Mommy and I are one") enhanced the effectiveness of behavior therapy. Extending their findings into the realm of clinical practice, these authors suggest how their concepts and results can be utilized in the conduct of behavior therapy.

A variant of this model is to translate the concepts of both therapies into a common language such as that of cognitive psychology, as Marvin Goldfried (1982) has proposed elsewhere.

COMMONALITIES IN PSYCHOANALYTIC AND BEHAVIOR THERAPY (KAZDIN'S PROCEDURAL AND STRATEGY INTEGRATION)

Similar to efforts at translation of concepts from psychoanalytic to behavior therapy and vice versa is the search for commonalities between the two therapies in their general strategies for change or in their more specific procedures. Examples of proposed shared strategies in psychoanalytic and behavior therapies are the provision of a corrective emotional experience, the alteration of self-efficacy, or the amelioration of patients' demoralization (Kazdin, Chapter 5). At a somewhat less abstract level, both therapies may be seen as exerting their influence via patient–therapist relationship factors or through the opportunity to discuss one's problems.

Psychoanalytic or Behavior Therapy as Adjunctive (Rhoads's Models 1 and 2; Schacht's Model 3)

In this model, each therapy is employed to tackle different aspects of the same patient's behavior.

Behavior Therapy as an Adjunct

Both Rhoads and Salzman advocate the use of behavioral techniques at the start of or during the course of a psychodynamic treatment for such targets as heavy smoking, headaches, and phobias. (Salzman emphasizes the use of behavior therapy particularly for incapacitating symptoms that interfere with a patient's work). This can either be accomplished by the same therapist or by two different therapists who are proceeding in tandem. In the latter case, the behavior therapist may be treating, for example, the patient's headaches, whereas the psychoanalytic therapist is exploring the patient's separation anxiety. The therapist might even focus on the presenting complaint in a behavioral way at the very start of therapy, thereby gaining the patient's trust and cooperation. This, argues Rhoads, can open the door to a discussion of broader life-style problems that the patient may not have been willing to approach initially.

Psychodynamic Therapy as an Adjunct

Rhoads recommends the use of psychodynamic approaches and understanding as an aid in dispelling passive resistance to behavioral techniques. It is useful, he says, to have patients discuss their feelings about the assignments and how such feelings may reflect reactions to similar situations in their present and earlier life (e.g., reaction to the perceived authority of the therapist).

In a related form of adjunctive integration, psychodynamic understanding is brought to bear on what may be the underlying nature of a problem (e.g., a phobia) so that a behavioral technique such as systematic desensitization can be applied to the original feared object or situation rather than to its symbolic displacement (as understood psychoanalytically). Schacht (in his Model 5) refers to this as an "emergent therapeutic technique" in which the particular combination of the familiar elements produces a new hybrid.

Psychoanalytic and Behavior Therapies as Complementary (Rhoads's and Schacht's Model 4)

Rhoads and Wachtel refer to a combined therapy in which the therapist moves back and forth from one approach to the other, depending on which seems most necessary or useful at the time. Similarly, Schacht describes a synergistic model in which the two therapies focus on the *same* problems. An example is the behavioral treatment of obesity's proceeding apace with exploration of the dependency needs that are thought to underlie it. In general, alleviation of the symptom might enhance self-esteem and interpersonal relations, whereas exploration of the conflicts and developmental difficulties may aid cooperation with the weight loss program.

Theoretical Synthesis of Psychoanalytic and Behavior Therapies (Shacht's Model 6)

This level of integration aims at a theoretical synthesis leading to a different image of humans from that contained in either therapy. Wachtel (Chapter 2) has made the most formidable effort at integration in this mode in constructing "a frame of reference in which the ideas and the observations emanating from both broad approaches can find a coherent place." He attempts to take elements of each therapy and to combine them into a new synthesis with an accompanying conceptual structure that unites the two perspectives. He refers to this structure as "cyclical psychodynamics." Peoples' difficulties are described as viscious circles "in which neither impulse nor defense, neither internal state nor external situation are primary but are continually determining each other in a series of repeated transactions." This level of integration is surely the most ambitious because it includes both technical and theoretical elements.

INTEGRATION: ISSUES AND OBSTACLES

Several authors take issue with one or more of these proposals for integration and see them as detracting from, rather than adding to, the conceptual advances of each therapy or to its efficacy. Others, although recognizing the potential merit of integration, express reservations about the extent of its possibility or desirability. A third group sees the value of debate about integration, insofar as it forces a careful look at what these two therapies represent and in this way serves heuristically to broaden and deepen our thinking about psychotherapy and its future directions. We turn now to the individual arguments about integration presented in these chapters. The reader is referred to the commentaries and rejoinders for further discussion of these issues.

Nature of Evidence or Data

There is a controversy alluded to in several chapters about what constitutes data and evidence in the psychoanalytic and behavior therapies. For Franks (Chapter 8), behavior therapy conforms to the canons of evidence of behavioral science but psychoanalysis does not. Thus, the proponents of behavior therapy insist on parsimony, testable predictions, quantifiable observables, objectivity, and where possible, the hypothetico-deductive method. The practitioners of psychoanalysis, on the other hand, employ a method more akin to the hermeneutic approach used in literary and historical scholarship (Messer & Winokur, Chapter 3; Wachtel, Chapter 2). In the hermeneutic approach, one strives to construct meaning out of a diversity of phenomena to aid the emergence of hidden meanings. One seeks the coherence, consistency, and harmony of the parts underlying the seeming disparity—like fitting together pieces of a puzzle. Any one piece only makes sense in the context of the adjoining pieces, and together they offer a "narrative fit" and "narrative truth" (Spence, 1982). Salzman (Chapter 11, this volume) points out that psychoanalysis is a psychological and not a physical science and that quantifying data in the manner of the physical sciences is simply inappropriate for this unique, subjective discipline. Because of such differences in rules of evidence, Franks concludes that psychoanalytic and behavior therapies are inherently nonintegratable, at least at the conceptual level. Wachtel and Messer and Winokur, on the other hand, point to the value of each therapy's partaking of the other's method as a way of enriching clinical understanding and theory building even if each therapy retains its own predominant and preferred approach to data.

Empiricism

From the empirical point of view, the fact that neither psychoanalytic therapy nor behavior therapy has demonstrated its superiority in outcome studies has provided a climate for efforts at integration (Kazdin, Chapter 5). Because the empirical base for the theory of change encompassed in each therapy is relatively weak, however, one may simply add weakness to weakness rather than strength to strength in attempting to integrate the two therapies. For example, "symptom substitution" (a psychoanalytic concept) and "response substitution" (a behavioral concept), which both refer to changes that treatment can bring about, are laden with conceptual problems and ambiguities that are difficult to resolve empirically. (Franks also points out that symptom substitution has meaning only within a psychoanalytic context and is not the same as response substitution in a behavioral framework). Furthermore, although each may help to explain certain consequences of therapy, neither concept helps to explain a phenomenon such as response covariation in which alterations of one area of behavior are likely to be associated with multiple, clustered changes in other areas. Trying to integrate such concepts, Kazdin notes, would pose substantial problems and would not help elucidate, in this instance, the basis for the particular response covariations that have been reported.

The emphasis on empirical research as the arbiter of the usefulness of integration is summed up by Kazdin (Chapter 5) as follows:

> An integrationist approach aimed at generating a new type of research, rather than at prompting conceptual harmony, heightens the prospect for genuine advances. But the principal goal must be kept in mind. Efforts toward integrationism must be evaluated on the basis of their empirical yield rather than on the compatibility of the different views that are achieved. If the empirical yield is viewed as the ultimate criterion, no doubt many existing theoretical notions will be discarded and others will be retained or modified. Ultimately, integrationism is likely to lead to a new position that does not lobby for conceptual harmony but for heightened empiricism.

Transference

For Merton Gill (Chapter 6), the major stumbling block to integration is the effect that active behavioral intervention has on the therapist's ability to analyze the transference—the sine qua non of psychoanalysis. He contends that such interventions lessen the ability of the analyst to point to the patient's perceptions of him or her as coming from their own prior expectations. Furthermore, the analytic atmosphere of neutrality will be upset and will unduly affect the patient's free associations. A regimen of systematic desensitization or assertion training is bound to affect the patient's associations strongly in what Gill suggests would be a very different and not especially helpful way. The greater emphasis on external situations that such interventions necessitate would, for example, lessen the cognitive regression necessary to meet the goals of psychoanalysis. By contrast, Wachtel contends that one can, indeed, analyze the transference reactions of the client to behavioral techniques, notwithstanding the strong stimulus provided by such intervention.

To the extent that an analytically oriented therapy is not centrally concerned with the analysis of transference nor sets the goal of characterological change, the integration of behavioral ingredients becomes more possible, according to Gill.

Visions of Reality

On a more molar and less clinical level, the values and visions of each therapy have been explored, and the differences noted are seen as setting limits to integration. Messer and Winokur (Chapter 3) draw on Northrop

Frye's mythic forms—comic, tragic, romantic, and ironic—to compare the theory, therapeutic process and relationship, and desired outcomes in psychoanalytic and behavior therapies. Although they see considerable discrepancy between the two *theories*, especially in the tragic and ironic modes, they acknowledge that between the more cognitively oriented behavior *therapies* and the neo-Freudian and ego-psychological viewpoints, compatibility is somewhat greater.

In the realm of *process*, they see psychoanalytic therapy as laden with tragic, romantic, and ironic elements and behavior therapy as more exclusively comic. Psychoanalytic therapy, they say,

> follows a tragic structure: suffering, self-knowledge, and inner reconciliation; its content is characterized by a romantic interest in the unconscious, dreams, and childhood, and its style by a romantic attitude to uncertainty and unpredictability, mixed with an ironic sense of the need for detachment in the face of ambiguity and contradiction. Behavior therapy tends to follow an experimental structure, a comic interest in social skills and social reconciliation in a format and style marked by precision and specificity.

Here, too, Messer and Winokur point to trends in psychoanalytic therapy away from the tragic vision and toward the comic that brings it and behavior therapy closer together.

Both Messer and Winokur and Kazdin refer to the importance in psychoanalytic and behavior therapies of the therapeutic relationship; yet each acknowledges the difference in emphasis in the two therapies. In psychoanalytic therapy, the relationship is an arena for exploring the client's difficulties, and empathy is central, whereas in behavior therapy, a positively toned therapist–client relationship in which sympathy is more central is viewed as necessary for enlisting cooperation with the behavioral procedures.

Although psychoanalytic therapists emphasize inner reconcilation and tolerance of feelings, and behaviorists, social reconciliation and removal of negative affects in gauging outcomes, both share an interest in positive interpersonal relationships, better functioning at work and play, and enhanced self-esteem. Kazdin, however, emphasizes the primacy in behavior therapy of behavior change and in psychodynamic therapy the primacy of elaborating the client's subjective experience.

Messer and Winokur conclude that the question of integration reduces to one of trade-offs: Each therapist has to give up something of the vision and values of his or her preferred approach to be a comfortable bedfellow of the other. Some therapists will willingly pay the price for such a love match, whereas others will emphasize the singular virtues of their approach and insist on separate beds.

Styles of Knowledge

Behavior therapists typically view clients from an external standpoint—knowing them "from the outside"—and they largely employ analytic and scientific thinking in explaining their clients' problems (Messer and Winokur, Chapter 3). In fact, clients are encouraged to think scientifically, that is, in a rational, logical way. Although there is, likewise, a certain degree of intellectual detachment in the way psychoanalytic therapists operate, to a greater extent than behavior therapists they attempt to project themselves into the clients' subjective world and to acquire knowledge of them through empathy and intuition—knowing them "from the inside." Messer and Winokur also view the behavior therapist as favoring a demonstrative, "tough-minded" way of reasoning in which truth is found in what can be pointed to, that is, demonstrated readily before one's eyes. The psychoanalytic therapist is more likely to employ a dialectical ("tender-minded") way of reasoning in which meaning is generated and emerges through discourse.

Messer and Winokur point to a trend among some behavior therapists in the direction of dialectical thinking and of poetic and intuitive ways of knowing, and they also point to an interest by some analysts in data generated through controlled research and systematic observation outside the consulting room that, in turn, can affect how they conduct therapy. Although they see the trends as offering some prospects for innovative integration, they also suspect that one aspect limiting integration is the predilection of individual therapists for one or the other way of knowing their clients and of reasoning about them.

Determinism

Psychoanalytic and behavior therapies encompass strongly deterministic points of view, and it is partly because of the difficulties and limitations of this philosophy that adherents of one model of therapy are looking to another for stimulation, enrichment, and possible integration (Mahoney, Chapter 10). The "billiard ball determinism" that characterizes these two therapies involves separating objects and experiences into classes or discrete events and then contending that one class is dependent on or associated with the other in a linear way that involves two-dimensional exchanges of energy. There are three differences in the form, however, in which determinism expresses itself in psychoanalytic and behavior therapies. The proponents of psychoanalysis endorse a "deep" form of determinism in which the locus of change is in the core aspects of personal functioning that are unconscious; for proponents of behaviorism, the locus is in those aspects of human behavior that are most publicly observable and conscious. Second, although psychoanalytic and behavior therapies employ mechanical metaphors to describe change (hydraulics vs. linear movement), the former aims at balance among psychic components, whereas the latter aims at manipulating environmental contingencies. On a third dimension of comparison, the psychoanalyst adopts a passive and pessimistic approach to human behavior, whereas his or her behavioral counterpart is more decidedly active and optimistic about change. That is, Freud believed that our abilities to choose and regulate consciously are weak, whereas Skinner emphasized our power to control.

Mahoney views billiard ball determinism as a major constraint on psychoanalytic and behavior therapies. He hopes that as the practitioners of each school move beyond it and devote more attention to areas such as choice, will, and intentionality, something new, but as yet unspecified, will result. Thus, he predicts the emergence of new therapies that will be reliant on a new metatheory regarding change, rather than convergence or integration of the present therapies that are based on determinate order causality. One might say then that he regards the debate over integration as heuristically useful for generating new ideas but not as a valuable or practical goal for which to strive.

Is Knowledge Unitary or Pluralistic?

The struggle for integration and the debate about its prospects raises the question of whether unity of knowledge is, in the most general and abstract terms, possible and desirable. Schacht points out that there are some scholars who see the search for unity and integration as either a necessity or even a duty. Others argue that heterogeneity of knowledge cannot be avoided and, furthermore, that it should not be avoided. This controversy is closely connected to the question of whether in science we *discover* what is in nature—which is assumed to be totally connected in one unitary reality—or whether we imaginatively *create* and *construct* what is out there, a corollary of which is that our grasp of reality can only be pluralistic and that integration, therefore, is a chimera.

Schacht goes on to illustrate that the knowledge-as-unitary and knowledge-as-discovery positions lead to the effort to integrate psychoanalytic and behavior therapies because the assumption is that nothing is ultimately irreconcilable. By contrast, the pluralistic view considers the obvious contradictions and differences in these two therapies as support for basic diversity in nature. Furthermore, this view regards such diversity as desirable because it serves as an impetus to the creation of new knowledge. Alternately, one can view the unitary and pluralistic positions in a dialectical manner and conclude that knowledge is best served by the existence of creative tension between the two poles which brings us back to the opening paragraph of this chapter. If we do not have a definitive and straightforward answer to the question "Is integration possible?"—what we more modestly may have accomplished in this volume is a small step in the advancement of knowledge by virtue of the clash or exchange of viewpoints. What we hope for from a dialectical exchange in which thesis and antithesis meet is not an ultimate solution but another dialectic pointing in new directions that generate yet other possibilities for the theory and practice of psychoanalytic and behavior therapies or their successors.

REFERENCES

Goldfried, M. (Ed.). *Converging themes in psychotherapy.* New York: Springer, 1982.
Meeks, J. E. *The fragile alliance.* New York: R. Krieger, 1980.
Spence, D. *Narrative truth and historical truth.* New York: W. W. Norton, 1982.

Author Index

Italic numbers indicate pages where complete reference citations are given.

Subject Index

MIX
Papier aus verantwortungsvollen Quellen
Paper from responsible sources
FSC® C105338

If you have any concerns about our products,
you can contact us on
ProductSafety@springernature.com

In case Publisher is established outside the EU,
the EU authorized representative is:
Springer Nature Customer Service Center GmbH
Europaplatz 3, 69115 Heidelberg, Germany

Printed by Libri Plureos GmbH
in Hamburg, Germany